Principles of Biomedical Ethics

Principles of Biomedical Ethics

SECOND EDITION

TOM L. BEAUCHAMP   JAMES F. CHILDRESS

New York   Oxford
OXFORD UNIVERSITY PRESS
1983

Library of Congress Cataloging in Publication Data
Beauchamp, Tom L.
  Principles of biomedical ethics.
  Bibliography: p.   Includes index.
  1. Medical ethics.   I. Childress, James F.
II. Title.   [DNLM: 1. Ethics, Medical. W 50 B372p]
R724.B36   1983   174′.2   82-18816
ISBN 0-19-503285-3
ISBN 0-19-503286-1 (pbk.)

Printed in the United States of America

Printing (last digit): 9 8 7 6 5 4 3 2

**To
Georgia, Ruth, and Don**

I can no other answer make but thanks,
And thanks, and ever thanks.

Twelfth Night

Preface

This edition retains the structure and general lines of argument of the first, but virtually every page has been thoroughly revised. In addition, significant new stretches of material have been introduced near the end of Chapter 4, at several points in Chapter 7, and throughout Chapters 3 and 8. Appendix I, which contains case material, has undergone extensive reworking. Instead of the 29 cases found in the first edition, there are now 35 cases, of which 14 are new. Appendix II, which contains codes, oaths, and federal guidelines, and the bibliography have been updated.

We owe a considerable debt of gratitude to several persons who assisted in the day-to-day preparation of this edition. Mary Ellen Timbol, Wanda Proffitt, and LaRea Frazier prepared the manuscript copy with great skill and efficiency. Mary Ellen Timbol and James B. Tubbs proofread the entire work, and the latter assisted in numerous other ways. Other valuable assistance was provided by Cathleen Kaveny, Linda Kern, Timothy Hodges, Margaret Pumper, Frederic Hoffman, and Steven Dalle-Mura. Without their dedicated and conscientious efforts the second edition would likely have been long delayed.

We also wish to express our appreciation to Jeff House and Ellie Fuchs, two superb editors at Oxford who have worked with us through both editions. We must also thank the many people who have offered constructive criticisms regarding arguments in the first edition or proposed changes in the second edition. In particular, we thank Rick O'Neil, Robert Veatch, Sara Fry, R. B. Brandt, and Ruth Faden, but many others, including our students in various courses, have also earned our deep appreciation.

Washington, D.C.   T. L. B.
Charlottesville, VA   J. F. C.
December 1982

Preface to the First Edition

This book offers a systematic analysis of the moral principles that should apply to biomedicine. Many books in the rapidly expanding field of biomedical ethics focus on a series of problems such as abortion, euthanasia, behavior control, research involving human subjects, and the distribution of health care. Rarely do these books concentrate on the principles that should apply to a wide range of biomedical problems—including but not limited to the aforementioned problems. As a result, the moral judgments involved in one dilemma may appear to be unconnected to the moral judgments in others. Such a disjointed approach often relies on the discussion of cases, with little attention to the principles that both create and illuminate the dilemmas. As noted by a character in Tom Stoppard's play, *Professional Foul,* "There would be no moral dilemmas if moral principles worked in straight lines and never crossed each other." Only by examining moral principles and determining how they apply to cases and how they conflict can we bring some order and coherence to the discussion of these problems. Only then can we see that there are procedures and standards for deliberation and justification in biomedical ethics that parallel those in other areas of human activity.

We understand "biomedical ethics" as one type of *applied ethics*—the application of general ethical theories, principles, and rules to problems of therapeutic practice, health care delivery, and medical and biological research. In our discussions of ethical theory per se, we offer analyses of levels of moral deliberation and justification and of the ways two major approaches—utilitarian and deontological theories—interpret principles, rules, and judgments (Chapters 1–2). The systematic core of the book (Chapters 3–6) presents four fundamental moral principles—autonomy, beneficence, nonmaleficence, and justice. Here we analyze the meaning, weight, and implications of these principles, as well as their interrelationships. The next chapter (7) sketches the principles of truthfulness and confidentiality, as well as some of the role responsibilities that frequently come into conflict for health care professionals and researchers. The final chapter (8) examines ideals, virtues, and integrity—other important ingredients of the moral life. We say that Chapters 3–6 constitute the systematic core of the book because these chapters are intended to provide an integrated framework of principles through which diverse moral problems may be handled. If there is either an incompleteness of principles or an ad hoc quality to the selection of these four principles, then we have not fully achieved our goals in this book.

Because biomedical ethics is *applied* ethics, it is essential to examine a wide variety of actual cases involving medical practice, health care delivery, research, and public policy. A systematic analysis of moral principles would otherwise be disembodied and useless. Thus, in our treatment of ethical theories and principles, we also discuss actual cases. Such cases not only illustrate principles and their conflicts, they also provide a way to explicate and to test the principles. And, as we know from the history of law and morals, hard cases sometimes lead to a modification of the principles themselves.

In Appendix I we present twenty-nine detailed cases. At various points in the text we discuss these cases in relation to moral principles. Virtually all these cases are based on actual occurrences, and most were originally reported by medical professionals. They are intended to be as representative of current problems as possible. Several cases are drawn from the law, not because law and morality are coextensive, but because legal decisions commonly appeal to moral principles and rules, or raise issues that must be handled at least in part by moral deliberation. Other cases not presented in the Appendix are used as illustrations in the text. (For teachers of biomedical ethics who wish to supplement these cases, Robert Veatch's *Case Studies in Medical Ethics* offers a number of similarly constructed cases.)

Even a comprehensive treatment of the principles of biomedical ethics cannot indicate all their important applications. We have been selective, and we have tended to concentrate on typical and representative issues and cases. Because of limitations of space, we have not included cases, for example, of transsexual surgery, in vitro fertilization, psychosurgery, or behavior modification. However, we believe that our framework of principles can illuminate such cases.

One major difficulty in a book of this sort is to define and then address the appropriate audience. Our intended audience includes health care professionals such as physicians and nurses, research investigators, policy makers in biomedicine, and students preparing for such roles who are interested in how ethical theories bear on their activities. Our intended audience also includes philosophers, theologians, and students in philosophy and religious studies who are interested in how their reflections on ethical theory relate to biomedicine. For such a mixed audience, it is necessary to eliminate or at least to define technical terms from each specialty. We have tried to presuppose only minimal acquaintance with philosophy, theology, and medicine—merely what the average aware person even on the college level could be expected to possess. Above all we have kept in mind teachers and students who will use this book in the classroom. We have tried to write as clearly and as concisely as possible, with ample cases and examples to clarify the theoretical points. In several cases in Appendix I, we have not, however, eliminated or defined all technical medical terms. In most instances, the gist of the case will be clear, and when we discuss the case in the text, we restate relevant points in nontechnical language.

Although our discussions and cases mainly refer to problems encountered by physicians and researchers, we intend our analyses to be pertinent to other health care professionals and policy makers as well. Consider nursing, for example. Most of the issues that we raise may be redescribed in virtually identical terms for nurses and other members of a health care team. The same moral principles and rules govern nurses as well as physicians. By explicating the presuppositions and implications of such principles and rules, we thus hope to illuminate nursing no less than medicine. What is special about nursing from a moral standpoint is the question of authority and power on the health care team. Special moral dilemmas for nursing may arise from power conflicts. Such conflicts frequently involve disagreements about moral principles and judgments;

but again these disagreements may occur among members of the same profession as well as among members of different professions. In any event, when the nurse has to decide whether to continue to cooperate on a health care team, whether to follow a doctor's instructions, etc., the relevant moral principles and rules for the decision are identical to those for doctors. Similar points could be made about other specialties. Thus, our general analysis of ethical principles is designed to apply to the whole range of biomedicine and health care delivery. (Appendix II is composed of several professional codes, declarations, and regulations derived from ethical and policy reflections within such specialty professions.)

Ethics as the systematic examination of the moral life is designed to illuminate what we ought to do by asking us to consider and reconsider our ordinary actions, judgments, and justifications. While we rarely find knockdown arguments in debates about applied ethics, such debates are subject to rational analysis. However—to paraphrase Aristotle—we can only expect the precision and degree of certainty appropriate to the subject matter. Sometimes the answers cannot be as tidy as we might wish.

T.L.B.
J.F.C.

Washington, D.C.
December 1978

Acknowledgments

Every book has its history, and every author incurs debts of gratitude. In 1976 the authors and Dr. Seymour Perlin, a psychiatrist then at the Kennedy Institute of Ethics and now at the George Washington University School of Medicine, frequently discussed the need for a systematic analysis of the *principles* that should govern a wide range of decisions affecting biomedicine. These discussions led the three of us to embark on the project that eventuated in this book. Our original intention was to produce a jointly authored analysis by a philosopher, a religious ethicist, and a physician. Although Dr. Perlin was prevented from participating in the actual writing because of other commitments, he did complete an anthology with Beauchamp on related matters, and he made important contributions in the early stages of this book. We are grateful to him for his inspiration and enthusiastic support.

Since 1976 the authors have had a range of professional experiences that partially compensate for the absence of a physician on the writing team. In each instance they received assistance that led to changes in this book. First, they assumed primary responsibility for the ethical theory portion of the Kennedy Institute Intensive Bioethics Course, which is held each summer for 50–60 scientists, physicians, nurses, and other health care professionals. In addition, Childress has offered two seminars for physicians and other health care professionals under the auspices of the National Endowment for the Humanities and has taught in several workshops at the Hastings Center. During this same period of time, Beauchamp served as staff philosopher for the National Commission for the Protection of Human Subjects of Biomedical and Behavioral Research (N.I.H.), as a lecturer and consultant to dialysis and transplant societies composed of physicians and nurses, and as a Chautauqua lecturer on these subjects for college teachers under the auspices of the National Science Foundation and the American Association for the Advancement of Science. These experiences, in conjunction with seminars, lectures, and consultations in a variety of clinical and research settings at Georgetown and elsewhere, have made us sensitive to the concrete problems that must be faced by health care professionals. We still have much to learn, but we hope that we have been able to depict realistically and sympathetically many dilemmas faced by these professionals and by their patients and subjects.

This is a jointly authored book in every sense of the term. Although each author initially had primary responsibility for certain chapters, both authors rewrote substantial parts of every chapter and take responsibility for the whole, which at every point bears their dual imprint, whether by conviction or by compromise. The interaction that permitted this collaboration was facilitated by the Kennedy Institute of Ethics, which offers maximal freedom and stimulation to pursue such projects and which brings together medical practitioners and health care professionals, as well as philosophers, theologians, and lawyers. We are grateful to various colleagues—particularly to André Hellegers, Director of the Kennedy Institute, and to LeRoy Walters, Director of the Center for Bioethics at the Institute, for making this setting so attractive. In addition, we are indebted to the Kennedy Foundation for its support of the Kennedy Institute and to Sargent Shriver and Eunice Kennedy Shriver for their personal interest and encouragement.

Writers who influence the authors of books can sometimes go unnoticed because readers customarily look only to chapter and footnote references for such influences. In the present book, however, two hidden sources deserve special mention. First, no footnotes to Gerald Dworkin appear in the first section of Chapter 3 on Autonomy. Nonetheless, one of his unpublished manuscripts heavily influenced some parts of this section. This has since been published as "Moral Autonomy," in H. Tristram Engelhardt, Jr. and Daniel Callahan, eds., *Morals, Science and Sociality*

(The Hastings Center, 1978). Second, the work of the National Commission for the Protection of Human Subjects was carried on almost coextensively with the writing of this book. The deliberations of this body led us to think through old and new problems more carefully. Several commissioners, particularly Donald Seldin, M.D., Al Jonsen, Ph.D., and Patricia King, J.D., influenced the development of the book. Both of us at different times had the good fortune to teach law school seminars with Professor King, and we are also indebted, to her for the perspectives gained from this exposure.

Among the several people who read full drafts of the manuscript, Dr. Joanne Lynn of the George Washington University School of Medicine, Dr. Joan Sieber, a psychologist at the Kennedy Institute and the California State University, Hayward, and Dr. Martin Benjamin of the Philosophy Department at Michigan State deserve special mention for their thorough and valuable commentaries. We are grateful to them and to others who offered criticisms and suggestions.

Several members of the Kennedy Institute staff aided us immeasurably. Our research assistants, James J. McCartney and Dorle Vawter, contributed in numerous ways by checking references, reading proofs, and making helpful suggestions regarding style and substance. In addition, McCartney wrote a number of cases for Appendix I; others who graciously provided cases are identified in footnotes to this Appendix. William Pitt prepared the index with his customary attention to detail. The library staff at the Institute, particularly Doris Goldstein and Betsy Walkup, supplied many references and materials, frequently on short notice. Most importantly, we are grateful to Mary Baker, executive secretary par excellence, who did most of the administrative organization and typing, assisted by Mary Ellen Timbol. We cannot exaggerate our gratitude to Mrs. Baker, whose cheerfulness, friendship, diligence, and remarkable abilities make our various activities easier and more fruitful.

Finally, Beauchamp wishes to express personal debts of gratitude to Ruth Faden of the Johns Hopkins University School of Hygiene and Public Health and the Kennedy Institute and to Don Seldin of the University of Texas Medical School (Southwestern). Sometimes it is impossible to distinguish special friendships from influential professional relationships, and this distinction was never more difficult to make than in the case of his association with these two remarkable individuals. The portion of this book contributed by Beauchamp is dedicated to these cherished friends. Childress expresses his deepest gratitude to his wife, Georgia, to whom he dedicates his portion of this book, and to his sons, Fred and Frank, for contributions that relate to, but also go well beyond, this book. They are an unfailing source of support and joy for him.

Contents

Principles of Biomedical Ethics

1

Morality and Ethical Theory

Moral dilemmas and moral reasoning

People in varied roles frequently face difficult decisions. Consider this example: Two California judges must reach a decision about a possible violation of medical confidentiality. A man killed a woman after confiding to a psychiatrist his intention to commit the act. The psychiatrist attempted unsuccessfully to have the man committed, but because of patient/physician confidentiality did not communicate the threat to the woman when the commitment attempt failed. This case eventually reached the California Supreme Court. The judge who writes the majority opinion in the case holds that "When a therapist determines, or pursuant to the standards of his profession should determine, that his patient presents a serious danger of violence to another, he incurs an obligation to use reasonable care to protect the intended victim against such danger." This obligation would include notification of the police and possibly a direct warning to the intended victim. The judge argues that although physicians generally ought to observe the protective privilege of medical confidentiality, the principle must yield in this case to the "public interest in safety from violent assault." The judge contends that rules of professional ethics have substantial public value but, nonetheless, matters of greater importance, such as the protection of persons from violent assault, can override them. In the minority opinion, a second judge disagrees with this analysis. He argues that doctors violate patient rights when they fail to observe rules of confidentiality. If it were common practice to break these rules, the fiduciary nature of the patient/doctor relationship would begin to erode. Patients would lose confidence in psychiatrists and would refrain from divulging critical information to them. Violent assaults would actually increase as a result, because mentally ill persons would not seek psychiatric aid.

This case (# 1 in Appendix I) can be read as a straightforward moral dilemma (as well as a legal dilemma) because both judges cite strong moral reasons to support their quite opposite conclusions. But what makes this or any situation a moral dilemma or quandary? In dilemmatic situations, the reasons on each side of a problem are weighty ones, and none is in any obvious way the right set of reasons. If one acts on either set of reasons, one's actions will be desirable in some respects but undesirable in others. It would be ideal, although impossible, to act on all the reasons, for each is, considered by itself, a good reason. If there is a conflict between moral obligation on the one hand, and self-interest or personal inclination on the other, we do not usually consider the situation as presenting a moral dilemma. *Moral* dilemmas arise when one can appeal to moral considerations for taking each of two opposing courses of action. If moral reasons compete with nonmoral reasons, difficult questions can be posed (for example, why be moral?) without creating a *moral* dilemma. Some situations, however, clearly involve moral dilemmas. They take the following forms:[1] (1) Some evidence indicates that act X is morally right, and some evidence indicates that act X is morally wrong, but the evidence on both sides is inconclusive. Abortion, for example, is sometimes said to be "a terrible dilemma" for women who see the evidence in this way. (2) It is clear to the agent that, on moral grounds, he or she both ought and ought not to perform act X. For example, some have viewed the intentional cessation of lifesaving therapies in the case of comatose patients as dilemmatic for this reason.

This book examines moral *deliberation* and moral *justification* in biomedicine. When trying to determine which course of action is right (i.e., morally justified), or even obligatory, reasons proper to justification also may be used in deliberation. Thus, the reasons present in moral deliberation are justifying reasons because they express the conditions under which an action is believed to be morally justified. However, they may not be sufficient actually to justify an action in a particular situation, for there may be similarly compelling reasons not to act in that fashion.

Our approach to moral reasoning by deliberation and justification can be diagrammed in the form of hierarchical tiers or levels:

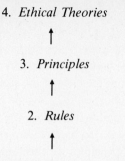

4. *Ethical Theories*

↑

3. *Principles*

↑

2. *Rules*

↑

1. *Particular Judgments and Actions*

According to this diagram, judgments about what ought to be done in particular situations are justified by moral rules, which in turn are justified by principles, which ultimately are justified by ethical theories. For example, a physician who refuses to perform an abortion may hold that it is morally wrong to kill an innocent human being intentionally. When pressed, the physician may justify the moral rule against killing an innocent human being by reference to a principle of the sanctity of human life. Finally, the particular judgment, the rule, and the principle may all be justified by an ethical theory—a theory that for many people may be only implicit and inchoate. ("Justified by" here has the meaning of "supported by." A *claim* to justification is not always a successful or fully adequate justification.)

Although our diagram may be oversimplified, its design indicates that in moral reasoning we appeal to different reasons of varying degrees of abstraction and systematization. Let us start with the lowest level and move upward. A *judgment* expresses a decision, verdict, or conclusion about a particular action (or, as we will see in Chapter 8, a character trait). Although the precise nature of the distinction between rules and principles is controversial, *rules* state that actions of a certain kind ought (or ought not) to be done because they are right (or wrong). A simple example is, "It is wrong to lie to a patient." *Principles* are more general and fundamental than moral rules and serve as their foundation or source of justification. The principle of respect for persons thus may support several moral rules of the "it-is-wrong-to-lie" sort. Finally, *theories* are bodies of principles and rules, more or less systematically related. They include second-order principles and rules about what to do when there are conflicts. Utilitarian and deontological theories, as we shall see in the next chapter, are important examples of ethical theories. Following William Frankena, we will refer to all these levels or tiers, but especially to principles and rules, as "action-guides."

Moral judgments involve applications of general action-guides to concrete situations, but such moral judgments also commonly rely upon factual beliefs about the world as well. For instance, if we hold that policy X is wrong because it imposes unjustified risks on a group of people, we presuppose certain beliefs about the facts of the situation. Similarly, judgments about the justifiability of abortion may depend not only on moral rules and principles, but also on factual beliefs about the nature and development of the fetus. It is thus a mistake to assume that moral disputes involve only conflicts between moral principles or their application, rather than conflicting factual interpretations. Nonmoral elements can play a decisive role in disputes over what morally ought and ought not to be done. As we will see in Chapter 6, for example, many disagreements about the allocation of health dollars to preventive and educational programs do not turn on principles of justice (as some related debates do), but rather on factual claims of whether such measures actually prevent illness or promote health.

Broad scientific, metaphysical, or religious beliefs often underlie our interpretation of a situation in which we must act. In addition, we may invoke these convictions to vindicate certain theories and action-guides (as for example, in the tradition of natural law). Thus, moral debate about a particular course of action may stem not only from disagreement about the relevant moral action-guides and the interpretation of factual information, but also from disagreement about the correct scientific, metaphysical, or religious description of the situation.

Consider as an example a debate involving various moral justifications and a complex interplay between moral action-guides and descriptive, nonmoral beliefs. In several exchanges, Paul Ramsey and Richard McCormick have urged different policies concerning the involvement of children in research.[2] They focus on research that does not offer potential medical benefit to the subjects involved, although it may ultimately benefit others. McCormick holds that it is morally permissible under some conditions to use children in such "nontherapeutic" research. His general rule is that this form of research is justified only if it involves minimal or negligible risk and if there is proxy (second-party) consent—providing, of course, that the research is also scientifically acceptable. His basic principle, which supports this rule, is one of justice: We all ought to bear certain burdens, usually of a minimal sort, for the common good. Such minimal or negligible burdens are not purely charitable, because they are demanded by justice. Thus, in McCormick's view, both adults and children ought to consent to participation in certain forms of research under appropriate conditions as a matter of justice.

McCormick further argues that parents (and other proxies) may legitimately consent for children to participate in nontherapeutic research where the child *ought* to consent (if the child could consent) because of a moral obligation. A judgment that it is morally acceptable to use children in nontherapeutic research would, for McCormick, depend on factual beliefs about the probable benefit and risks of the research; for example, if the risks are more than minimal or negligible, the research is never justified. In addition, McCormick's ethical theory, a version of natural-law thought, depends on certain factual beliefs about human tendencies that allow him to derive principles and rules about what people ought to do. These tendencies, including the human inclination toward community, are ultimately grounded for McCormick in metaphysics and theology: God has created man with tendencies toward certain values.

By contrast, Paul Ramsey holds that we should never use any child in nontherapeutic research. This rule is supported by a (deontological) principle of respect for persons: We should never treat people merely as means to some other end. To use human subjects who cannot consent in nontherapeutic research violates their integrity; it treats them merely as means to the end of scientific knowledge. Because participation in research involves the use of one's body, Ramsey holds that participation is a matter of charity, not justice, even if the risks are only minimal or negligible. We cannot be charitable for other people by enlisting them in research without their informed and voluntary consent. One of Ramsey's grounds for the principle of respect for persons is a theological interpretation of covenant-fidelity. Whether the risks of research are minimal or negligible is irrelevant under Ramsey's principles and rules. Because children are unable to give informed and voluntary consent, it is morally wrong to use them in nontherapeutic research, regardless of the risk-benefit ratio. Furthermore, in contrast to McCormick's view that research is of critical importance and perhaps even mandatory for the society and for individuals, Ramsey tends to view research as seeking benefits that the society is not obligated to pursue.

Although several other points in this debate are noteworthy, what has been said is sufficient to illustrate the complex interrelations both among tiers of moral justification and between action-guides and factual beliefs. This debate indicates that disputes over acts and policies often involve complex disagreements about factual beliefs, as well as about moral rules and principles. As this debate also suggests, it is necessary to distinguish a reason's *relevance* to a moral judgment from its *adequacy*. Relevant reasons are not always sufficient to support a moral judgment. An agent's appeal to a level or tier of justification may be relevant to a position the agent defends, but insufficient in the end to justify that position. Determining adequacy as well as relevance is one task of ethical theories.

Ethical theories and biomedical ethics

Which action-guides are worthy of moral acceptance and for what reasons? *General normative ethics* is the field of inquiry that attempts to answer these questions. It is constituted by what are called ethical theories in our levels of justification. Such theories, which are studied in detail in Chapter 2, seek to formulate and to defend a system of fundamental moral principles and rules that determine which actions are right and which are wrong. These action-guides are presumably valid for everyone. Ideally, any such ethical theory will include a complete set of ethical action-guides and will defend them as universally valid. However, numerous ethical questions would remain unanswered even if a fully satisfactory ethical theory were to be developed. For example, what do the various principles and rules imply for the concrete decisions people must make in everyday life? An attempt to apply these action-guides to different problem areas can be labeled *applied normative ethics*. The term "applied" is used because one applies general ethical principles and rules to illuminate and resolve specific moral problems. For example, one might appeal to principles of justice and utility in order to discuss moral dilemmas involved in the allocation of scarce medical resources, abortion, or the use of human subjects in biomedical research.

In addition to normative ethics, either general or applied, there are at least two *nonnormative* approaches to morality. First, there is *descriptive ethics*, the factual investigation of moral behavior and beliefs. Anthropologists, sociologists, psychologists, and historians determine whether and in what ways moral attitudes and codes differ from society to society. They study different beliefs and practices regarding sexual relations, professional codes of ethics, the treatment of the dying, the nature of consent obtained from patients, and the like. Second, there is the field of *metaethics*. This approach to morality, which has been warmly embraced by numerous philosophers in this century, involves analysis of the meanings of crucial ethical terms such as "right," "obligation," "virtue," and "responsibility." Students of metaethics also analyze the logic of moral reasoning, including the nature of moral justification.

Descriptive ethics and metaethics can be grouped together because both are nonnormative; that is, they do not attempt to provide prescriptive action-guides. They attempt to establish what factually or conceptually *is* the case, not what ethically *ought* to be the case.[3] Only in passing do we take positions in this book on problems of descriptive ethics and metaethics. For example, we operate descriptively in trying to determine what professional medical codes say about certain issues. Even so, our ultimate interest is whether the codes' prescriptions are *defensible*. We also occasionally deal in metaethics. For example, our discussion later in this chapter of the distinction between moral and nonmoral action-guides is metaethical. However, both descriptive and metaethical approaches are secondary to normative ethics throughout this book. Accordingly, when we use the term "ethics" without qualification, we shall mean normative ethics, either general or applied.

We focus on applied normative ethics because, in biomedical ethics, we are applying general moral action-guides to biomedicine. ("Biomedicine" is a short-hand expression for science, medicine, and health care.) Biomedical ethics is thus comparable to political ethics and business ethics. The term "bioethics," which is sometimes used to describe our area of interest, can be misleading. It suggests that we are dealing with an independent field, rather than with the *application* of general moral principles to an area of human activity. This usage may obscure the applicability of the action-guides to different activities such as politics and business as well as science, medicine, and health care.

Although the origin of systematic work in biomedical ethics is fairly recent, many issues in this applied field have been debated for decades and, in some cases, for centuries. While philosophers and especially theologians have long engaged in these debates, the most influential reflection on problems of biomedical ethics has evolved in professional codes of medical ethics and codes of research ethics. (For example, see Appendix II.) Such codes include highly specific rules that apply to persons in professional roles. These codes appeared in Western medicine in ancient Greece and have been constantly refined over the centuries. Their rules specify normative standards for situations likely to arise in the practice of medicine, in health care, and in research. It is important, then, to distinguish between general moral codes, which govern whole societies and apply to everyone alike, and more particular moral codes, which govern groups such as doctors, nurses, advertising agents, electrical engineers, and lawyers.

A general moral code proposed for or operative in a society consists of fundamental moral principles and rules. The code should not include so many principles, rules, and exceptions to rules that many members of the society cannot grasp or remember them. An example of a rule in a general moral code is "Whenever you have promised to do something, then you have an obligation to to it." By contrast, a special or professional moral code emphasizes derivative moral rules that specify obligations and duties for a particular group, such as physicians. These moral rules are justified by reference to more general and fundamental principles and rules, which may not be explicitly identified in the codes themselves. Such codes will not be effective if their rules are too numerous or too complex. Some of their rules, however, will be more professional and technical than those in the general moral code. The following is an example of a moral rule in the current code of the American Medical Association (AMA): "Once having undertaken a case, the physician should not neglect the patient, nor withdraw from the case without giving notice to the patient, the relatives, or responsible friends sufficiently long in advance of withdrawal to permit another medical attendant to be secured." We may view this rule as a specification of one of the principles that the AMA espouses in its Principles of Medical Ethics: "A physician shall respect the rights of patients. . . ." (See Appendix II.) This rule is also clearly derived from the rule of fidelity or promise-keeping in the general moral code.[4]

In order to indicate the advantages and disadvantages of professional codes, something should be said first about professions themselves. According to Talcott Parsons, a profession is "a cluster of occupational roles, that is, roles in which the incumbents perform certain functions valued in the society in general, and by these activities, typically earn a living at a full-time job."[5] For this reason, sociologists often characterize professional obligations as "role norms." Professions control entry into their occupational roles by certifying that candidates have developed the requisite body of skills and knowledge. In addition to attempting to ensure professional competence, professions typically specify and enforce certain responsibilities and obligations, so that those who enter into a relationship with members of the profession can trust them.[6] A professional code represents an articulated statement of role morality *as seen by the members of the profession*. It is distinguished from sets of standards imposed by external bodies such as governments. Sometimes codes also will specify rules of etiquette and role responsibilities that hold between members of the profession. (For example, an earlier AMA code instructed physicians not to criticize a fellow physician previously in charge of a case, and it urged them to offer professional courtesy.)

Professional codes are beneficial if they serve effectively to express moral principles and rules in the special relationships they govern. Their function is to promote trust and confidence within professional relationships so as to encourage professional activities performed for socially valued ends, such as the care of the sick. No doubt some professional codes oversimplify moral requirements or claim more completeness and authority than they actually possess. They may lead professionals to think that everything morally required has been done if the rules of the code have been followed. Such weaknesses of codes, however, may be outweighed by their value in controlling moral conduct. A more serious question concerns whether the codes specific to biomedicine express all the important principles and rules. For example, most of the medical codes have much to say about the implications of some principles, such as nonmaleficence and beneficence, and about some rules, such as confidentiality. However, they have little if anything to say about the implications of other important principles and rules, such as veracity, autonomy, and justice, which have been the subject of much contemporary philosophical discussion.[7]

Some of these relatively neglected principles and rules have played more prominent roles in two recent developments. First, some groups, including the American Hospital Association, have formulated statements of patients' rights that invoke such principles as autonomy and veracity. These statements, in effect, are codes of proper professional conduct for a wide range of health professionals, including physicians. They differ from earlier codes in that they focus on the rights of those receiving health services rather than on the obligations of health professionals. Different substantive emphases are also noteworthy: Whereas earlier codes tended to be paternalistic by affirming the professional's judgments about harms and benefits for the patient, these recent statements of rights stress the patient's autonomy.[8]

Second, in addition to codes formulated by consumer groups, several regulations and guidelines have been promulgated by government agencies. While much work in biomedical ethics has been limited to or has primarily focused on *individual* conduct—such as what a physician should or should not do to a patient—numerous questions of *public policy* also surround biomedicine. Consider issues about research, for instance. Since the Nuremberg Code of 1947, the United States government has promulgated several guidelines for research involving human subjects. In 1974, Congress created the National Commission for the Protection of Human Subjects of Biomedical and Behavioral Research to recommend guidelines to the Secretary of the Department of Health, Education, and Welfare (now the Department of Health and Human Services).[9] Their conclusions and lengthy recommendations, along with other government policies pertaining to biomedicine, raise questions about the proper relation between government and professional groups in formulating standards and controlling conduct. Many of these questions are at least partly moral in nature.

But what is meant by "public policy," and how is it connected to ethics? According to one recent author, "Public policy is whatever governments choose to do or not to do."[10] As such, public policies often involve the following actions: (1) regulation (such as prohibition of an activity) and (2) the allocation and distribution of both social benefits (such as services and goods) and social burdens (such as taxation). In this book we will deal briefly with selected problems of public policy: For instance, we will consider whether the government should prohibit active euthanasia, regardless of conclusions reached by individuals and health professionals. We will also inquire whether certain patterns of allocating health resources are more just than others.

The same principles and rules that apply to ethical issues in biomedicine also apply to public policies regarding biomedicine. However, it is rarely possible to move assuredly from a judgment that *act* X is morally right (or wrong) to a judgment that *policy* Y is morally right (or wrong). Numerous factors, such as the symbolic value of law and the cost of enforcement, must be considered. Thus, the judgment that an act is morally wrong does not necessarily lead to the judgment that the government should prohibit it, or even refuse to allocate funds for it. For example, it is possible to hold that sterilization or abortion is morally wrong without holding that the law should prohibit it or even deny government funds to women who otherwise could not afford these procedures. Nor does the judgment that an act is morally acceptable in some circumstances imply that the law should permit it. For example, it is possible to hold that *acts* of active euthanasia are morally justified in circumstances where patients face uncontrollable pain and suffering, and yet to hold simultaneously that the government should prohibit active euthanasia because it is not possible to design a permissive *law* that would prevent abuses.

Tests of ethical theories

Several general tests can be used to determine the adequacy of ethical theories. It is possible that no ethical theory will satisfy all of these tests, but we do and should appeal to them when trying to determine which theories or elements of theories are acceptable. It will suffice for the moment just to identify these tests. When analyzing and assessing ethical theories in subsequent chapters, we will amplify these tests as we use them.

First, an ethical theory should be as clear as possible, as a whole as well as in its parts. A clear theory is easier to understand and apply than an unclear one, and it is always appropriate to criticize a theory for its lack of clarity.

Second, an ethical theory should be internally consistent and coherent. At the very least, this test means that parts of a theory should not be inconsistent with each other—indeed they should be mutually supportive. Ralph Waldo Emerson dismissed a foolish consistency as "the hobgoblin of little minds," but a theory that is internally inconsistent or incoherent is to that extent unacceptable. Indeed, it is questionable that such a "theory" could really count as a theory, because it would not yield similar results when used by different people or even by the same persons in different but relevantly similar circumstances.

Third, a theory should be as complete and comprehensive as possible in listing moral principles and rules and their interactions. There should be no major gaps or holes in the theory.

Fourth, simplicity is a virtue of theories. For example, a theory should have no more principles and rules than are necessary, and certainly no more than people are able to remember and to apply without confusion.

Fifth, a theory must be able to account for the whole range of moral experience, including our ordinary judgments. We participate in morality on a daily basis by making decisions, reaching judgments, and offering reasons in the name of morality. Ethical theories must build on, systematize, and criticize our ordinary concepts and beliefs.

Our moral experience and moral theories are dialectically related. We develop theories to illuminate experience and to determine what we ought to do, but we also use experience to test, corroborate, and criticize theories. If a theory yields conclusions totally at odds with our ordinary judgments—for example, if it allows human subjects to be used merely as means to the ends of scientific research—we have reason to be suspicious of that theory and to search for another. But in many matters of morality, we may be uncertain whether the theory is in error and needs to be modified or even rejected, or whether our ordinary judgments are mistaken. As Joel Feinberg suggests, our procedure is similar to the dialectical reasoning that occurs in courts of law:

If a principle commits one to an antecedently unacceptable judgment, then one has to modify or supplement the principle in a way that does the least damage to the harmony of one's particular and general opinions taken as a group. On the other hand, when a solid well-entrenched principle entails a change in a particular judgment, the overriding claims of consistency may require that the judgment be adjusted.[11]

The cases found in Appendix I are used throughout this volume to "modify or supplement" the principles proposed, and likewise the principles can serve to modify judgments about the cases. Because judgments and principles are themselves among the tiers of justification, the relations between the different tiers obviously follow a similar pattern.

Although other tests could be formulated, these are the most important for analyzing and appraising various theories. As we will see in subsequent chapters, a theory may receive a high score on the basis of one test, but a low score on the basis of another test. In Chapter 2, utilitarianism is depicted as relatively consistent, coherent, simple, and comprehensive, but its critics claim that it is in tension with our ordinary judgments, especially our judgments about just actions and policies. By contrast, utilitarian critics of some deontological theories commonly agree that such theories are consistent with our ordinary judgments, but they insist that these ordinary judgments at least occasionally should be modified by a more consistent, coherent, simple, and comprehensive theory.

Moral and nonmoral action-guides

What makes some dilemmas and judgments—and not others—moral? That is, by what criteria can we say that any given normative standard is properly moral rather than religious, legal, or political? This question is not merely theoretical; it has practical significance. For instance, in 1974, Congress charged the National Commission for the Protection of Human Subjects of Biomedical and Behavioral Research "to conduct a comprehensive investigation and study to identify the *basic ethical principles* which should underlie the conduct of biomedical and behavioral research involving human subjects."[12] The National Commission then attempted to determine during its deliberations whether, and how, ethical principles can be distinguished from, for example, legal principles.

Many people believe that they can recognize moral action-guides when they encounter them, but it may be very difficult to distinguish moral and nonmoral considerations in controversies about cases. Consider, for example, debates about Case #22. Infant Doe was born with Down's syndrome and other complications that prevented food from reaching the stomach. An operation probably could have saved the baby's life, but the parents and the physicians, ultimately with the permission of the courts, allowed the baby to die. Supporters of this decision might hold that parents have the right to make such a decision, that the infant would have been better off dead than alive, or that the burdens of caring for the infant would have been too great for the family. Opponents of the decision might claim that the infant had a right to life, that the infant could have anticipated a reasonably good quality of life and thus would have been better off alive than dead, or that the state should help families with such burdens rather than allowing them to withhold treatment from defective newborns.

Several contemporary philosophers have tried to identify criteria by which we can distinguish moral and nonmoral considerations in such disputes. They have concentrated on three main conditions of moral action-guides. The first two conditions are formal: They refer to the form, not the particular content, of moral judgments, rules, and principles. Because they do not pertain to content, they would (if used alone) allow more action-guides to be counted as moral than the third condition would allow.

According to the first condition, moral action-guides are whatever a person or, alternatively, a society accepts as *supreme, final,* or *overriding* in judgments about actions. Unless this condition of overridingness is combined with other conditions, it permits almost anything to count as moral if a person, or a society, is committed to its overriding pursuit. For example, a person's primary commitment to scientific knowledge could be considered that person's morality. While we often say that a person or a society has a morality because of an acknowledgement of some supreme set of action-guides, it is difficult to hold that supremacy is either necessary or sufficient for morality. It is not *sufficient*, because other conditions such as our second one (universalizability) appear to be indispensable. Thus, we cannot say that *every* overriding action-guide counts as moral. Furthermore, to hold that supremacy is a *necessary* condition of morality is to prejudge the weight that moral action-guides should have in our deliberations when they conflict with political, legal, and religious action-guides. We cannot with certainty say that moral considerations, by definition, must outweigh or override all other considerations in competition with them. Nothing about morality itself makes such a demand.

A second and widely accepted condition for moral action-guides is *universalizability*, which requires that all relevantly similar cases be treated in a similar way. This formal condition may be a necessary condition of moral thinking, but it is insufficient to distinguish moral judgments from other action-guiding judgments that also meet this requirement. Many universalizable action-guiding propositions are not moral—for example, "Always train your dogs before they are six months old." The important point is that a judgment that an act is right (or wrong) commits the person who makes it to the same conclusion in relevantly similar circumstances. If a person holds that act X is right and act Y is wrong, but cannot point to any significant differences between them, the person is not making a moral judgment.

The practical significance and the limits of the principle of universalizability (which, as we will see in Chapter 6, can also be formulated as the principle of formal justice) can be seen in the deliberations and recommendations regarding fetal research of the aforementioned National Commission for the Protection of Human Subjects of Biomedical and Behavioral Research. (1) The Commission affirmed that in cases of experimentation *in utero*, the fetus to be aborted and the fetus to be brought to term should be treated as equals. It held "that the woman's decision for abortion does not, in itself, change the status of the fetus for purposes of protection. Thus, the same principles apply whether or not abortion is contemplated; in both cases, only minimal risk is acceptable."[13] (2) The Commission was otherwise divided, however, because similar treatment is not identical treatment. "Minimal risk" for a fetus who will be brought to term is different from "minimal risk" for a fetus who will be aborted, if we assume that the woman will not change her mind. For example, the injection of a drug that crosses the placenta might not injure a fetus aborted within two weeks after the injection, but it might injure a fetus two months after the injection. Thus, the Commission agreed that the principle of universalizability (in this case, a principle of equal treatment) is applicable to fetal research. Yet Commission members disagreed about what this principle implies for research involving differently situated fetuses.

This disagreement points up an important qualification that must be made about the notion of a universalizable moral principle. Universalizability has sometimes been explicated in moral treatises as if it meant that all moral principles apply universally to everyone alike and never apply exclusively to restricted groups—irrespective of moral traditions and moral disagreements. If this were so, then American views about the treatment of defective newborns and about access to health care resources would have to be the same as Chinese views—or some group's views would have to be declared simply mistaken. Universalizability need not, however, entail that only one moral system of principles and rules is correct and universally applicable regardless of the social context. Rather, universalizability makes a formal point about the logic of moral judgment: Any moral judgment, because moral, must, for any person who accepts the judgment, apply universally in *relevantly similar circumstances*. All of the parties in the dispute about Infant Doe may have been willing to make the same judgments about similar defective newborns.

Some philosophers have also proposed a third criterion of morality, one with moral *content*. They argue that it is necessary for a moral action-guide to have some direct reference to the *welfare of others*. This condition of other-regardingness excludes egoistic principles, for example, from the realm of moral action-guides; and it would also exclude certain religious action-guides. But clearly most principles and rules of interest in biomedicine, whether moral or not, involve some direct reference to human welfare. Most of the considerations offered by defenders and opponents of the decision in the case of Infant Doe meet this condition. Also, the contention that moral action-guides must have some reference to the welfare of others does not indicate that the welfare of *all* parties must receive the same weight. For example, if someone argued for a policy of massive, high-risk, nontherapeutic research on prisoners for the benefit of society, we could not count that recommendation as *nonmoral* merely because it would sacrifice some individuals for the sake of others. It would, however, be *immoral* according to most ethical theories.

In order to determine the grounds on which this policy and many other policies and acts could be held as immoral, we shall now turn to an examination of major ethical theories and their moral principles, rules, and judgments.

Notes

1. See John Lemmon, "Moral Dilemmas," *Philosophical Review* 71 (1962): 139–58.
2. Paul Ramsey, *The Patient as Person* (New Haven: Yale University Press, 1970), pp. 1–58, "The Enforcement of Morals: Nontherapeutic Research on Children," *Hastings Center Report* 6 (August 1976): 21–39, "Children as Research Subjects: A Reply," *Hastings Center Report* 7 (April 1977): 40–42; and Richard McCormick, S. J., "Proxy Consent in the Experimental Situation," *Perspectives in Biology and Medicine* 18 (Autumn 1974): 2–20, "Experimentation in Children: Sharing in Sociality," *Hastings Center Report* 6 (December 1976): 41–46. See also William E. May, "Experimenting on Human Subjects," *Linacre Quarterly* 41 (November 1974): 238–52; Robert J. Levine, *Ethics and Regulation of Clinical Research* (Baltimore: Urban and Schwarzenberg, 1981); the National Commission for the Protection of Human Subjects of Biomedical and Behavioral Research, *Report and Recommendations: Research Involving Children* (Washington, D.C.: U.S. Department of Health, Education, and Welfare, 1977), especially Chapter 8; and current federal regulations regarding research (excerpts in Appendix II).
3. For various reasons it is controversial whether such a sharp distinction can be drawn between metaethics and normative ethics. See for example Philippa Foot, "Goodness and Choice", and J. R. Searle, "How to Derive 'Ought' from 'Is'," in *The Is/Ought Question*, ed. W. D. Hudson (London: Macmillan, 1969).
4. Earlier a version of the rule prohibiting the neglect of patients appeared in the AMA Principles of Medical Ethics (1957); while it also appeared in a proposed revision of the Principles, it was dropped from the final version. It now appears in the Opinions of the Judicial Council of the AMA; many of these opinions function as rules. See *Current Opinions of the Judicial Council of the American Medical Association* (Chicago: American Medical Association, 1981); Bruce Nortell, "AMA Judicial Council Activities," *Journal of the American Medical Association* 239 (April 3, 1978): 1396–97; and Robert M. Veatch, "Professional Ethics: New Principles for Physicians?" *Hastings Center Report* 10 (June 1980): 16–19.

5. Talcott Parsons, *Essays in Sociological Theory*, rev. ed. (Glencoe, Ill.: The Free Press, 1954), p. 372.
6. *The American Medical Association Code of Ethics* of 1847, largely adapted from Percival's *Medical Ethics* (1803), was to a great extent a response to a crisis in public confidence. See Donald E. Konold, "History of the Codes of Medical Ethics," *Encyclopedia of Bioethics*, ed. Warren T. Reich (New York: The Free Press, 1978). Professional ethics may be formal or informal and may or may not be backed by sanctions held by a disciplinary body. Medicine is characterized by both formal codes and disciplinary bodies, but some other health professions lack disciplinary structure and sanctions (e.g., social workers).
7. See Sissela Bok, "The Tools of Bioethics," in *Ethics in Medicine: Historical Perspectives and Contemporary Concerns*, eds. Stanley Joel Reiser, Arthur J. Dyck, and William J. Curran (Cambridge, Mass.: MIT Press, 1977), pp. 137–41.
8. See George J. Annas, *The Rights of Hospital Patients: The Basic ACLU Guide to a Hospital Patient's Rights* (New York: Avon Books, 1975). For a discussion of the evolution of medical codes, see *Encyclopedia of Bioethics*, "History of the Codes of Medical Ethics."
9. See Public Law 93-348 and various publications of this Commission. See also the several volumes published by the President's Commission for the Study of Ethical Problems in Medicine and Biomedical and Behavioral Research.
10. Thomas R. Dye, *Understanding Public Policy*, 2nd ed. (Englewood Cliffs, N.J.: Prentice-Hall, 1975), p. 1.
11. Joel Feinberg, *Social Philosophy* (Englewood Cliffs, N.J.: Prentice-Hall, 1973), p. 34. Chaim Perelman writes, "in morals absolute preeminence cannot be given either to principles—which would make morals a deductive discipline—or to particular cases—which would make it an inductive discipline. Instead, judgments regarding particulars are compared with principles, and preference is given to one or the other according to a decision that is reached by resorting to the techniques of justification and argumentation." *The New Rhetoric and the Humanities: Essays on Rhetoric and its Applications* (Boston: D. Reidel Publishing Co., 1979), p. 33.
12. Public Law 93-348, emphasis added. See note 9 above. For a discussion of some of the issues and major positions, see James F. Childress, "The Identification of Ethical Principles," *Journal of Religious Ethics* 5 (Spring 1977): 39–68. We often use the term "moral" and "ethical" interchangeably, although some distinctions can be drawn between them. Cicero apparently formed the Latin word *moralis* (from *mores*) to translate the Greek term *ethikos*. Etymologically their meanings are similar and stress manners, character, and customs. Contemporary usage suggests some rough but not very precise distinctions between them. "Ethics" often refers to reflective and theoretical perspectives, while "morality" often refers to actual conduct and practice. Our use of the terms "ethics" and "morality" in this book respects this rough distinction, although we use the adjectives "moral" and "ethical" interchangeably.
13. The National Commission for the Protection of Human Subjects of Biomedical and Behavioral Research, *Report and Recommendations: Research on the Fetus* (Washington, D.C.: U.S. Department of Health, Education, and Welfare, 1975), p. 66.

2

Utilitarian and Deontological Theories

A well-developed ethical theory provides a framework of principles within which an agent can determine morally appropriate actions. But in light of the tests we developed in the previous chapter, which ethical theory is most satisfactory? In this chapter, we shall concentrate on the two types of ethical theories that have received the most attention in recent years: utilitarian and deontological theories.

The classical origins of utilitarianism are found in the writings of David Hume (1711–76), Jeremy Bentham (1748–1832), and John Stuart Mill (1806–73). Utilitarianism is only one of several ethical theories that gauge the worth of actions by their ends and consequences. These theories are sometimes said to be consequentialist or teleological (derived from the Greek term *telos*, meaning "end"). They hold that morally right actions are determined by the nonmoral value, such as pleasure, friendship, knowledge, or health, produced by their performance. The value is said to be *nonmoral* because it is the general goal of such human activities as art, athletics, and academics, and thus is not a distinctly moral value as is, for example, fulfilling a moral obligation. A common feature of these theories is that duty and right conduct are subordinated to what is good, for right and duty are defined in terms of goods or that which produces goods.

By contrast, deontological theories (derived from the Greek term *deon*, meaning "duty") deny precisely what teleological theories affirm. Their classical origins are more diverse and include, for example, some religious ethics that concentrate on divine commands. However, the ethical theory of

Immanuel Kant (1734–1804) is generally regarded as the first unambiguous formulation of a deontological ethical theory. Deontologists maintain that the concept of duty is independent of the concept of good and that right actions are not determined exclusively by the production of nonmoral goods. Whereas the teleologist (and thus the utilitarian) holds that actions are determined to be right or wrong by only one of their features, viz., their consequences, the deontologist contends that even if this feature sometimes determines the rightness and wrongness of acts, it does not always do so. Other features of an act are also relevant, e.g., the fact that it involves telling a lie or breaking a promise. In this chapter we consider these two general approaches to ethics as ways to account for rightness and wrongness in biomedical ethics. Rather than considering the many different versions of teleological theories, we focus on the most prominent version, utilitarianism.

Utilitarianism

While the term "utilitarianism" is familiar to most of us, its popular usage can be confusing and misleading. It is said, for example, to be the theory that "the end justifies the means." It is also said to be the view that "we ought to promote the greatest good of the greatest number." Since "utility" is commonly translated as "usefulness," this theory is sometimes said to be the view that what is right is what is most useful. In some respects each of these popular characterizations is accurate, but utilitarianism is considerably more sophisticated and refined than such characterizations suggest. In this book the term "utilitarianism" refers to the moral theory that there is one and only one basic principle in ethics, the principle of utility. This principle asserts that, in all circumstances, we ought to produce the greatest possible balance of value over disvalue for all persons affected (or the least possible balance of disvalue if only bad results can be brought about).

An example of utilitarian thinking is the following: It is universally agreed that physicians should minimize the costs for and suffering of their patients. This obviously does not mean that physicians should never charge fees to patients or should never allow any suffering or risk of harm to patients. But it does mean that whenever there is a choice between different but equally efficacious methods of treatment, patients' benefits should be maximized and their costs and risks minimized. Any other approach would rightly be regarded as an unethical practice. This example and many similar ones from everyday life—such as designing a family budget to meet the family's needs or creating a new national park in a wilderness region—reflect a utilitarian method of calculating what should be done by balancing resources and comparing the actual needs of everyone affected. According to this method, any decision is justified if it produces more good than any alternative would.

Utilitarians do not believe this method of calculating imposes something alien or even unusual on the moral life. They think that utilitarianism simply renders explicit and systematic what is already implicit in ordinary deliberation and justification. The utilitarian believes that such reasoning is dominant both in individual actions and in public policy. Case #33 in the Appendix discusses a 1980 policy decision announced by the twelve lay trustees of the Massachusetts General Hospital. These trustees voted not to permit heart transplants at that institution "at the present time" because "in an age where technology so pervades the medical community, there is a clear responsibility to evaluate new procedures in terms of the greatest good for the greatest number." They had decided that the costs of heart transplantation would probably outweigh its benefits. This is a splendid example of the way a utilitarian approach has filtered down from a philosophical system into practical policy decisions affecting medicine.

While this discussion reflects elementary utilitarian thinking, there are disputes among utilitarians concerning how the theory is best characterized, as well as disputes over which values are most important. Some grasp of these internal disputes is required to understand utilitarian ethics.

The concept of utility

We have seen that all utilitarians share the conviction that human actions are to be morally assessed in terms of their production of maximal nonmoral value. But how are we to determine what value could and should be produced in any given circumstance? Utilitarians agree that ultimately we ought to look to the production of what is intrinsically valuable rather than extrinsically valuable. That is, what is good in itself and not merely what is good as a means to something else ought to be produced. For example, neither undergoing nor performing an abortion is considered by anyone to be intrinsically good. However, many people would sometimes consider it extrinsically good as a means to another end, such as the restoration of an ill woman to a state of health. Utilitarians believe that we ought to seek certain experiences and conditions in life that are good in themselves without reference to their further consequences, and that all actions are ultimately to be gauged in terms of these intrinsic values. Most utilitarians would include health and freedom from pain among such values. From the utilitarian perspective, the whole point of the institution of morality is to promote such human values by maximizing benefits and minimizing harms.

An intrinsic value, then, is a value in life we wish to possess and enjoy just for its own sake and not for something else it produces. Without such values, the things we pursue as means to other things would lose their value. If, for example, a surgical procedure restores a person to a state of health, but he or she does not value health, then it is hard to understand why the surgical procedure is valuable to that person. The value of most procedures in medical practice and research derives from some other basic value, such as health. Sometimes, of course, a single item can possess both intrinsic and extrinsic value. For example, new knowledge about nuclear-powered, artificial hearts (see Case #32) may be intrinsically valuable to scientific investigators, but it may also be extrinsically valuable for thousands of (future) patients. Health also can be extrinsically good, as a means to the end of an enjoyable and productive life. Still, the main task for utilitarians is to provide an acceptable theory that explains why things are intrinsically good, and that develops categories of such goods.

Within utilitarian theories of intrinsic value a major distinction is drawn between hedonistic utilitarians and pluralistic utilitarians. Bentham and Mill are referred to as hedonistic utilitarians because they conceived utility entirely in terms of happiness or pleasure—two very broad terms that here may be taken as synonymous. Bentham, for example, viewed utility as that aspect of any object or event whereby it tends to produce different pleasures in such forms as benefit, advantage, good, and the prevention of pain.[1] Mill went to considerable lengths not to be misunderstood on the matter of what "happiness" means. He insisted that happiness does not refer to "a continuity of highly pleasurable excitement," but rather encompasses a realistic appraisal of the pleasurable moments afforded in life, whether they take the form of tranquillity or passionate excitement.[2] The principle of utility for Bentham and Mill thus demands courses of action that produce the maximum possible happiness in the broad sense of the term employed by these philosophers. That is, an action ought to be performed if the sum of the happiness of all affected individuals would be maximized by the performance of that action.

Mill and Bentham knew, of course, that many human actions do not appear to be performed merely for the sake of happiness. For example, they were aware that highly motivated professionals—such as research scientists—can work themselves to the point of exhaustion for the sake of knowledge they hope to gain, even though they might have chosen different and better routes to happiness and pleasure. Mill's explanation of this phenomenon is that such persons are initially motivated by pleasure. They are at that time interested either in prestige or in money, both of which promise pleasure. Along the way, however, either the pursuit of knowledge becomes itself productive of happiness or else such persons never stop associating their hard work with the money or prestige they hope to gain (despite their not actually deriving much, if any, pleasure from it). Mill also believed that there are qualitatively different kinds of pleasure, some worth cultivating more than others because they are intrinsically more valuable. This claim proved difficult to sustain, but Mill's problems with it cannot be considered here. The main point is that for some utilitarians, including two of its leading proponents, happiness or pleasure is the single form of intrinsic value, even though it may be analyzed into many different subtypes.

Later utilitarian philosophers have not looked favorably on this monistic conception of intrinsic value. They have argued that other values besides happiness possess intrinsic worth; among these values are friendship, knowledge, courage, health, beauty, and perhaps even certain moral qualities. According to G. E. Moore, who defended this view, even some states of consciousness can be valuable apart from their pleasantness.[3] The idea that there are many kinds of intrinsic value eventually received widespread acceptance among utilitarians. Its proponents held that the greatest aggregate good, as well as all moral rightness or wrongness, is to be assessed in terms of the total range of intrinsic value ultimately produced by an action.

However, in recent philosophy, economics, and psychology, neither the approach of the hedonists nor that of the pluralists has prevailed. Both approaches seem inadequate for purposes of objectively aggregating widely different interests in order to determine where maximal value and, therefore, right action lies. The major alternative approach is to appeal to individual *preferences*. For this approach, the concept of utility refers not to experiences or states of affairs, but rather to an individual's actual preferences, as determined by his or her behavior. To maximize a single person's utility is to provide what that person has chosen or would choose from among the available alternatives. This approach rejects both hedonistic and pluralistic views of intrinsic value. What is intrinsically valuable is what individuals prefer to obtain, and utility is thus translated into the satisfaction of those needs and desires that individuals choose to satisfy.

This modern approach to value has seemed to many preferable to its predecessors for two main reasons. First, recent disputes about hedonism and pluralism have proved interminable, sometimes ideological, and in the view of many, irresolvable. One's choice of a range of values seems deeply affected by personal experiences—a problem preference utilitarianism perhaps avoids in that personal preference is part of the theory. Second, to make utilitarian calculations, it is necessary in some way to measure values. In the monistic theory espoused by Bentham and Mill, for example, we must be able to measure pleasurable and painful states and then compare one person's pleasures with another's in order to decide which is greater. Yet, it is uncertain what it means to measure and then compare the values of pleasure, health, and knowledge—or any value at all, for that matter. As Alasdair MacIntyre observes, "The happiness which belongs peculiarly to the way of life of the cloister is not the same happiness as that which belongs peculiarly to the military life. For different pleasures and different happinesses are to a large degree incommensurable."[4] It does make sense, however, to develop a utility scale that numerically measures strengths of individual and group preferences. This approach has proved fruitful in recent discussions of health economics, to take just one of many examples.

The preference approach nonetheless is not trouble-free. A major problem of utilitarianism arises when individuals have what are, according to ordinary views about morality, morally unacceptable preferences. For example, if a skillful researcher derived supreme satisfaction from inflicting pain on animals or on human subjects in experiments, we would condemn and discount this person's preference and would seek to prevent it from being actualized. Utilitarianism based on subjective preferences is an acceptable theory only if a range of acceptable preferences can be formulated. This task has proven difficult, and may even be inconsistent with the preference approach, because human value is logically tied to preferences in the theory.

The main utilitarian response is that unacceptable desires can be distinguished. On the basis of past experience, some utilitarians maintain, we can know which preferences undermine utilitarian social objectives by creating conditions adverse to the production of human value. Such desires would then not be permitted to count in the utilitarian calculus. Thus, we would refuse to acknowledge preferences to taunt and abuse aged citizens, not only because these preferences obstruct the preferences of the aged, but because more generally such preferences destroy or undermine the achievement of human value (themselves determined by firmly established preferences). Such preferences thus deserve no status whatever in a calculus of goods. This account is presumably consistent with preference utilitarianism because both preferences and the principle of utility are sources of value. The principle of utility simply excludes some preferences on more general utilitarian grounds. However, whether this exclusion of preferences *is* consistent in a theory based upon preferences is debatable.

If utilitarianism could be fully worked out along the lines we have envisioned, it would give us a definite procedure for making moral choices. We would first calculate, to the best of our knowledge, the consequences that would result from our performance of the various actions open to us. In making this calculation we would ask how much value and how much disvalue—as gauged by the preferences of those affected by our actions— would result in the lives of all affected, including ourselves. Once we have completed all these calculations for all relevant courses of action, we are morally obliged to choose the action that maximizes intrinsic value (or minimizes intrinsic disvalue) for all affected parties. Knowingly to perform any other action is to take a morally wrong course.

It would be easy to overestimate the demands of this moral theory. While we must always attempt to make accurate measurements of the preferences of others, this seldom can be done because of our limited knowledge and time. Often in everyday affairs we must act on severely limited knowledge of the consequences of our actions. The utilitarian does not condemn any sincere attempt to maximize value merely because the consequences of the attempt turn out to be less than maximal. What is important, morally speaking, is that one conscientiously attempts to determine the most favorable action. Because common sense and careful deliberation will ordinarily suffice for these calculations, utilitarians cannot be accused of demanding more than we can do, as some critics have alleged.

Act and rule utilitarianism

The next distinction to be considered is between act and rule utilitarians. For all utilitarians the principle of utility is the ultimate source of appeal for the determination of morally right and wrong actions. Controversy has arisen, however, over whether this principle is to be applied to particular *acts* in particular circumstances in order to determine which act is right *or* whether it is to be applied instead to *rules* of conduct that themselves determine which acts are right and wrong. Using the scheme of ascending levels of justification introduced in Chapter 1, we may outline how utilitarians attempt to justify moral actions and, at the same time, illustrate how act and rule utilitarians differ:

Rule Utilitarianism	*Act Utilitarianism*
Principle of Utility	Principle of Utility
↑	↑
Moral Rules	Particular Judgments and Actions
↑	
Particular Judgments and Actions	

According to the schema on the left, the rule utilitarian justifies actions and judgments by appealing to rules such as "Do not steal" and "Do not lie," which in turn are justified by appeal to utility. An act utilitarian simply skips the level of rules and justifies actions by appealing directly to the principle of utility.

The act utilitarian considers the consequences of each particular act, while the rule utilitarian considers the consequences of generally observing a rule. Accordingly, the act utilitarian asks, "What good and evil consequences will result from this action in this circumstance?" and not "What good and evil consequences will result from this sort of action *in general* in these sorts of circumstances?" The act utilitarian may see rules such as "You ought to tell the truth" as useful rules of thumb in guiding human actions, but not as prescriptions. According to this species of utilitarian, the question is always "What should I do now?" and not "What has proved generally valuable in the past?" Act utilitarians take this position because they think observance of a general rule such as truthtelling would not on some occasions be for the general good.

For this latter reason, act utilitarians regard rule utilitarians as unfaithful to the demands of the principle of utility. This principle requires that we maximize values or, in the traditional formulation, "do the greatest good for the greatest number." But there are circumstances in which abiding by a generally beneficial rule will not prove most beneficial to the persons involved, even in the long run. Why ought a rule be obeyed in individual cases if obedience will not maximize value? A contemporary utilitarian, J. J. C. Smart, has argued that the rule utilitarian cannot reply to this criticism that it would be better that everybody should obey the rule than that nobody should. This objection fails, according to Smart, because there is a third possibility between never obeying a rule and always obeying it—viz., that it should *sometimes* be obeyed.[5] For example, physicians do not always tell the truth to their patients. They sometimes withhold information and even lie. Perhaps they invoke the legal doctrine of therapeutic privilege as a justification for their action, but they nonetheless violate general moral rules of truthfulness. They do so because they think it is better for the patient and for all concerned, and they do not think their act really undermines the moral rules. Smart's objection seems in the end reducible to the empirical prediction that we will be better off in the moral life if we sometimes obey and sometimes disobey rules, because this selective obedience will not erode either moral rules or our general respect for morality. Rules are stabilizing but dispensable guides in the moral life; that is, they are useful rules of thumb, but they are not valid for all circumstances.

An example of act-utilitarian thinking emerged in a case of research in the social sciences. (See Case #3 in Appendix I.) In order to observe homosexual behavior, a sociologist posed as a lookout for male homosexuals using isolated public facilities (so-called "tearooms"). His desire to provide a thorough study of this form of lifestyle led him to record the automobile license plate numbers of the participants so that he could subsequently locate their residences. By misrepresenting himself as a researcher pursuing a different and innocuous kind of study, he gained entrance to their homes and obtained data on family background, marital status, and the like. This research methodology has been heavily criticized not only because it put the subjects studied at risk (because the police might have obtained damaging data, including license plate numbers), but also because it involved outright deception, including a set of lies to gain entrance to private homes. In other words, it violated a number of standard moral rules prohibiting deception, lying, invading privacy, and placing other persons at risk. The sociologist involved defended his work on act-utilitarian grounds. He argued that his study would provide a valuable understanding of the motives and general behavioral patterns of those who perform homosexual acts—and also that it would help others appreciate the social pressures that can lead to homosexual activity. In short, he attempted to justify the violation of standard moral rules by appeal to the valuable and otherwise unattainable goals of his research.

Act utilitarianism has been subjected to sharp criticism in recent moral philosophy—justifiably, in our view. One major theoretical reason for its rejection relies on examples of intuitively wrong but undetectable actions. For example, suppose a physician kills by an undetectable means his rapidly deteriorating dialysis patient, who would have died in two to three months anyway, on the grounds that the patient's death would maximize utility in the circumstances. Now imagine a second physician who performs the identical action under the identical circumstances, except that the action is detected. It would seem that, according to act utilitarianism, the second action is morally wrong, whereas the first is not necessarily so. The first action plausibly does maximize utility in the circumstances. After all, the dialysis patient has little life left and is a severe financial and psychological burden to his family. In addition, the first doctor does not suffer the consequences of public criticism or even imprisonment. In the second case, however, the doctor does suffer imprisonment, and the families of both the patient and the physician may suffer the embarrassment, guilt, and anguish that usually accompany such events.

This conclusion of act utilitarianism strikes many as odd and unacceptable, for at least two reasons. First, the killing (if wrong) seems to be equally wrong in both cases; the second action does not appear more blameworthy simply because of a chain of unpleasant consequences. Second, we are inclined to say that the consequences of the physician's action, apart from the immediate consequence for the victim, are disconnected from our *moral* assessment of the action as wrong. Act utilitarianism seems to make certain extraneous consequences such as imprisonment not only relevant when they should be irrelevant, but relevant in such a way that they should change our assessment of the moral value of the action.

A similar and by now standard form of counterexample to act utilitarianism is captured in the following imagined sequence of events: Suppose that you are mountain climbing with your closest friend, a person whom you admire and respect, and from whom you have received many favors. Now suppose you lose your grip on a rope while he is descending a sheer cliff. He falls. By the time you reach him he is dying. In these dying moments he asks that you make a secret promise to him, and you agree. He reveals a great financial secret he has been harboring. Through years of hard work and careful investments he has hoarded a million dollars. He asks you to deliver this money to an uncle who has helped him in the past. But you know that this uncle is a very rich gambler and will eventually squander the money. No one else knows about either the promise or the secret cash. On act-utilitarian principles, it would appear that you should not carry out your promise to your dying friend. You could surely put the money to much better use by giving it to charitable institutions. You would not disappoint the man to whom you made the promise because he is dead. Nor would you weaken faith in the socially useful institutions of promise-making and promise-keeping.

The point of these counterexamples is to show that act utilitarianism is inconsistent with our common convictions about moral rightness, or what might be called the common moral consciousness. We saw in Chapter 1 that one test of an ethical theory is its congruence with these common, but well-considered, ethical convictions. The rule utilitarian would agree with this objection from common morality on the basis of the utility of the rule of promise-keeping in general. The act utilitarian would reply that although promises usually should be kept in order to maintain a climate of trust, this consideration fails to apply in cases where more good is produced by breaking the promise, which, in any event, is not public.

Arguments that similarly stress utilitarian consequences have been used to justify research into private behavior and the use of confidential information. A defense of those practices has been constructed on the basis of predictions about the likely consequences of curtailing research into private behavior or of prohibiting the research use of confidential information. The argument is that beneficial consequences for public health or some other public good are possible only through research methods that in some respects "invade" privacy. Methods of data collection in epidemiology, for example, may in some cases violate participant rights to privacy and confidentiality, yet alternative procedures may not be available or affordable.[6] The act utilitarian willingly admits this inconsistency with ordinary moral convictions in all such cases, but responds that we need to revise our ordinary convictions, not to discard act utilitarianism.

Act utilitarianism certainly challenges our ordinary convictions, as Case #34 nicely indicates: It features two Harvard professors who became interested in facts and policies pertaining to high blood pressure in American society. These investigators wanted to determine the most cost-effective way to tackle the problem of controlling hypertension in the American population. As they developed their research, they discovered that, rather than launching a community-wide campaign, it is more cost-effective to treat three classes of persons in the attempt to reduce the general public health problem of high blood pressure: (1) younger men, (2) older women, and (3) those patients with very high blood pressure. When they combined these findings with other findings that large-scale, public screening and informational programs are not medically effective (and not cost-effective), they concluded that:

A community with limited resources would probably do better to concentrate its efforts on improving adherence of known hypertensives, even at a sacrifice in terms of the numbers screened. This conclusion holds even if such proadherence interventions are rather expensive and only moderately effective, and even if screening is very inexpensive. . . . Finally, screening in the regular practices [of physicians] is more cost-effective than public screening.

This recommendation, if acted on by the government, would exclude the poorest sector of the country, which is also in greatest need of medical attention, from the benefits of high blood pressure education and management. Public screening would be sacrificed in order to do a larger good for the whole community; only persons known to have high blood pressure and already in contact with a physician about their problem would be recontacted. These investigators were concerned because there seemed to them to be a possible injustice in excluding the poor and minorities by a public health endeavor aimed expressly at the economically better-off sector of society. Yet their statistics were very compelling: No matter how carefully planned the efforts, nothing worked except programs directed at those already in touch with physicians. They knew that in light of other health needs, there would be no new federal allocations of public health money to control high blood pressure. Yet it would take massive new allocations even to begin to affect the poorer sections of society. These investigators therefore recommended what they explicitly referred to as a "utilitarian" set of criteria for allocation. This is the most difficult kind of case presented by act utilitarianism for testing our ordinary moral convictions.

The objections thus far considered are exclusively directed to act utilitarianism and cannot be used without modification to refute the rule utilitarian. According to rule utilitarians, rules themselves have a central position in morality and cannot be disregarded merely because of the exigencies of particular situations. Because of the substantial contributions made to society by the general observance of rules such as truthtelling, the rule utilitarian would not compromise them in a particular situation. Such a compromise would threaten the integrity and existence of the rule itself. For example, the act of a physician who withheld information from a patient would be immoral unless he or she were able to justify it by appeal to a moral rule strong enough to override the rule requiring that the truth be told. Such rules are selected in the first instance because their general observance would maximize social utility better than alternative rules or no rules. For the rule utilitarian, then, the conformity of an act to a valuable rule makes the action right, whereas for the act utilitarian the beneficial consequences of the act alone make it right.

A relevant example of rule-utilitarian thinking is found in Case #1 in the Appendix. In this case, which we discussed in Chapter 1, a woman was killed by a man who had previously confided to a psychiatrist his intention to kill her. The psychiatrist did attempt to have the man committed but, on grounds of patient/physician confidentiality, did not communicate the threat to the woman when the commitment attempt failed. The majority opinion in the case holds that if a patient presents considerable physical danger to another person, there is an ensuing obligation on the part of the psychiatrist to use reasonable care to protect the intended victim. This could possibly include giving the endangered individual a direct warning. Justice Tobriner goes on to argue that "public policy" in such matters is based on the relative importance of rules—in this case rules protecting confidentiality and rules protecting persons from violent assault. The judge not only appeals to the public importance of observing rules, but on utilitarian grounds holds that rules of confidentiality are less important than rules protecting persons from violent assault.

The opinion of Justice Clark, the dissenting judge in this case, expresses rule-utilitarian thinking as well. He reasons as follows:

Policy generally determines duty. . . . Overwhelming policy considerations weigh against imposing a duty on psychotherapists to warn a potential victim against harm. While offering virtually no benefit to society, such a duty will frustrate psychiatric treatment, invade fundamental patient rights, and increase violence.

After this paragraph the judge lists a series of consequence-centered reasons supporting a firm rule of confidentiality regarding information transmitted to psychiatrists. Not observing such a rule, he argues, would cause irreparable harm to "the very practice of psychiatry" and would even deter people from seeing psychiatrists. Although the judge does not expressly invoke utilitarian ethical theory in support of his views, his opinion is a fine example of rule-utilitarian reasoning.

While many rule utilitarians justify various rules by their consequences, some rule utilitarians propose that we consider the utility of *whole codes or systems of rules* rather than independent rules. Among the defenders of different versions of this position are David Hume, the eighteenth-century Scottish philosopher, and R. B. Brandt, a contemporary American philosopher.[7] According to this approach, the rightness or wrongness of individual acts is determined by reference to moral rules that have a place in a general code or system of rules. The system is assessed as a whole in terms of its overall consequences. It is necessary to consider the consequences of moral rules not as *independent* rules, but as parts of an entire network of rules. By again using the scheme of ascending levels of justification introduced in Chapter 1, we may illustrate this version of rule utilitarianism:

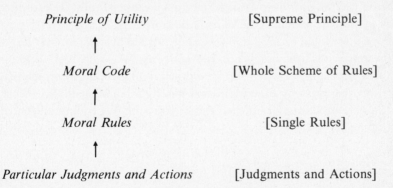

Principle of Utility	[Supreme Principle]
↑	
Moral Code	[Whole Scheme of Rules]
↑	
Moral Rules	[Single Rules]
↑	
Particular Judgments and Actions	[Judgments and Actions]

While this whole-code approach resembles simple rule utilitarianism, it allegedly has additional advantages. Most importantly, proponents claim that we are more likely to be able to maximize utility across an entire society with a whole system of rules than merely with single rules, each isolated from the consequences of other rules in the system. It would be difficult to motivate individuals in society to conform to rules if they were individually tested for their consequences, and we rarely think of morality in this way. Most of us accept a morality that determines a whole way of life, and we generally think of morality as a system of integrated principles and rules, none of which stands in isolation.[8] It may be that *traditional* moral rules already endorsed in society will (for utilitarian reasons) be a better set of rules than some *ideal* set, but this obviously depends on the particular features of social circumstances.

It is important to note, in concluding this section, that from the rule utilitarian's perspective no rule (and hence no moral action) is ever absolutely wrong in itself, and no rule in the system of rules is absolute and unrevisable. A rule's acceptability in the system of rules depends strictly on its consequences. Even rules against killing may be revised or substantially overturned. There has, for example, been considerable discussion in recent biomedical ethics of the possibility that seriously defective newborn infants should be killed rather than merely "allowed to die," as is now the practice in some cases. (See Case #22 in the Appendix.) The rule utilitarian argues that we should support rules *permitting* such killing if the rules would maximize value; but the rule utilitarian also insists that instead there should be rules *against* such killing if those rules would maximize value. To some this utilitarian approach seems shocking and outrageous, because in theory it would permit radical shifts in our present system of moral rules. But utilitarians are not impressed by this "conservative" objection. They point to the reason why we now have the rules we do have. Specifically, we presently do not permit the killing of newborn infants because of the adverse consequences that would be produced for many affected by such actions. But if this unhappy series of consequences did not generally occur, then the utilitarian would see no reason *in principle* why such killing should be prohibited. Such cases indicate why utilitarianism is strictly a consequentialist theory and also why utilitarians view their theory as responsive to unprecedented social change.

Deontological theories

We have seen that a teleological or consequentialist theory holds that the right is a function of the good, specifically of intrinsically valuable ends or consequences. Within such a theory one determines what should be done by asking whether an act or class of acts would probably produce the greatest possible balance of good over evil. By contrast, deontological theories (sometimes called formalist theories) hold that some features of acts other than, or in addition to, their consequences make them right or wrong. They insist that the concept of right or duty is not wholly derivative from the concept of good. In Case #4, where a therapist deceives a patient by substituting a placebo, a deontologist would consider both the feature of deception itself (not merely the effects of the deception) and the therapist's motives. For many deontologists deception is a wrong-making characteristic regardless of its consequences. As we shall see, a deontologist need not hold that deception or any other type of action is absolutely wrong and never justifiable. However, to qualify as a deontologist, one must hold that at least some acts are wrong and others right independent of their consequences. In deontological systems right-making characteristics such as fidelity to promises and contracts, gratitude for benefits received, truthfulness, and justice determine right acts and duties.

Versions of deontology

Different deontological theories compete with each other, as well as against teleological theories. It is possible to analyze these theories from several perspectives. First, we could explore the different ways deontologists try to vindicate their judgments that certain acts are right or wrong. Some moralists in religious traditions appeal to divine revelation (e.g., to God's promulgation of the Ten Commandments), while others appeal to natural law, which they contend can be known by human reason. Some philosophers, including W. D. Ross, find intuition and common sense sufficient. Still others, such as John Rawls, derive their principles from a hypothetical social contract by asking which principles rational contractors would adopt if they were placed behind a "veil of ignorance" and thus blinded to their talents, abilities, and conceptions of the good life.[9] To analyze and assess these and other warrants for moral judgments would lead us into the thickets of metaethics (theories of the meaning and justification of ethical terms), and this pursuit would be an unnecessary detour. Most of the principles and rules that we will consider are accepted by most deontological theories and can also be discovered in the "common morality."[10]

Second, like utilitarian theories, deontological theories may be *monistic* or *pluralistic*. A *monistic* deontological theory holds that there is a single principle or rule from which all other rules or judgments about duty and about right and wrong can be derived. Thus, a deontologist could affirm a single basic principle such as love, or respect for persons, or "the Golden Rule," and then derive rules such as truthtelling and fidelity from it. A contemporary example appears in Alan Donagan's *The Theory of Morality.* Donagan tries to locate the "philosophical core" of the morality of the "Hebrew-Christian tradition," or the part not dependent upon explicitly theistic beliefs. He identifies the fundamental principle of this common morality: "It is impermissible not to respect every human being, oneself or any other, as a rational creature."[11] Donagan believes that it is possible to derive all other moral principles and rules of the common morality in the Hebrew-Christian tradition from this fundamental principle.

Donagan is clearly indebted to Immanuel Kant's classic proposal of a single "categorical imperative" for testing all maxims of action. As an example of Kant's thesis, consider a person who desperately needs money and knows that he will not be able to borrow it unless he promises to repay it in a definite time, even though he also knows that he will not be able to repay it within this period. He decides to make a promise that he knows he will break. According to Kant, when we examine the maxim of his action— "When I think myself in want of money, I will borrow money and promise to pay it back, although I know that I cannot do so"—we discover that it cannot pass the basic test of the categorical imperative, according to which maxims must be *universalizable.* This test of universalizability is richer and more complicated than the formal test of universalizability that we introduced in Chapter 1.

To be universalizable, according to Kant, a maxim must be capable of being conceived and willed without contradiction as a universal law. The above maxim about misleading promises cannot be *conceived* as a universal law, for it would contradict itself. As Kant writes,

"How would things stand if my maxim became a universal law?" I then see straight away that this maxim can never rank as a universal law of nature and be self-consistent, but must necessarily contradict itself. For the universality of a law that everyone believing himself to be in need can make any promise he pleases with the intention not to keep it would make promising, and the very purpose of promising, itself impossible, since no one would believe he was being promised anything, but would laugh at utterances of this kind as empty shams.[12]

Some maxims that can be *conceived* as universal nonetheless cannot be *willed* without contradiction. Consider, for example, the maxim of a person who is well-off but refuses to help those who are struggling. According to Kant, an agent cannot, without contradiction, will that his maxim of refusing to help become universal law, for he might be in need of others at some point, and he would certainly want their help.

Although few philosophers would hold, as Kant appears to, that the universalizability of a maxim is both necessary and sufficient for determining its acceptability, most concur that it is a necessary condition of the validity of ethical judgments, rules, and principles. Kant himself may actually have had more than one basic principle, since the several formulations he offers of the categorical imperative are not clearly equivalent. In any case, neither Kant nor others who have proposed monistic theories have worked out a compelling account of a single fundamental principle.

Pluralistic deontologists, by contrast, affirm more than one basic rule or principle. For example, W. D. Ross, a prominent twentieth-century deontologist, held that there are several basic and irreducible moral principles, such as fidelity, beneficence, and justice. While this pluralistic approach may at first glance appear more plausible than monistic approaches because it is closer to our ordinary judgments, it encounters the difficulty—as Ross recognized—of what to do when these principles or rules come into conflict. Case #2 provides an example of this problem. A physician has to determine whether to tell the truth or to break a confidence. He cannot do both, yet each of the two principles or rules commands his allegiance. The pluralistic deontologist may give us little guidance about which rules or principles take priority in such cases of conflict. For example, Ross held that the principle of nonmaleficence (noninfliction of harm) takes precedence over the principle of beneficence (production of benefit) when they come into conflict, but he gave no answer about the priorities among the other principles except to say that several duties (such as keeping promises) have "a great deal of stringency." Finally, he quoted Aristotle: "the decision rests with perception."[13] While we intuit the principles, according to Ross, we do not intuit what is right in the situation; rather we have to find "the greatest balance" of right over wrong. However, if a pluralistic deontological theory does not provide some ordering of its principles and rules or some method of determining the relative weight of moral claims, it offers little guidance in many hard decisions.

One major recent attempt to overcome some of these difficulties of pluralistic theories is John Rawls's *A Theory of Justice*, which arranges general principles of justice (not the whole of morality) in a serial or lexical order. Such a lexical order reduces the need for a pluralistic deontologist to appeal to intuition or to balance every single principle against every other principle. As already noted, Rawls argues that rational contractors behind the "veil of ignorance" in a fair bargaining situation would accept the following principles of justice: (I) the principle of equal liberty, (IIa) the difference principle (which permits inequalities in the distribution of social and economic goods only if those inequalities will benefit everyone, especially the least advantaged), and (IIb) the principle of fair equality of opportunity. According to Rawls, it is not necessary or permissible to balance these principles because we have to satisfy (I) before we can consider (IIa) or (IIb). Thus, the principle of equal liberty has absolute weight relative to the second principle. And within the second principle, (IIb) has priority over (IIa). Rawls does not, however, propose that this sort of ordering can be extended to cover all moral principles.[14]

Finally, just as there can be act and rule utilitarianism, deontologists may focus on *acts* or on *rules* that cover classes of acts. Few philosophers or theologians have tried to defend act deontology, though traces of it can be seen here and there. It has been held, for example, that an individual can immediately and directly perceive what he or she ought to do by intuition, conscience, or faith in God's revelation and grace. (Someone might advise a physician—"Just follow your conscience!") But act deontology is problematic for several reasons. We do not have firm grounds for confidence in our own or others' intuition, conscience, or faith to perceive right and wrong in the situation—particularly in the light of immediate pressures, lack of time for deliberation, and the power of self-interest to distort perception. Furthermore, to judge that a particular act is wrong in the situation is implicitly to appeal to a rule. *If* we are making a moral judgment when we say that act X is wrong, we are saying that all relevantly similar acts in similar circumstances are wrong. To say it is wrong to lie to a patient who asks a direct question about his prognosis is to say that it is wrong to lie in all similar circumstances. Such a statement is at least an incipient rule.

As we will see later in this chapter, in the section on rules, the act deontologist as well as the act utilitarian may recognize some "rules." But neither will accept those rules as rigidly prescriptive. For the act utilitarian, "rules" are suggestive generalizations from past experience that alert us to possible consequences of acts; they are not binding, either absolutely or even in most circumstances. For the act deontologist, "rules" may identify what people have previously viewed as intuitively required, as dictated by conscience, or as commanded by God in particular situations. Such "rules" do not, however, bind the agent in new situations, because intuition, conscience, or God may prompt new decisions. Act utilitarianism is more plausible than act deontology because, at the very least, it requires agents to try to *calculate* the good that might be produced by alternative actions. In act deontology, the agent's response to the situation is more mysterious.

For *rule deontologists*, the heart of morality is a set of binding principles and rules that classify acts as right, wrong, obligatory, or prohibited. Kant,

for example, held that several rules could be derived from the basic categorical imperative. According to Ross, there are several independent duties
that can be stated as rules or principles. Some of these duties rest on one's
previous acts. For example, promises and implicit promises give rise to
duties of *fidelity*. And one's previous wrongful acts engender duties of
reparation. Other duties rest on the previous acts of other persons. When
they render services to us, for example, we have duties of *gratitude*. Ross
goes on to develop duties of *self-improvement, nonmaleficence, beneficence,*
and *justice*. Several of these duties will be central in later chapters. At the
moment we only want to indicate how one version of rule deontology
regards some classes of acts as right or wrong independent of their consequences.[15]

Rule deontology is widely represented in contemporary biomedical ethics.
Frequently, major opponents are best characterized as rule deontologists
whose disputes hinge on which principles or rules are primary or more
stringent. For example, Paul Ramsey is a rule deontologist who believes that
various principles and rules can be derived from love or covenant-fidelity;
those derivative principles and rules include the sanctity of life. Because of
this principle, it is permissible to override even a competent patient's refusal
of livesaving medical treatment. Thus, Ramsey recognizes the legitimacy of
strong paternalism (which we discuss in Chapter 5). By contrast, both
Robert Veatch and H. Tristram Engelhardt, Jr. defend the priority of the
principle of liberty: A competent patient has the right to refuse even lifesaving medical treatment. Both Veatch and Engelhardt thus oppose any
strong paternalism. But when Veatch and Engelhardt consider the allocation
of health care resources, Veatch argues for the priority of the principle of
equality and Engelhardt for the priority of the principle of liberty (i.e.,
noninterference with people's property, even to tax them to cover the health
needs of others). In both sorts of conflicts—over refusal of lifesaving medical
treatment and over justice in the allocation of health care resources—the
method of analysis used by these rule deontologists would be opposed by act
utilitarians such as Joseph Fletcher,[16] although the practical results may in
some cases be the same.

Deontology as an ethical theory

What are some of the major characteristics, as well as the strengths and
weaknesses, of deontological theories as compared to utilitarian theories?
First, utilitarians hold that only one moral relationship between persons is
fundamental: the relationship of benefactor and beneficiary. All other im-

portant human moral relationships are derivative. Deontologists, however, take various relationships between people as more or equally basic. For them it is not sufficient to say that we should maximize the good and that each person counts as one and only one. They claim that we do not encounter other people merely as depositories of good, as beneficiaries, each one counting as one and only one; rather, we are related to them in various ways by their and our previous acts. For example, the physician does not confront each sick person merely as someone needing attention and care. If the physician has already been treating a patient, the relationship to that person is different from the relationship to another person who appears at the office door at the same time with the same ailment. The physician makes an implicit commitment to a patient by taking care of the patient and generally does not have the right to abrogate that relationship merely in order to maximize good for others. The texture of the moral life thus seems to deontologists richer and more complicated than any utilitarian model suggests, for numerous relationships with others have special moral significance: parent and child, friend and friend, promisor and promisee, as well as physician and patient. Parents assume certain obligations to their children, and the children incur certain obligations to their parents. It is not the case, of course, that utilitarians deny such relationships. The disagreement here is that deontologists think such relationships do not merely rest on a utilitarian foundation. They believe that such relationships have independent moral significance.

A second and closely connected point concerns the role of past actions in our moral assessments. Utilitarianism seems to have little room for the past in moral judgments, because of its orientation toward the present and the future. If utilitarianism considers the past from a moral standpoint, it is only because paying attention to the past appears to be important for present and future consequences. For example, to reward people for their past accomplishments tends to encourage them and others to act in similar ways in the present and the future, just as punishment discourages negative behaviors. But for a rule deontologist such as Ross, the mere fact that one has performed certain acts in the past by itself creates certain obligations, quite independent of the consequences in general for human relationships. If I have made a promise, for example, I have an obligation to fulfill it that is independent of the consequences of doing so.

The debates of a few years ago concerning kidney dialysis illustrate these points about the moral significance of interpersonal relationships and past actions. Some utilitarians held that we should distribute this scarce, life-saving resource by choosing (after the appropriate medical and psychiatric judgments) the patients who shoulder the greatest social responsibilities and those who would probably be the most productive for society. However, these utilitarians usually applied this standard only to *admission* to dialysis. With a few exceptions, they held that once a commitment has been made to a patient, it would be morally improper to remove that patient from the machine to make room for a more qualified patient, one who would probably contribute comparatively more to society. Utilitarians were not willing to call for a reassessment every few weeks or months of all the patients on, and candidates for, dialysis. Of course, the rule-utilitarian view underlying this unwillingness is that a rule calling for faithfulness to those to whom we have made implicit if not explicit commitments will ultimately maximize good. To justify this rule, one could argue that a practice of frequently reassessing patients and breaking commitments to some of them would probably destroy the morale of all patients and thereby reduce the program's success rate. The rule deontologist, however, would concentrate directly on the commitment itself, apart from the consequences of respecting that commitment. Here, as elsewhere, the rule utilitarian and the rule deontologist may wind up holding similar or even identical rules, but for apparently different reasons.

Third, utilitarianism conceives the moral life in terms of means-to-ends reasoning. It asks: "What is our objective?" and "How can we most effectively and efficiently realize the objective of the production of the greatest possible good?" This conception of the moral life in terms of means to ends relates well to such empirical sciences as economics. Deontologists, by contrast, hold not only that there are standards independent of the ends for judging the means, but that it is a fundamental mistake to conceive the moral life in terms of means and ends—a matter of the wrong starting point. Why? In part, because it seems to deontologists to presuppose a greater capacity to predict and control than we actually have. Deontologists also insist that the utilitarian model of choosing effective and efficient means to good ends fundamentally distorts the moral life. Antony Flew reflects this deontological view: "To do one's duty, or to discover what it is, is rarely if ever to achieve, or to find a way to achieve, an objective. Rather and typically, it is to meet, or to find a way to meet, claims; and also, of course, to eschew misdemeanors. Promises must be kept, debts must be paid, dependents must be looked after; and stealing, lying, and cruelty must be avoided."[17] From this view we are not merely agents who initiate acts for good ends; we also directly encounter the claims of others. Our responsibilities to others are more varied and more specific than the responsibility to promote good and prevent harm.

Fourth, the deontologist's standard, and perhaps most attractive, objection is that utilitarianism can lead to morally unacceptable conclusions. One test of moral theories, as we saw earlier, is their congruence with our ordinary moral convictions. Deontologists pose this situation against act utilitarians: Suppose we have two acts, A and B, which appear to yield the same utilitarian score when we balance their respective good and evil results. The scales appear to be perfectly balanced. But suppose that A involves lying to a patient, while B does not. In the end, the result is the same: The patient can be expected to get well. The consistent act utilitarian must say that the acts are equally right. Now suppose that act A, which involves lying to a patient about his or her condition, is preferable on utilitarian grounds because it offers a greater chance of success in restoring the patient's health while act B, which does not involve lying, has a slightly smaller chance of success. According to act utilitarianism, A is right and obligatory and the physician should therefore lie to the patient because it is in the patient's interest. (This assumes, of course, that one can reliably predict in the circumstances that other consequences—such as a loss of confidence in the physician—will *not* eventuate.) The deontologist claims that in both cases act utilitarianism leads to morally unacceptable judgments.[18]

Perhaps the rule utilitarian can avoid these difficulties by holding that a fuller analysis of the consequences, including the remote or long-term consequences, leads us to assign greater weight to the rule of truthtelling. But while rule utilitarianism thus appears to be more congruent with our ordinary judgments, it does not, according to many critics, adequately account for claims of justice, which most people believe are valid apart from the consequences of adopting rules or principles of justice. For example, consider the issue of fairness in bearing the burdens of some common enterprise such as conserving water in a crisis. One possible (perhaps unrepresentative) utilitarian view is, "If a person happened to know that nearly everybody else was in fact going to make a sacrifice that no one wants to make, and if he knew that, as a result, a similar sacrifice by him was not really essential for the public welfare, then he need not make it."[19] If he has good grounds for thinking that his act will not be known (and emulated) by others and that the enterprise will in no way suffer from his using water, he would have no obligation to conserve water on some act- and rule-utilitarian systems. Nevertheless, according to some interpretations of our ordinary judgments about fairness, this person acted unfairly and wrongly, regardless of the consequences. Such a case indicates that our sense of fairness or justice may not be reducible to utility.[20]

On balance, which ethical theory is to be preferred? For one author of this volume rule utilitarianism is more defensible than any deontological theory, while for the other, rule deontology is more acceptable than any form of utilitarianism. We come to these different conclusions after testing the various theories for their consistency and coherence, their simplicity, their completeness and comprehensiveness, and their capacity to take account of and to account for our moral experience, including our ordinary judgments. Still, for each of us, the theory that we find more satisfactory is only slightly preferable, and no theory fully satisfies all the tests.

Whether one takes the utilitarian or deontological standpoint no doubt makes a great deal of difference at many points in the moral life and in moral reflection and justification. Nevertheless, the differences can easily be over-emphasized. In fact, we find that many (not all) forms of rule utilitarianism and rule deontology lead to *identical* rules and actions. It is possible from both utilitarian and deontological standpoints to defend the *same rules* (such as truthtelling and confidentiality) and to assign them roughly the same weight. These standpoints draw even closer if utilitarians take a broad view of the values supporting the rules and consider a wide range of direct and indirect, immediate and remote consequences of classes of acts, while deontologists admit that moral principles or rules such as beneficence and nonmaleficence require us to maximize good and minimize evil outcomes.

At least one substantial theoretical difference would remain, however. The rule utilitarian believes that the principle of utility justifies the other principles and rules, which have their point and rationale in the prediction that they will maximize utility over time. By contrast, the rule deontologist believes that some principles and rules are justified apart from utility and that they are binding even if they cannot be reliably predicted to maximize utility. While the rule deontologist may hope and perhaps even expect that such principles and rules will maximize good, that hope or expectation does not *justify* the principles and rules. The rule deontologist may believe that having moral rules will maximize utility, but will not believe that we can determine which rules we ought to have only by considering their utility.

Such theoretical differences *can* of course have practical significance and can even produce radically different points of view. For example, we shall see throughout this volume that utilitarians tend to support a wide variety of types of research involving human subjects on grounds of the social benefits of the research. Deontologists, by contrast, tend to be skeptical of much of this research on grounds of its actual or potential violation of principles of autonomy and respect for persons. Roughly this difference of approach characterizes the debate between McCormick and Ramsey found in Chapter 1 (although McCormick cannot be safely classified as a utilitarian).

An indication that those utilitarians and deontologists who accept a conception of the moral life as rule-governed can and sometimes do develop similar or even identical rules—rather than fragment into disagreement—is found in the writings of Richard B. Brandt, a contemporary utilitarian philosopher. As we have seen, he argues that morality should be conceived as an ideal code consisting of a set of rules that guides the members of a society to maximize utility. While Brandt appeals to utilitarian reasoning to justify rules in the code, the following statement is revealing:

[The best code] would contain rules giving directions for recurrent situations which involve conflicts of human interests. Presumably, then, it would contain rules rather similar to W. D. Ross's list of prima facie obligations: rules about the keeping of promises and contracts, rules about debts of gratitude such as we may owe to our parents, and, of course, rules about not injuring other persons and about promoting the welfare of others where this does not work a comparable hardship on us.[21]

That Brandt appeals to utility and that Ross appeals to intuition to ground an identical set of rules is a significant difference on the level of ethical theory, but it may turn out to be a trivial difference when it comes to what we ought to do as a matter of moral rightness and how we should judge our actions and those of others.

Moreover, within what we would consider the most adequate rule-utilitarian theory and the most adequate rule deontology, moral agents have to face some of the same issues: What should we do when rules come into conflict? What shall we do when we cannot realize all the claims upon us or all the goods that we seek? How can we resolve these competing demands? The fact that no presently available rule utilitarianism or rule deontology adequately resolves all moral conflicts perhaps points to their incompleteness. But this incompleteness may reflect more the complexity and even the tragedy of the moral life than any failures of the theories.

The observation that even the most adequate moral systems are substantially incomplete may seem odd, for we argued in Chapter 1 that one test of any moral theory is its "completeness and comprehensiveness." Our present point is that no available moral system *fully* satisfies the ideal set forth by this criterion. In reference to consequentialist theories, Alan Donagan has correctly observed that "In all the vast and imposing body of work on consequentialist moral theories, there are many sketches and projects for constructing moral systems. But none has been constructed."[22] This assessment, we suggest, applies as well to deontological theories. The most complete and comprehensive of the latter theories tend to be on special subjects, such as justice, rather than providing a comprehensive account of the moral life. (Some would contest these claims in the cases of Kant and others.)

It is quite possible that the moral life is so diverse that no theory can stand up to the completeness test even though a theory may capture some specific domain of that life, such as our conception of "justice" or our conception of "the public interest." Yet each of the broad general ethical theories that we have examined arguably offers a valuable *perspective* from which to view morality. Perhaps we can best appreciate the contributions made by these theories by extracting what is insightful and rejecting what fails the tests set out in Chapter 1. This will be our approach in the ensuing sections of this book.

The place of rules

Many utilitarians and deontologists, as we have seen, find that the moral life requires various rules. They thus reject "situation ethics," which may take either act-deontological or act-utilitarian forms. Although there are several versions of situation ethics, many of its proponents hold that there is a single fundamental principle such as utility, love, or obedience to the divine command, and that all the moral agent has to do is discern the meaning of that principle in the situation. Thus, the agent asks what would serve the greatest good for the greatest number, what would be the most loving deed, or what God commands at the moment, without relying on intermediate rules that connect the basic principle and the situation. In defending a rule-governed concept of morality, we have implicitly rejected situation ethics by giving several reasons for favoring rule utilitarianism and rule deontology. These theories are viable in light of the tests set out in Chapter 1, while all forms of situation ethics must face insurmountable problems of coordination, cooperation, and trust. The following encounter between act utilitarians in a medical setting, as envisioned by G. J. Warnock, expresses some salient reasons for rejecting all act and situation theories:

Suppose that I, a simple Utilitarian, entrust the care of my health to a simple Utilitarian doctor. Now I know, of course, that his intentions are generally beneficent, but equally that they are not *uniquely* beneficent towards me. Thus, while he will not malevolently kill me off, I cannot be sure that he will always try to cure me of my afflictions; I can be sure only that he will do so, *unless* his assessment of the "general happiness" leads him to do otherwise. I cannot of course condemn this attitude, since it is the same as my own; but it is more than possible that I might not much like it, and might find myself put to much anxiety and fuss in trying to detect, at successive consultations, what his intentions actually were. But conspicuously, there are two things that I could not do to diminish my anxieties: I could not get him to promise, in the style of the Hippocratic Oath, always and only to deploy his skills to my advantage; nor could I usefully ask him to disclose his intentions. The reason is essentially the same in each case. Though he might, if I asked him to, promise not to kill me off, he would of course keep this promise only if he judged it best on the whole to do so; knowing that, I could not unquestioningly rely on his keeping it; and knowing *that*, he would realize that, since I would not do so, it would matter that much less if he did not keep it. And so on, until his "promise" becomes perfectly idle. Similarly, if I ask him what his intentions are, he will answer truthfully only if he judges it best on the whole to do so; knowing that, I will not unqualifiedly believe him; and knowing *that*, he will realize that, since I will not do so, it will matter that much less if he professes intentions that he does not actually have. And so on, until my asking and his answering become a pure waste of breath. And this is quite general; if general felicific beneficence were the only criterion, then promising and talking alike would become wholly idle pursuits. At best, as perhaps in diplomacy, what people said would become merely a part of the evidence on the basis of which one might try to decide what they really believed, or intended, or were likely to do; and it is not always obvious that there is much point in diplomacy.[23]

Situational theories of ethics can recognize rules, of course; but they treat all rules as mere *summary rules* or *rules of thumb* that are expendable in decisionmaking, because they merely summarize the wisdom of the past by expressing better and worse ways to handle recurring problems. Such rules assist deliberation, but can be set aside at any time according to the demands of the situation. For example, an investigative reporter seeking facts about a potential political scandal might "have to" lie and break laws governing privacy and confidentiality; yet from the perspective of a situational theory, the reporter's acts may be justifiable because of the importance of the story. Moral and legal action-guides are thus treated as rules that may direct but do not prescribe with authority what we ought to do. Such rules illuminate but do not bind. A rule of thumb in baseball is "Don't bunt on third strike," but in some situations it would be advisable for the batter to bunt despite having two strikes. The rule is jettisoned when it does not serve us well. For act deontology, act utilitarianism, and all situational theories, moral rules approximate this rule of thumb in baseball.

We have argued against this view of moral rules. Even if some moral rules may resemble rules of thumb (e.g., some rules in professional codes), others are more binding, e.g., the rules that prohibit murder, rape, and cruelty. It is therefore important to consider whether some rules are not only *binding*, but *absolute*—that is, rules that cannot be overridden under any circumstances. Obviously, there are good reasons for being suspicious of such a view of moral rules. It undermines the freedom and discretion of moral agents (rightly emphasized in act theories), and an overly rigid adherence to rules can produce moral victims. Even if it is not true that everything depends on the consequences, it seems undeniable that in some cases, such as emergencies, the consequences of following some moral rules would be so terrible that those rules should be overridden.

Nevertheless, we have to face the possibility that some moral rules are virtually exceptionless or absolute: (a) Some rules that refer to traits of character whose development and expression are always good may be absolute. To exhort a physician colleague to "Be caring" or "Be a loving physician" or "Be conscientious" is to call for the development and expression of traits of character that are good. Of course, one may obscure the important aspects of one's responsibilities by misconstruing or too narrowly construing the demands of care, love, or conscientiousness. (In the final chapter we will examine traits of character and virtues.) (b) Some rules of action formulated to include all exceptions may be absolute. An example might be, "Always obtain the informed consent of your competent patients except in emergency or low-risk situations." There might still be considerable debate about what constitutes an "emergency" or a "low risk," but the rule would be absolute if *all* exceptions could be included. (c) Finally, some rules that do not specify exceptions may also be virtually absolute. If "murder" is taken to mean "unjustified killing," then its prohibition would be absolute; and the prohibition of cruelty can be considered absolute if the term means "Do not inflict suffering for the sake of suffering." In medical contexts, especially in some therapeutic settings, there might at first appear to be exceptions to this second prohibition; but if a therapist intentionally makes a patient suffer so that the patient will become angry and assume responsibility for his decisions, this act does not fall under the prohibition of cruelty, since the infliction of suffering is strictly a means to the valuable end of assuming responsibility.

These examples indicate that the debate about whether some rules can be defended as absolute hinges in part on the definition of moral terms such as "murder," "cruelty," and "lying." Suppose Nazi soldiers investigating a hospital in Germany in the late 1930s had asked the administrator whether there were any Jewish patients in the hospital. If the administrator insisted that the hospital had no Jewish patients, although he knew there were in fact several, how should we describe this exchange and, in particular, the administrator's statement? Consider two possibilities: (1) The administrator's statement is a *lie*, but the lie is justified because it is intended to save the lives of innocent patients. (2) The administrator's statement is not a lie, because his questioners have no right to the truth. In (1) "lying" may be defined as intentionally telling a person what one believes to be untrue in order to deceive him or her. In (2) "lying" may be defined as not giving the truth to a person to whom it is due. The first involves a "neutral and relatively definite description" of lying, while the second involves a "nonneutral and relatively indefinite description."[24] The first definition indicates what counts as lying or truthtelling, but not how much moral weight lying or truthtelling has. The second definition, however, indicates how much lying or truthtelling counts, but not what is to count as lying or truthtelling. Although the second approach holds that lying is always wrong, it leaves open the question when the truth is *due* someone. The first approach could stress that the moral life often involves doing the "lesser of two evils." It may sometimes be necessary to lie in order to prevent a worse evil. Proponents of the second approach may stress the harmony rather than the conflict among various principles and rules once we appreciate their meaning and thus their range of applicability.

The importance of the meaning of central moral terms may be illustrated as follows: In Case #2, a father decided that he did not want to donate a kidney to his five-year-old daughter. His reasons are complex, and they include an uncertain prognosis for his daughter who had been on chronic renal dialysis for three years. He asked the physician to tell the other family members that he was not histocompatible, because he feared that the truth would lead to recriminations against him and would wreck the family. The physician informed the family that "medical reasons" prevented the father from being a donor. One could hold that the physician told a lie by intentionally deceiving the wife, but that it was justified because of the evil it prevented. Or one could hold that it was justified because, in a conflict of duties, the protection of confidentiality takes precedence over telling the truth to another "patient," and the father had entered into a relationship of confidentiality with the physician. Or one could hold that the "lie" was justified not because there was a stronger competing duty, but because the physician had no duty to tell the wife the truth. Because what transpired between the father and the physician was confidential, the wife had no right to that information; hence, deceiving her was not even an act of lying. In this analysis, we have not eliminated the possibility of holding that the statement to the wife was an unjustified lie. The present point is merely that different approaches to moral dilemmas and rules may hinge on different understandings of the relevant moral terms, such as "lying," as well as on their weight and stringency.

In addition to conceiving of moral rules as rules of thumb or absolute rules, a third and very important possibility is to conceive them as *binding*, but not absolutely so. W. D. Ross has usefully distinguished prima facie duties from actual duties. He uses the phrase "prima facie duty" to indicate that duties of certain kinds are on all occasions binding *unless* they are in conflict with equal or stronger duties. One's *actual duty* in the situation is determined by an examination of the weight of all the competing prima facie duties. Duties such as beneficence and promise-keeping are not absolute, because they can be overridden under some conditions. Yet they are more than rules of thumb. Because they are always morally relevant, they constitute strong moral reasons for performing the acts in question, although they may not always prevail over all other prima facie duties. One might say that they count even when they do not win.

For example, Ross considers nonmaleficence—noninfliction of harm—as a prima facie duty. (Indeed all of the moral principles taken as primary in this book state prima facie duties in Ross's sense.) While it is plausible, as we have seen, to hold that murder is absolutely prohibited because of the meaning of "murder," it is not plausible in most moral theories to hold that killing is absolutely prohibited. Even the prohibition against killing in the Ten Commandments is more accurately translated as the prohibition of "murder" or "unjustified killing," since the Hebrew people recognized justified killing in self-defense, in war, and as a form of punishment. Killing human persons nonetheless is prima facie wrong, because it is an act of maleficence. To call "killing" prima facie wrong, then, is to say that insofar as an act involves killing, it is wrong.

Because acts have many features, other features besides killing may lead to moral conflicts. The duty not to kill someone, for example, may come into conflict with the duty of justice, which includes protecting innocent persons from aggression. The duty not to kill may also come into conflict with the duty of beneficence, the duty to benefit others—as mercy killing illustrates. It is not clear that killing a person in order to alleviate that person's pain would always be wrong, as the case of a person trapped in a burning wreck illustrates. Indeed, W. D. Ross's view that nonmaleficence always has priority over beneficence is a dubious general thesis. The point to notice about prima facie duties, however, is that insofar as an act involves killing, it has a wrong-making feature. It is always prima facie wrong and always actually wrong unless justified by another overriding prima facie duty. Yet killing may be the only way to meet some other prima facie duties; and, if so, then killing can even become an actual duty.

To choose a different example, if lying is prima facie wrong, the fact that a physician deceives a patient by giving a placebo (see Case #4) is a moral reason against the action. One traditional formulation of the rule for truth-telling in medical matters is, "When you are thinking of telling a lie, ask yourself whether it is simply and solely for the patient's benefit that you are going to tell it. If you are sure that you are acting for his good and not for your own profit, you can go ahead with a clear conscience."[25] From the Kantian perspective it would be impossible to *universalize* this rule without contradiction. Another difficulty is that this rule always gives beneficence priority over both truthtelling and respect for autonomy when there is a conflict. It also fails to recognize the weight of the duty not to lie in the medical context, for it would authorize any lie for benevolent motives. But if, as we think, the duties of veracity and respecting autonomy are strong, then lying must be the most acceptable alternative in a situation in order to be justified.

Furthermore, when a prima facie duty, such as veracity, is outweighed or overridden, it does not simply disappear or evaporate. It leaves what Robert Nozick calls "moral traces."[26] The agent should not only approach such a decision conscientiously, but should also experience regret and perhaps even remorse at having to infringe this duty. The duty's "moral traces" should also lead the agent to seek to minimize the effects of the infringement. For example, in the case (#4) in which a therapist deceives a patient by giving a placebo, the deception, which in this case will later become known, will harm the patient's self-conception and his confidence in and reliance upon the therapists—just as Warnock envisions in the aforementioned "simple utilitarian" example. Other moral rules and principles require conscientious efforts to minimize such risks. At the very least, the overridden duties of veracity and respect for autonomy should require the therapist to give an explanation and an apology to the patient.

The argument in this section thus culminates in a strong endorsement of rule-based moral theories, but we note in conclusion some inherent limits of any rule-based morality (beyond those problems we noted in discussing the prima facie and absolute interpretations of rules). First, it can be quite unclear whether a case falls under a rule. For example, it may be unclear whether a physician's disclosure to a patient is or is not deceptive under the circumstances, and hence any rule that simply and unqualifiedly bans deception in the patient-physician relationship cannot determine one's precise moral obligation in all circumstances. Indeed, the strongest argument advanced by situational theories is that rules can be so abstract or unclear in their applicability that we are forced to call upon non-rule resources. We agree that rules can conflict without mediating rules being available to resolve the conflict, and that there will be times when we are uncertain as to whether a rule applies. But this concession does not commit us to situation ethics. To recognize the importance of casuistry, of *applying* principles and rules to particular cases, is not to deny the binding principles and rules themselves.

Second, these rules are not constructed to take account of competing factors (including nonmoral factors) that no moral system could ever fully account for. Family responsibilities, religious convictions, and professional obligations may all on occasion compete with moral obligations. Life in all its particularity is like that (as act theories rightly, to this extent, insist), and no system of rules can make these problems vanish. It scarcely follows that we can or must dispense with general action-guides or treat all of them merely as rules of thumb. Without general rules, judgments about right and wrong can rarely if ever be made in particular circumstances. The question to be asked is where discretion rightly enters and how such rules are to be understood and applied, not whether they apply at all.[27]

Rights

Throughout our discussion we have used terms like "right," "wrong," "obligatory," "obligation," and "duty." We have examined how principles and rules in both deontological and utilitarian theories establish our duties and obligations, as well as the rightness and wrongness of our acts. It may seem odd that we have not employed the language of *rights*, since so many moral controversies in biomedicine and public policy involve debates about such rights as a right to die or a right to reproduce. For example, controversies about abortion often pit the woman's right of privacy or right to determine the use of her body against the fetus's right to life. In discussions of health care delivery, proponents of a broad extension of medical services often appeal to the "right to health care," while opponents commonly appeal to the "rights of the medical profession." We have witnessed an explosion of rights language in numerous contexts, from biomedicine to foreign policy— as debates about international "human rights" exemplify. Indeed, our moral, political, and legal debates often appear to presuppose that no arguments or reasons can be persuasive unless they can be couched in the language of rights.

Rights language is especially congenial to the liberal individualism pervasive in our society. From Thomas Hobbes and John Locke to the present, liberal individualists have employed the language of rights to make their moral, social, and political arguments. Our Anglo-American legal tradition has broadly incorporated this language. In the tradition of liberal individualism, the language of rights has sometimes served as a means to oppose the status quo, to assert claims that demand recognition and respect, and to force social reforms. Historically it was instrumental in securing certain freedoms from established orders of religion, society, and state—e.g., freedom of the press. Although statements of fundamental rights are shared across many societies, they are not universally accepted. Indeed, some languages, such as ancient Hebrew and Greek, do not have equivalent expressions for our terms "a right" or "rights." Nevertheless, rights language is important, not only because of its symbolic significance in our society, but also because it plays a legitimate role in ethical theory. It is difficult, however, to determine the status and content of those rights that deserve recognition.

Most recent writers in ethics recognize that "rights" should be defined in terms of claims. In our framework, rights are best understood as justified claims that individuals and groups can make upon others or upon society. A right is thus analogous to property that one holds and over which one has discretion. Legal rights are claims that are justified by legal principles and rules, and moral rights are claims that are justified by moral principles and rules. A moral right, then, is a morally justified claim or entitlement—i.e., a claim or entitlement validated by moral principles and rules.[28] Just as obligations and duties may take many different forms (such as religious, legal, and moral obligations and duties), rights may be justified by different forms of principles and rules. For example, in dealing with the abortion issue, the Supreme Court had to determine whether the Constitution and the law embodies legal rights relevant to this issue. Because of the nature of its inquiry, the court did not confront the question of moral rights, except by implication. However, even the court recognized that moral rights and legal rights often are similar and sometimes even identical.

Are the claims designated "rights" absolute? Here we need to recall the prima facie *duties* discussed in the previous section on rules. We noted that duties are not absolute but instead make strong moral demands that may be validly overridden by more stringent competing demands in particular circumstances. The same conflicts can occur among rights—as we noticed about the fetus's right to life and the woman's right to privacy. Even the right to life cannot be plausibly maintained to be absolute, irrespective of competing claims or social conditions, as is evidenced by common moral judgments about killing in war and killing in self-defense. We have only a right not to have our life taken without sufficient justification, not an absolute right to life. This and any right can be legitimately exercised and can create actual duties on others only when the right overrides rights that compete with it. Thus, rights claims are also prima facie claims. However, philosophical and practical controversy rages not only about the weights of rights—whether they are prima facie, absolute, or only relative—but also about their meaning, their scope, and the conditions of their possession— e.g., whether fetuses and animals qualify as rights holders. (We will touch on some of these questions in subsequent chapters, although we will concentrate on duties.)

Some philosophers distinguish the *violation* of a right from the *infringement* of a right.[29] "Violation" refers to an *unjustified* action against a right, while "infringement" refers to a *justified* action overriding a right. When a (prima facie) right is justifiably overridden, it is therefore infringed but not violated. Just as prima facie principles and rules stating duties do not disappear when they are justifiably overridden, so rights do not disappear when they are infringed. They continue to have an impact on the action, often by requiring that the infringement proceed in certain ways (for example, if a right of noninterference is overridden, it still requires that the least restrictive alternative be used) or by requiring an explanation and even compensation to the right holder. Even though the right holder has only a prima facie right, he or she retains that right even if it is justifiably overridden or infringed.

It follows from the analysis thus far that rights express morally valid demands on human conduct. Relatedly, we believe there also exists what David Braybrooke calls "a firm but untidy correlativity" between obligations and rights, a relation that makes it possible to analyze both obligations and rights in terms of principles and rules.[30] According to the doctrine of the "logical correlativity" of obligations and rights, a right entails that someone else has an obligation to act in certain ways.[31] For example, if a physician agrees to take John Doe as a patient and commences treatment, he incurs an obligation to Doe that he does not have toward strangers, and Doe has certain rights against the physician. There are rights to a certain standard of care and rights in care—such as the right to refuse treatment. We thus could analyze the moral issues in the relationship between the physician and Doe either by examining the physician's duties or by examining the patient's rights, because the doctrine of the logical correlativity of rights and obligations holds that it is possible to start from a right and infer a correlative obligation, and vice versa. It indicates that we can secure the same moral content from either standpoint, that of the right or of the obligation. However, the doctrine does not tell us whether obligations are ultimately grounded in rights or vice versa, and we take no stand on this issue here.

While the doctrine of the logical correlativity of rights and duties is generally sound, there is a generalized use of "requirement," "obligation," and "duty" that sometimes appears not to imply correlative rights. For example, we sometimes refer to "duties" or "requirements" of love, charity, and self-sacrifice that do not seem to be restatable in terms of rights. It seems awkward in most instances to hold that one person can claim another person's love or charity as a matter of right. The problem is that some so-called duties and obligations express what we ought to do in the light of ideals and supererogatory actions, such as those of heroes and saints, that are somewhat inappropriately labeled *moral requirements* (probably because they are morally *demanding*). More likely, they express self-imposed duties not strictly required by morality—as when we believe that we *ought* to contribute substantially to charity, even though morality does not strictly require it. We will discuss such ideals and self-imposed requirements in the final chapter.

John Stuart Mill usefully approached this problem by employing the distinction between duties of perfect obligation and duties of imperfect obligation: "Duties of perfect obligation are those duties in virtue of which a correlative *right* resides in some person or persons; duties of imperfect obligation are those moral obligations which do not give birth to any right."[32] Mill goes on to indicate that duties of perfect obligation are duties of justice that entail rights, while duties of imperfect obligation belong to other spheres of morality: "Justice implies something which is not only right to do, and wrong not to do, but which some individual person can claim from us as his moral right. No one has a moral right to our generosity or beneficence, because we are not morally bound to practice those virtues towards any given individual."[33]

Both rule utilitarianism and rule deontology, as obligation-oriented theories, can incorporate the language and substance of rights. This claim may appear somewhat surprising, since some utilitarians have vigorously opposed certain conceptions of rights, and many of the strongest supporters and theoreticians of individual rights have operated within deontological frameworks. Indeed, in ordinary moral discourse, we frequently set the rights of individuals and groups in opposition to social utility. Nevertheless, it follows from the doctrine of the logical correlativity of rights and obligations that both rule utilitarianism and rule deontology are logically committed to rights as well as to obligations.[34]

An illustration of this claim is found in Ronald Dworkin's argument about the possibility of rights within a rule-utilitarian political theory, an argument that also holds for moral theory:

A political theory might provide for a right to free speech, for example, on the hypothesis that the general acceptance of that right by courts and other political institutions would promote the highest average utility of the community in the long-run. . . . If the theory provides that an official of a particular institution is justified in making a political decision, and not justified in refusing to make it, whenever that decision is necessary to protect the freedom to speak of any individual, without regard to the impact of the decision on collective goals, the theory provides free speech as a right.[35]

Rights, according to our use of the logical correlativity thesis, may serve as constraints or "trumps" within either rule utilitarianism or rule deontology. In rule utilitarianism, they are justified by their likely contributions to utility, and Mill defended rights of autonomy and liberty in precisely these terms (as we shall see in subsequent chapters). In a deontological framework, rights are likely to be based on respect for persons, autonomy, or some similar nonutilitarian principle; rights express and embody those principles, and are not merely instrumental to the maximization of good consequences. Of course, there will be disputes about whether certain claims qualify as "rights," about their scope, and about their relative weight, but these particular disputes will probably be no more frequent or intractable between rule utilitarians and rule deontologists than among defenders of one of these two general approaches to ethical theory.

An important distinction thus far neglected is between positive rights and negative rights. As Joel Feinberg writes, "A *positive* right is a right to other persons' positive actions; a *negative* right is a right to other persons' omissions or forebearances. For every positive right I have, someone else has a duty to *do* something; for every negative right I have, someone else has a duty to *refrain* from doing something."[36] Examples of both sorts of rights can be found in biomedical practice and research. If there is a right to health care, it is a positive right to goods and services, grounded in the principle of justice, while the right not to be operated on without one's consent is a negative right, grounded in the principle of autonomy. The liberal individualist tradition has generally found it easier to justify negative rights, especially those that call for noninterference with liberty, than positive rights; but the recognition of welfare rights has extended the range and power of positive rights. Positive rights may be directed against other individuals or against the society as a whole.

Much confusion in moral discourse about public policies governing biomedicine can be traced to a failure to distinguish positive rights from negative rights. One example comes from the controversy surrounding the Supreme Court decisions on abortion.[37] Some who contend that the abortion decisions are contradictory fail to see that the Court recognized a negative right in 1973 and refused to recognize a positive right in 1977. In *Roe* v. *Wade* and *Doe* v. *Bolton* (1973), the Court ruled that a woman's right to privacy, especially in relation to her physician, gives her a right to abort her fetus within certain limits. If the decision is made within the first trimester of the pregnancy, the state may not intervene. The state, however, may regulate abortions for the protection of maternal health in the second trimester; and in the third trimester it may even prohibit abortions, except in cases of a threat to the mother's life or health. The constitutionally protected right of privacy is here construed as a negative right. It identifies a sphere of general noninterference and limits state interference to certain specified circumstances. This right was interpreted in the *Danforth* decision (1976) to exclude a husband's veto of his wife's and her physician's decision to terminate her pregnancy. Again, the Court recognized a right of noninterference.

Many people apparently thought that the Court had also recognized a positive right—i.e., a right to have aid and assistance from the state or others in abortions. They were therefore surprised that the Court in 1977 ruled that the federal and state governments do not have to provide funds for nontherapeutic abortions; governments do not have a duty to provide such funds, and pregnant women who are seeking nontherapeutic abortions do not have a right to financial assistance. The Court's reasoning is consistent: It affirms a negative right in one decision and denies a positive right in another. Although it is possible to argue that the Court *should* have found a positive right as well as a negative right, there is no inconsistency over rights.

Opponents of the most recent decisions may, however, charge that these decisions embody a different order of inconsistency in that they affirm a positive right to financial assistance for bringing a pregnancy to term while they deny a positive right to the services necessary to terminate a pregnancy. Some opponents contend that abortion and birth are two legitimate alternative ways to deal with the condition of pregnancy. One of the strongest arguments for the view that the legislature morally ought to provide funds for poor women who seek abortions appeals to a principle of justice (cf. Chapter 6): It is unfair not to assist poor women in obtaining abortions, if other women can easily obtain them; and it is unfair for the society to try to salve its conscience about abortion by forcing poor women to complete pregnancies that others can terminate or by forcing them to seek inexpensive and risky abortions in unsafe surroundings.

This abortion controversy, and rights claims more generally, may also be analyzed by reference to the distinction between the statements (1) "X has a right to do Y" and (2) "X acts rightly in doing Y." The distinction is between "rights" (or "a right") and "right conduct," as well as between "rights" and their "right exercise."[38] Sometimes when we say that a person has a right to do X, we mean that he or she does not do wrong in performing X. But often our statement that someone has a right to do X implies nothing about the morality of the act; it means only that we believe others have no right to interfere with the act. Thus, one can affirm that a woman has a moral or a legal right to have an abortion without affirming that she acts rightly in those circumstances. A society might create a legal right to abortions because of pervasive and distressing consequences of criminal prohibition (e.g., women seek illegal abortions under unsafe conditions); and one might argue that there is a moral right to an abortion for the same reasons. Nevertheless, it is not inconsistent to say that a woman who has this legal and moral right to have an abortion is not acting rightly in having an abortion. Perhaps her reasons are not strong enough to warrant an abortion, or perhaps she acts on false information. To say that she has a right is merely to say that no one has valid grounds to intervene in her decision.

As the controversy over abortion makes clear, many disputes that plague obligations and duties reappear in discussions of rights. For example, is there a right of privacy, and does the fetus have a right to life? How much weight do we assign to these different rights? When they come into conflict, which (prima facie) right takes precedence? Answers to these questions, which may finally be unanswerable to everyone's satisfaction, can only come through systematic reflection on moral principles and rules, including a careful examination of particular duties, obligations, and rights that allegedly have the weight of morality behind them. We shall examine such principles and rules in subsequent chapters.

Notes

1. Jeremy Bentham, *An Introduction to the Principles of Morals and Legislation* (New York: Hafner Publishing Co., 1948). Cf. Principle I.3.
2. John Stuart Mill, *Utilitarianism, On Liberty, and Essay on Bentham,* ed. with an Introduction by Mary Warnock (New York: New American Library, 1974), pp. 256–78.
3. G. E. Moore, *Principia Ethica* (Cambridge: Cambridge University Press, 1962), pp. 90f.
4. Alasdair MacIntyre, *After Virtue* (Notre Dame, Ind.: University of Notre Dame Press, 1981), p. 62.
5. J. J. C. Smart, *An Outline of a System of Utilitarian Ethics* (Melbourne: University Press, 1961), and "Extreme and Restricted Utilitarianism," *Philosophical Quarterly* VI (1956), as reprinted in *Contemporary Utilitarianism,* ed. M. Bayles (Garden City: Doubleday Anchor Books, 1968), especially pp. 104ff in the latter source.
6. See R. Jay Wallace, Jr., "Privacy and the Use of Data in Epidemiology," in *Ethical Issues in Social Science Research,* ed. Tom L. Beauchamp, et al. (Baltimore, Md.: Johns Hopkins University Press, 1982), pp. 274–91; see also, Leon Gordis and Ellen Gold, "Privacy, Confidentiality, and the Use of Medical Records in Research," *Science* 207 (January 11, 1980): 153–56.
7. David Hume, *A Treatise of Human Nature,* ed. L. A. Selby-Bigge (Oxford: Oxford University Press, 1888). Book III, Parts I and II, especially pp. 494–500. Richard B. Brandt, "Toward a Credible Form of Utilitarianism," in *Contemporary Utilitarianism,* ed. Bayles, pp. 143–86. Brandt's later views are found in his *A*

Theory of the Good and the Right (Oxford: Clarendon Press, 1979), especially Chapters 14 and 15.

8. Moral code utilitarianism also may provide a way of circumventing a prominent objection against the act/rule distinction that has been advanced by David Lyons in *Forms and Limits of Utilitarianism* (Oxford: Clarendon Press, 1965). He argues that whatever would count for an act utilitarian as a reason for *breaking* a rule would count equally for a rule utilitarian as a good reason for *emending* a rule—and hence the two come in practice to the same theory. It would be very difficult and perhaps impossible to emend an entire code with the frequency with which a rule could be validly broken by act utilitarians.

9. See W. D. Ross, *The Right and the Good* (Oxford: Clarendon Press, 1930) and *The Foundations of Ethics* (Oxford: Clarendon Press, 1939); and John Rawls, *A Theory of Justice* (Cambridge, Mass.: Harvard University Press, 1971).

10. Utilitarians face a similar problem: Because they derive the concept of duty or right from the concept of good, it is necessary for them to define and determine what is good before they can make judgments about right and wrong. They too have various ways of defining and determining what is good, including a psychology of human desires (Mill) and intuition (Moore). For our purposes it is not essential that we examine different metaethical theories.

11. See Alan Donagan, *The Theory of Morality* (Chicago: University of Chicago Press, 1977), p. 66.

12. Immanuel Kant, *Groundwork of the Metaphysic of Morals*, translated by H. J. Paton (New York: Harper and Row, Harper Torchbooks, 1964), pp. 90–91.

13. Ross, *The Right and the Good*, pp. 22, 41–42.

14. Rawls, *A Theory of Justice*, Pars. 8, 11, 46 (especially pp. 302–303) and 51 (especially pp. 339–40).

15. See Ross, *The Right and the Good* and *The Foundations of Ethics*.

16. See Ramsey, *The Patient as Person* (New Haven: Yale University Press, 1971), and *Ethics at the Edges of Life: Medical and Legal Intersections* (New Haven: Yale University Press, 1978); and Veatch, *Death, Dying and the Biological Revolution* (New Haven: Yale University Press, 1976) and *A Theory of Medical Ethics* (New York: Basic Books, 1981). For an analysis of Ramsey and Veatch, see James Childress, "Ethical Issues in Death and Dying," *Religious Studies Review* 4 (1978): 180–88. Among Engelhardt's various writings, see Karen Lebacqz and H. Tristram Engelhardt, Jr., "Suicide and the Patient's Right to Reject Medical Treatment," in *Death, Dying and Euthanasia*, eds. Dennis J. Horan and David Mall (Washington: University Publications of America, 1977), pp. 669–705, and Engelhardt, "Health Care Allocations: Responses to the Unjust, the Unfortunate, and the Undesirable," in *Justice and Health Care*, ed. Earl E. Shelp (Dordrecht, Holland: D. Reidel Publishing Co., 1981), pp. 121–37. Another major deontologist in biomedical ethics is Charles Fried. See his *Medical Experimentation: Personal Integrity and Social Policy* (New York: American Elsevier Publishing Co., 1974) and *Right and Wrong* (Cambridge, Mass.: Harvard University Press, 1978).

17. Antony Flew, "Ends and Means," in *The Encyclopedia of Philosophy*, ed. Paul Edwards (New York: Macmillan and Free Press, 1967), vol. II, p. 510.

18. See William Frankena, *Ethics*, 2nd ed. (Englewood Cliffs, N.J.: Prentice-Hall, 1973).

19. This example is quoted from Richard B. Brandt, *Ethical Theory* (Englewood Cliffs, N.J.: Prentice-Hall, 1959), p. 404. Brandt mentions the view only to reject it.

20. See Lyons, *The Forms and Limits of Utilitarianism.*

21. "Toward a Credible Form of Utilitarianism," in *Contemporary Utilitarianism*, ed. Bayles, p. 166.

22. Alan Donagan, *The Theory of Morality*, p. 191.

23. G. J. Warnock, *The Object of Morality* (London: Methuen and Co., 1971), p. 33.

24. Donald Evans, "Paul Ramsey on Exceptionless Moral Rules," *American Journal of Jurisprudence* 16 (1971): 184–214. See also Sissela Bok, *Lying: Moral Choice in Public and Private Life* (New York: Pantheon Books, 1978), pp. 13–16.

25. Richard C. Cabot quotes one of his teachers to this effect. See Cabot, "The Use of Truth and Falsehood in Medicine: An Experimental Study," *American Medicine* 5 (1903): 344–49, as reprinted in *Ethics in Medicine: Historical Perspectives and Contemporary Concerns*, eds. Stanley Joel Reiser, Arthur J. Dyck, and William J. Curran (Cambridge, Mass.: MIT Press, 1977), p. 213.

26. See Robert Nozick, "Moral Complications and Moral Structures," *Natural Law Forum* 13 (1968): 1–50.

27. In Stephen Toulmin's vigorous article, "The Tyranny of Principles" [*Hastings Center Report* 11 (December 1981): 31–39], it is unclear whether he is opposed to principles and rules *as such* (as his language sometimes implies) or only to *absolute* principles and rules (as his argument generally seems to indicate). For a defense of casuistry, or "clinical ethics," see Albert R. Jonsen, Mark Siegler, and William J. Winslade, *Clinical Ethics* (New York: Macmillan, 1982). But such "clinical ethics" can only be done within principles and rules, which it applies to clinical situations, even though the principles and rules do not always provide clear answers. There is then room for discretion.

28. See Joel Feinberg, *Social Philosophy* (Englewood Cliffs, N.J.: Prentice-Hall, 1973), p. 67. Feinberg prefers the narrower term "validity" to the broader term "justification," since validity "is justification of a peculiar and narrow kind, namely justification within a system of rules."

29. See Rex Martin and James W. Nickel, "Recent Work on the Concept of Rights," *American Philosophical Quarterly* 17 (July 1980): 172–74. See also the discussion of rights in Theodore M. Benditt, *Rights* (Totowa, N.J.: Rowman and Littlefield, 1982).

30. David Braybrooke, "The Firm but Untidy Correlativity of Rights and Obligations," *Canadian Journal of Philosophy* 1 (March 1972): 351–63.

31. Feinberg, *Social Philosophy*, p. 61.

32. Mill, *Utilitarianism*, p. 305.

33. *Ibid.* It is still largely undecided whether we should ascribe rights to nonpersons, such as trees and animals. We have a duty not to be cruel to animals, for example, but is it appropriate to ascribe rights to them? The answer to this question will obviously depend upon one's theory of rights and their foundation. According to one theory, only entities capable of having *interests* can have rights,

and therefore trees and vegetables cannot have rights. However, both animals and future generations can be said to have interests, and therefore they can be said meaningfully to have rights. See Joel Feinberg, "The Rights of Animals and Unborn Generations," in *Philosophy and Environmental Crisis*, ed. W. T. Blackstone (Athens, Ga.: University of Georgia Press, 1974).

34. Act utilitarians, by contrast, seem committed to the translation of rights into interests and needs in order to facilitate utilitarian calculation; but rule utilitarians need not resort to this maneuver. The utilitarian critique of natural rights offered by Bentham is well-known: "Natural rights is simple nonsense: natural and imprescriptible rights, rhetorical nonsense—nonsense upon stilts." That critique, however, was aimed at the epistemology of *natural* rights, not at all uses of the language of rights or at all developments of a theory of moral rights. Bentham's invectives were thus directed against "naturalistic" theories rather than "rights." Bentham, *Anarchical Fallacies*, in *The Collected Papers of Jeremy Bentham*, vol. 2, ed. John Bowring (Edinburgh, 1843), as reprinted in *Human Rights*, ed. A. I. Melden (Belmont, Calif.: Wadsworth Publishing Co., 1970), p. 32.

35. Ronald Dworkin, *Taking Rights Seriously* (Cambridge, Mass.: Harvard University Press, 1977), pp. 96–97. See also Richard Flathman's justification of the practice of rights in *The Practice of Rights* (Cambridge: Cambridge University Press, 1976).

36. Feinberg, *Social Philosophy*, p. 59. The distinction between positive and negative rights is usefully situated in the context of contemporary political affairs by Henry Shue, *Basic Rights: Subsistence, Affluence, and U.S. Foreign Policy* (Princeton: Princeton University Press, 1980), pp. 5ff, 35ff.

37. The relevant decisions are: *Roe* v. *Wade* 410 U.S. 113 (1973), *Doe* v. *Bolton* 410 U.S. 179 (1973), *Planned Parenthood of Missouri* v. *Danforth* 423 U.S. 52 (1976), *Beal,* v. *Doe* 432 U.S. 438 (1977), *Maher* v. *Roe* 432 U.S. 464, *Poelker* v. *Doe* 432 U.S. 519 (1977).

38. See A. I. Melden, *Rights and Right Conduct* (Oxford: Basil Blackwell, 1959).

3

The Principle of Autonomy

Diverse figures in philosophy, ranging from Kant, Mill, Nietzsche, and Sartre to Robert Paul Wolff, have held that morality requires autonomous persons. Their philosophies are different, however, because they select different themes from a family of ideas associated with autonomy: rights of individual liberty and privacy, free choice, choosing for oneself, being one's own person, creating one's moral position, accepting ultimate responsibility for one's moral views, and the like. These divergent interpretations suggest a need to examine the *concept* of autonomy before trying to develop a *moral principle* of autonomy and sketching its implications for biomedical ethics.

The concept of autonomy

The autonomous person

"Autonomy" is a term derived from the Greek *autos* (self) and *nomos* (rule, governance, or law) and was first used to refer to self-rule or self-governance in Greek city-states. The most general idea of personal autonomy is still that of self-governance: being one's own person, without constraints either by another's action or by psychological or physical limitations. The autonomous person determines his or her course of action in accordance with a plan chosen by himself or herself. Such a person deliberates about and chooses plans and is capable of acting on the basis of such deliberations, just as a truly independent government is capable of controlling its territories and policies. A person of diminished autonomy, by contrast, is controlled by or highly dependent on others and is in at least some respect incapable of deliberating or acting on the basis of such deliberations. Institutionalized populations such as prisoners and the mentally retarded have diminished autonomy. A form of psychological incapacitation affects the capacity of the retarded, while a severely restricted social environment limits the autonomy of prisoners.

The term "autonomy," as applied to individuals, is thus quite broad, for it can refer to *the person, the will*, or *action in society*; and both internal and external constraints can limit autonomy. Two figures in the history of philosophy have shaped our understanding of autonomy as, respectively, freedom of the will and freedom of action. These figures are Immanuel Kant (a rule deontologist) and John Stuart Mill (a utilitarian). In his *Groundwork of the Metaphysic of Morals* and other writings, Kant argued for his celebrated injunction that persons should always treat each other as autonomous ends and never merely as means to the ends of others. This principle of respect for autonomy expresses Kant's view of the *value* of autonomy: Persons are rational agents of unconditional worth who must not be treated merely as conditionally valued things incapable of choosing for themselves. In analyzing autonomy, Kant contrasted it with heteronomy (rule by other persons or conditions). To be autonomous is to govern oneself, including making one's own choices, in accordance with universalizable moral principles, i.e., principles that can be willed to be universally valid for everyone. Under "heteronomy," Kant included both external and internal determinations of the will, but *not* moral principles. While a moral rule does oblige one to act in accordance with it, one is only complying with a self-legislated rule. Actions from fear and impulse, as well as coerced actions, are obviously heteronomous, but Kant also regarded acting from desire and habit as heteronomous.

Whereas Kant was largely concerned about the moral autonomy of the *will*, Mill was more concerned about the autonomy—or, as he preferred to say, the individuality—of *action* and *thought*. In *On Liberty*, Mill argues that social and political control over individual actions is legitimate only if it is necessary to prevent harm to other individuals. He construes the principle of utility to permit all citizens to develop their potential according to their convictions, as long as they do not interfere with a like expression of freedom by others. The promotion of autonomous expression in his view maximizes the benefits of all concerned. Conformity to established patterns reduces individual productivity and creativity that, if developed, could benefit society. In his discussion, Mill holds that a person with true character is one of genuine individuality, whereas a person "without character" is controlled by an authoritative environment such as church, state, parents, or family. "Firmness and self-control" as well as "choosing a plan of life" are declared by Mill as essential to a proper framing of one's character. "The government of a strong will" he takes to be essential to this goal.[1]

Mill and Kant therefore had somewhat different objectives in treating the concept of autonomy. Mill was interested in the concept of *individual* autonomy or self-determination from a personal point of view. He argued that one's right to this form of self-determination is morally fundamental. Kant, by contrast, was interested in *moral* autonomy—the idea of giving oneself the moral law, or self-determination in accordance with morally valid principles. He argued that one morally ought to act in accordance with such principles. These two views are substantially different, for Kant regarded a purely individual action as outside the moral order.

For our purposes, Kant's main contribution to a theory of autonomy is his discussion of self-legislation: The reasons for actions by autonomous persons are their own reasons, and they are principled rather than arbitrary reasons. This notion of self-directed action based on a principle freely accepted by the agent (but not necessarily a valid universal principle) is the central ingredient of "autonomy" in the remainder of this chapter. "*Acceptance* by the agent" needs emphasis. Kant is often interpreted as holding that each individual person must *make* (author or originate) his own principles—a strained interpretation in light of Kant's view that purely personal or subjective principles are morally unacceptable. Moreover, this subjectivist perspective denies much that we know about the moral life, and thus we will understand Kant to mean only that each individual must *will the acceptance* of his or her principles. Finally, while Mill's views on autonomous action in many ways parallel Kant's, Mill's concerns about the tyranny of society led him to unrealistic ideals of detaching oneself from society in sovereign isolation. In our discussion of autonomy in this chapter, and subsequently in our treatment of paternalism in Chapter 5, we will see both the importance and the limits of these ideals.

In summary, the most general formulation of autonomy in the two theories thus far canvassed, and many others as well, is that a person is autonomous if and only if he or she is self-governing. Autonomy as governance in the absence of controlling constraints points to the individual able to legislate norms of conduct (Kant) and able voluntarily to fix a course of action (Mill). Only if these conditions are present is a person autonomous.

Respect for autonomy and the principle of autonomy

Being autonomous and choosing autonomously are not the same as being *respected* as an autonomous agent. To respect autonomous agents is to recognize their right to self-governance by affirming that they are entitled to such autonomous determination free of imposed limitations.

This conclusion follows directly from Mill's views on individualism and social liberty, but it also has important roots in Kant's thought. For Kant, respect for autonomy flows from the recognition that all persons have unconditional worth, solely as ends in themselves determining their destinies. To violate a person's autonomy is to treat that person merely as a means, because he or she is treated in accordance with rules not of his or her choosing. To reject that person's considered judgments or to preclude his or her freedom to act on those considered judgments is not to respect his or her autonomous personhood. For example, in Case #8 a surgeon withheld information about risks of surgery for an ulcer, and the patient consented. In this case, the surgeon failed to provide relevant information, and thereby limited the patient's autonomy. For Kant a moral relation between autonomous persons requires a *mutual* respect for autonomy, and this case raises interesting questions about whether a surgeon can have such a moral relation if he or she withholds information.

The moral prescription to respect the autonomy of persons can, for our purposes, be formulated as a *principle of autonomy* that should guide our judgments about how to treat self-determining agents. It follows from the views advanced by Mill that insofar as an autonomous agent's actions do not infringe upon the autonomous actions of others, that agent should be free to perform whatever action he or she wishes—even if it involves serious risk and even if others consider it to be foolish. Mill's exceptive clause ("insofar as . . .") is too complex, however, for a prima facie moral principle. Hence, we shall here understand the principle of autonomy as follows: *Autonomous actions and choices should not be constrained by others.* The principle of respect for autonomy should therefore be treated as a broad, abstract principle independent of restrictive or exceptive clauses such as "We must respect individuals' views and rights *so long as* their thoughts and actions produce no serious harms to other persons." The principle of autonomy, like all moral principles, has only prima facie standing. It asserts a right of noninterference and correlatively an obligation not to constrain autonomous actions—nothing more but also nothing less.

The principle of respect for autonomy thus neither determines what a person ought to be free to know or do *on balance*, nor what is to count as a valid justification for constraining autonomy. For example, in Case #5 a patient with an inoperable, incurable carcinoma asks, "I don't have cancer, do I?" The physician lies, saying, "You're as good as you were ten years ago." Because this lie denies the patient information he may want or need to determine his future course of action, it is clearly an infringement of the principle of autonomy. However, it may be (and here we state no opinion) that on balance the lie is justified by the principle of beneficence, which requires that we help others. (See Chapters 5 and 7 on this issue.) We shall later discuss valid ways to override the principle, as well as how to handle those occasions on which a rational agent expresses an autonomous wish to waive consent, delegate authority to others, or take his or her own life. That is, we shall discuss possibly valid restraints on autonomous actions—including, in Chapter 5, permissible *paternalistic* restraints. Whether or not there are limits to the valid expression of autonomy, Mill was right to insist that we have a strong prima facie moral obligation not to interfere with the autonomous actions of others, and correlatively that we have a right of noninterference with our own autonomous actions.

This same principle can be derived from a Kantian position: In evaluating the autonomous actions of others we ought to respect them as persons with the same right to their choices and actions as we have to our own. This principle is often referred to as the principle of respect for persons, because it demands respect for no other reason, utilitarian or otherwise, than that another individual is a person and therefore rightfully a determiner of his or her destiny. At the level of abstract moral principle, it is thus doubtful that the theories of Mill and Kant demand significantly different courses of action. Although Mill's view most obviously demands noninterference with autonomous expression, and Kant's view entails a moral imperative that certain attitudes of respect be framed, in the end these two profoundly different philosophies present similar views about what we are calling "the principle of autonomy."

We reiterate that the principle of autonomy should not be interpreted as too broad in scope. It does not apply to persons who are not in a position to act in a sufficiently autonomous manner—perhaps because they are immature, incapacitated, ignorant, coerced, or in a position in which they can be exploited by others. Infants, irrationally suicidal individuals, and drug-dependent patients are typical examples. The behavior of clearly nonautonomous persons may be validly controlled in order to protect them from harms that might result from such behavior, and the actions of substantially nonautonomous persons may also on some occasions be validly controlled. Those who defend autonomy have never denied that the latter forms of

intervention are justified, because they regard such actions as either wholly
or substantially nonautonomous. We will return to these matters when we
discuss paternalism in Chapter 5.

Meeting the demands of the principle of autonomy has often proved
difficult in clinical and research settings, partially because of the problem of
persons with compromised autonomy. Codes of professional ethics therefore
occasionally have mentioned the importance of respecting autonomy. For
example, the 1953 Code of Nursing Ethics of the International Council of
Nurses stated: "The religious beliefs of a patient must be respected." In 1973
this principle was updated to read as follows: "The nurse, in providing care,
promotes an environment in which the values, customs, and spiritual beliefs
of the individual are respected." Similarly, the American Hospital Association's "Patient's Bill of Rights" prominently turns on such considerations of
respect for autonomy. (The latter two codes are found in Appendix II to this
volume.)

Autonomy and authority

It is sometimes held that autonomy is inconsistent with the authority of
church, state, social groups, or individuals who function in special contexts
as authorities and who make decisions over the lives of autonomous agents.
This radical position rejects, for example, the legitimacy of governmental
implementation of restrictive public policies intended to protect and promote health. It also entails that medical authorities can never validly intervene in the lives of autonomous patients. One argument for this position is
that the autonomous person is one who determines his or her actions
through moral deliberation *totally unimpeded by any authority's controlling
influence.*[2] In this theory, because autonomous persons must act on their
own reasons, they should never submit to another person or authority
simply because the other utters an imperative. This thesis applies to physicians as authorities, to the authority of the state, and to divine commands. A
conflict between autonomy and all such authority necessarily results: It is a
necessary condition of authority that a person be obeyed merely because that
person occupies a position of authority; and it is a necessary condition of
autonomy that a person must refuse all controlling influence by authorities.[3]
Because this conclusion might seem to follow from the philosophies of both
Mill and Kant, it is worth considering whether autonomy is radically inconsistent with authority, as this theory suggests.

We think there is no fundamental inconsistency, because the operative
notions of autonomy and authority are eccentric and indefensible. Common

conceptions of nondictatorial political and social practices assume that the provision of justifying reasons is part of, not distinct from, the process of legitimate authoritative command. Dutiful citizens are not expected to comply with authoritative commands without provision of reasons and merely because authorities have spoken. The legitimacy of any command is contingent upon its not exceeding the limits set by those who delegated the authority to command in the first place—the autonomous citizens.

Moral principles too are not disembodied rules, cut off from their cultural setting. To interpret autonomy in morality as entailing the reign of subjective principles involves an inherent misunderstanding of both moral belief and ethical theory. This conception wrongly portrays moral principles as formulated by atomized "moral" agents disengaged from a cultural setting. Such a depiction harbors warped notions of both autonomy and morality. "Morality," as we understand the term, emerges from shared experiences and social arrangements (tacit or otherwise). By its nature morality is not individual-centered. That we *share* accepted principles in no way prevents them from being an individual's *personal* principles. Virtuous conduct, role responsibilities, acceptable forms of loving, charitable behavior, respect for persons, and many other moral views are individually *assumed*, but usually appropriated from established cultural arrangements.

It is hard to conceive how a principle could be a *moral* principle and stand outside minimal social arrangements. What would make such a principle more than the belief or policy of an individual? Could the moral requirement that we respect autonomy be a personal creation, or valid if accepted only by one single individual? And what of rules or codes of professional ethics? They clearly do not permit individual authorship. Does this fact somehow render them invalid?[4] In rejecting all social understandings of morality, one can, of course, be acting autonomously. It does not follow that because it is an autonomous action it is morally acceptable or even morally principled. Autonomy is compatible, on the one hand, with immorality, and, on the other hand, with moral authority and tradition. Autonomy is thus linked to reflective individual choice but not to rejection of authority or tradition.

This conclusion about the compatibility of autonomy and both delegated authority and moral tradition holds for medical contexts as well as for political ones. The authority assumed by medical professionals presents many difficulties about autonomy and consent in the medical setting. In Case #15 a sixty-eight-year-old patient (and physician by profession) asked that no further steps be taken to prolong his life, and entered this request in his case records. Nonetheless, he was revived by the hospital's emergency resuscitation team. Here the professional authority of the attending physician was used to override the patient's autonomous refusal—a classic conflict between two forms of authority.

We shall see that a number of paradoxes of autonomy emerge in medical contexts because of the condition of the subject, on the one hand, and the authoritative position of the medical professional, on the other. There will be a number of occasions (both here and in the section on paternalism in Chapter 5) where we may doubt that authority and autonomy are in fact compatible. These contexts will usually be ones where authority either has not been delegated or is itself questionable as an authority.

Informed consent

The voluntary consent of the human subject is absolutely essential.
    This means that the person involved should have the legal capacity to give consent; should be so situated as to be able to exercise free power of choice, without the intervention of any element of force, fraud, deceit, duress, over-reaching, or other ulterior form of constraint or coercion; and should have sufficient knowledge and comprehension of the subject matter involved as to enable him to make an understanding and enlightened decision. This latter element requires that before the acceptance of an affirmative decision by the experimental subject there should be made known to him the nature, duration, and purpose of the experiment; the methods and means by which it is to be conducted; all inconveniences and hazards reasonably to be expected; and the effects upon his health or person which may possibly come from his participation in the experiment. (*Nuremberg Code*, Rule 1; see Appendix II.)

The horrible stories of experimentation in concentration camps led to serious concern about the use of nonconsenting subjects in questionable and sometimes brutal experiments. Since the Nuremberg Trials the issue of informed consent has received more attention than any ethical issue in biomedical research involving human subjects. The Nuremberg Code cited above is one outcome, but controversies about informed consent have also arisen in other quarters. In Anglo-American law, for example, the doctrine of informed consent has gradually emerged from malpractice cases involving nonconsensual touching of the patient's body. Touching competent patients without consent has been found unacceptable in these cases, irrespective of considerations of the quality of care. Throughout this section we shall see how standards for medical *practice* have derived from case law and how standards for *research* have grown from their roots in both the Nuremberg Code and the Declaration of Helsinki.

Functions and justifications of informed consent

In recent years virtually all medical and research codes of ethics have held that physicians must obtain the informed consent of patients before undertaking significant therapeutic or research procedures. These consent measures have been designed largely to protect the autonomy of patients and subjects, but they serve other functions as well. Alexander Capron has helpfully identified several important functions.[5]

1. The promotion of individual autonomy
2. The protection of patients and subjects
3. The avoidance of fraud and duress
4. The encouragement of self-scrutiny by medical professionals
5. The promotion of rational decisions
6. The involvement of the public (in promoting autonomy as a general social value and in controlling biomedical research)

Capron correctly argues that informed consent serves each of these functions. However, both historically and contemporarily, two positions about *function and justification* have dominated the literature. One maintains that the purpose and justification for obtaining informed consent is to protect persons from various risks of harm. Those who subscribe to a justification based on *protection from harm* are inclined to protect patients whether or not it is the patient's choice that leads to an "unwise" assumption of a risk. The other position sees the purpose and justification for obtaining informed consent as respect for the autonomy of patients, by recognizing their rights to know and choose. Those who subscribe to a justification based on *protection of autonomy* are not inclined to protect patients against their choices, on grounds that such constraint would violate their autonomy. The aforementioned case (#15) of a patient (also a physician) who refused further steps to prolong his life, but was resuscitated nonetheless, may well be the result of these two different approaches applied in the clinical setting.

In this chapter we accept the view that the primary function of informed consent is the protection and promotion of individual autonomy. The communication between a health professional and a patient should prevent ignorance from constraining autonomous choice, whether ignorance is present from a lack of information or a lack of comprehension. Our theory therefore generates requirements of comprehension as well as disclosure. A protection-from-harm justification is based on the principles of nonmalefi-cence and beneficence, and is put in the most favorable light by legal requirements governing consent. The law of battery protects against inten-tional bodily invasions where there has been no consent whatever; and the law of negligence holds researchers responsible for inadequate disclosures that might lead to injury.[6] Informed consent provisions thus protect against battery and negligence, and can be justified on this basis in the law. Second-party consent, or consent on behalf of a person given by another, can be similarly justified. Nonetheless, this justification in terms of the principle of nonmaleficence does not seem *fundamental* to moral justifications of first-party consent. While a person's decision may indirectly function to prevent harm, the person may also autonomously choose a greater risk than others would choose for him or her. The principle of autonomy justifies allowing a person this option of accepting increased risk, and we therefore consider the protection of autonomy to be the primary function of informed consent regulations.

A third justification for informed consent is based on the principle of utility: Informed consent requirements will maximally protect and benefit everyone in society, including health professionals, patients, and the institu-tions of medical practice and research themselves. Rules of consent serve to protect and benefit patients and professionals, to allay public fears (especially about research), to encourage self-scrutiny by physicians and investigators, and to maintain a relation of trust between them. This justification is closely related to Capron's fourth and sixth functions.

Even though justifications based on utility and nonmaleficence are appro-priate for some consent requirements, the justifications based on autonomy recognize consent as valid *because* the consenting party is an autonomous person, with all the entitlements that status confers. Neither utility nor nonmaleficence leads to this strong conclusion, for both would justify not seeking consent in some circumstances—utility when it would not maximize the social welfare and nonmaleficence when no apparent harm would result. When informed consent is justified by the principle of autonomy, it is intro-duced, as Robert Veatch puts it, "not to facilitate social benefits, but as a check against them,"[7] for persons have rights to information and to consent that are independent of such considerations as immediate social utility and risk to patients or subjects.

This view has long-standing appeal in the law, where it is somewhat more fully developed than in writings on moral philosophy. Justice Cardozo's early statement (1914) in behalf of autonomy is well known: "Every human being of adult years and sound mind has a right to determine what shall be done with his own body; and a surgeon who performs an operation without his patient's consent commits an assault, for which he is liable in damages. . . . This is true except in cases of emergency."[8] An updated, and in some ways even stronger, statement is found in a landmark 1960 case, *Natanson* v. *Kline*, where it is asserted that

Anglo-American law starts with the premise of thoroughgoing self-determination. It follows that each man is considered to be master of his own body, and he may, if he be of sound mind, expressly prohibit the performance of lifesaving surgery, or other medical treatment.[9]

In short, the fact that we would often seek to obtain informed consent, even when it does not maximize immediate social utility and even when subjects and patients are not being protected against risk, indicates that autonomy is the basic justifying principle.

The ability of compromised patients to give such an autonomous, informed consent to clinical research or treatment is often doubtful, as Cases #12, #14, and #19 illustrate. Here seriously compromised patients must make vital decisions about treatment in far from ideal contexts for autonomous decisionmaking. In cases where we might fall into error, it seems best to err on the side of ethical conservatism: We should strive not to deny an important medical benefit when a person has not accepted or is incapable of knowledgeably accepting it, even if—after careful examination—we are uncertain about the validity of a consent or refusal. Of course this rule has its limits. The medical benefit might be the wrong choice for other reasons. Like other rules, this one is strictly prima facie.

The elements of informed consent

Whether first parties or second parties are in question, it is generally agreed that informed consent must be solicited whenever a procedure is intrusive, whenever there are significant risks, and whenever the purposes of the procedure might be questionable. However, the exact nature of these requirements and the elements that constitute informed consent are both subjects of dispute.

Medical and research codes, as well as federal regulations, have traditionally emphasized that the act of consent must be genuinely *voluntary* and that there must be adequate *disclosure* of information. However, there are several elements of informed consent, each presenting distinct issues. The information component of informed consent refers to adequate disclosure of information and adequate comprehension by patients or subjects of what is disclosed, while the consent component refers to a voluntary decision on the part of a competent person. But how much and what types of information must be imparted, and how well must it be understood? Is consent valid if it is given under conditions of social, institutional, or family pressure or if the consent is irresponsible? Beneath these questions is the need for a detailed analysis of the concept of informed consent that probes moral problems unique to each element. Accordingly, each of the following four elements is treated in this chapter:

I. Information Elements
    1. Disclosure of Information
    2. Comprehension of Information
II. Consent Elements
    3. Voluntary Consent
    4. Competence to Consent

It is widely presumed in literature on the subject that each of these four elements is a necessary condition not only of an *informed* consent, but of a *valid* consent as well. This assumption is understandable because informed consent *authorizes* others to act in certain ways, in the sense of giving them valid permission. However, that something is an informed consent need not entail that it is a valid permission, or vice versa. Such a broad generalization neglects problems of whether a consent is authoritative if informed (think of children) and informed if valid (think of waivers). Perhaps there can be a valid uninformed consent or an invalid informed consent. Perhaps the above elements are jointly *sufficient* conditions of an informed consent, rather than individually *necessary* conditions. These several possibilities should be kept in mind as each of the elements is studied.

We begin with the last of the four elements in the above chart.

Competence

The concept of competence

Competence to consent could perhaps be more appropriately described as a *presupposition* of informed consent than as an *element* of informed consent. In one primary use, "competence" is a psychological term referring to a precondition of acting voluntarily and apprehending information. It is fundamental in biomedical contexts, where certain physical and mental conditions render patients and subjects incapable—in psychological fact or in law—of informed consent or refusal. Obviously many conditions external to an agent may inhibit voluntary action, but many internal conditions may also limit voluntariness. It is usually the latter conditions that lead to questions about competence. For example, minors commonly are not capable of responsible actions, and mentally disabled persons present similar problems.

Judgments of competence always require a context. Depending on the context specified or assumed, one could be competent or incompetent to stand trial, to raise dachshunds, to write checks, or to lecture to law students about competence. While it is possible to speak of someone as *generally* incompetent, this judgment assumes the ordinary affairs of life as its context. Rarely do we judge a person incompetent with respect to every sphere of life, for we usually consider some particular kind of competence or incompetence, such as the competence to decide about treatment or to participate in research.

Judgments of competence and incompetence thus often apply to a limited range of decisionmaking, not to all decisions made by a person. Some persons who are legally incompetent may be competent to conduct most of their personal affairs, and vice versa. The same person's ability to make decisions may vary over time, and he or she may at a single time be competent to make certain practical decisions but incompetent to make others. For example, a person judged incompetent to drive an automobile may be competent to decide to participate in medical research, and may be able to handle simple affairs easily, while faltering before complex ones. In Case #9 a woman has been involuntarily hospitalized because of periods of confusion and loss of memory, but is competent most of the time to perform ordinary tasks. Health professionals and a court are called upon to determine whether this legally incompetent patient can be provided with an alternative medical therapy suitable to her situation. The notions of *limited* competence and *intermittent* competence thus have practical implications. They require a statement of the precise decisions a person can make, while avoiding the false dichotomy of "either competent or incompetent." Use of these notions should preserve maximum autonomy, for they justify intervention only in those areas where a person is substantially incompetent.

For practical and policy reasons, we often need cut-offs on the continuum from wholly competent to wholly incompetent. In competence judgments we are concerned with ability to perform at or above an established threshold on a performance continuum.[10] Any person below a certain level of abilities will be treated as incompetent. Except for the extreme end of "no ability," however, it is difficult in most contexts to avoid a great many cases of borderline incompetence. Moreover, if persons have been declared generally incompetent, it does not follow that they are incompetent to make some important decisions, including ones about medical treatment. The validity of their consent or refusal will depend in complex ways on the precise nature of their incompetence to consent and on the precise constraints characteristic of their conditions of life.

A case included in the Appendix (#10) illustrates the difficulties often encountered in attempting to judge competence. In this case, a man who generally exhibits normal behavior patterns is involuntarily committed to a mental institution because of bizarre actions prompted by his unorthodox religious beliefs. Because the man's religious beliefs lead to serious self-destructive behavior (pulling out an eye and cutting off a hand), he is judged incompetent, despite his generally competent behavior and despite the fact this his peculiar actions follow "reasonably" from his—many would say, equally peculiar—religious beliefs. While this troublesome case probably cannot be understood in terms of intermittent competence, analysis in terms of limited competence clearly seems appropriate.

Standards of competence

Perhaps the major question about competence in recent years centers on *standards*—especially legal standards—for its determination. The most promising headway toward a useful definition has come through criminal law and civil law, which specifically consider competence to make an informed choice. Legal standards cluster about various abilities to comprehend and process information and to reason about the consequences of one's actions. Lack of mental capacity, understood as sufficient rationality and intelligence, is central. A person is commonly said to be competent only if both capable of processing specifiable information and capable of choosing goals and the means to those goals as well as acting on reasonable decisions. But even in law competence is not a simple concept with an easily specified context. It has different content in discussions of property, estate, and business affairs. Several forms and standards for determining competence thus have been delineated to fit the context in which a judgment is needed.

Courts have disagreed on which of the following three properties is most crucial to a determination of competence:[11] (1) capacity to reach a decision based on *rational reasons*, (2) capacity to reach a *reasonable result* through a decision, or (3) the capacity to *make a decision* at all. Without attempting to distinguish all the arguments and possible reasons for adopting one or more of these three standards, it seems reasonable for our purposes to combine them as follows: A person is competent if and only if that person can make decisions based on rational reasons. In biomedical contexts this standard entails that a person must be able to understand a therapy or research procedure, must be able to weigh its risks and benefits, and must be able to make a decision in light of such knowledge and through such abilities, even if the person chooses not to utilize the information.

Case #12 could be used as a test for this general standard. In this case two seriously burned patients without any chance for survival are treated as competent. They are mentally alert, capable of conversation, and their decisions about treatment are taken seriously. Judging from the descriptions offered by the nurse and physician who wrote this case, these patients would be competent by the standard we have proposed. However, this judgment would be controversial.

Value-laden judgments of competence

A further problem is that a "competence" judgment can hide a significant value judgment about another person. A person who appears irrational or unreasonable to others might be declared incompetent in order that "treatment" can be provided. Such a declaration conceals a value judgment about what a rational person ought to consent to do, presented in the guise of an empirical determination of incompetence. Jeffrie Murphy has correctly observed that all theories of incompetence have troublesome borderline cases that present moral problems of assessment:

[T]he vast majority of cases that confront us will be borderline—cases in that greyish area between full competence and obvious incompetence. The real problem that will face us, then, is what to do in the borderline cases. When in doubt, which way should we err—on the side of safety or on the side of liberty? It is vital that we do not adopt analyses of "incompetence" or patterns of argument that obscure the obviously moral nature of this question.[12]

It is no simple *empirical* question whether a borderline person is or is not competent. If precise, nonevaluative criteria were available for making such determinations, the gray area would vanish. But since such criteria are not available, moral judgments and policy choices about what to do with possibly incompetent persons cannot be avoided.

Nevertheless, once the criteria for determining incompetence have been established, it is in principle an empirical question whether someone is competent or incompetent under those criteria. The difficult borderline cases should not obscure the empirical character of the inquiry into whether the person exhibits the set of requisite abilities (or some part of the set). To say that determinations of competence are empirical is not, however, to overlook the fact that the initial choice of criteria for determining competence is not an empirical matter. A choice of criteria *establishes* certain abilities rather than others as the requisite abilities, and only then can we empirically test for the abilities. For example, competence in diving, college debate, and surgery are established by well-entrenched, contextual criteria. However, those criteria could have been different than they are, and they still can and do shift over time. These criteria are selected on the basis of certain *shared values*; thus, empirical judgments of psychological competence are not *value free*.

Disclosure of information

Some medical and research codes discuss conditions under which a person can be said to have sufficient information to make an informed choice. Frequently listed as necessary items of disclosure are the following: contemplated procedures, alternative available procedures, anticipated risks and benefits, and a statement offering the person an opportunity to ask further questions and to withdraw at any time in the case of research. (See the presently operative federal regulations in the Appendix for a thorough list.) Several writers on the subject of informed consent have proposed additional or supplementary conditions—for example, statements of the purpose of the procedure, the uncertain risks involved, persons in charge, and, if research is involved, criteria for the selection of subjects. Such lists could be expanded indefinitely, but many possible inclusions are not applicable to all areas of medical research and practice. Expansive lists of conditions are sometimes appropriate, while in other contexts they would waste precious time and might even prove to be damaging to patients or subjects. Accordingly, it is more important to determine which primary moral standards should govern the disclosure of information. We shall concentrate on this topic.

Standards of disclosure

Many recent court cases have emphasized problems of a *standard* for adequate disclosure. Two general standards of adequate disclosures are in competition in the law as a result of these cases: the "professional practice standard" and the "reasonable person standard." A third standard, commonly called the "subjective standard," has also been proposed. These competing standards deserve careful scrutiny.

(A). THE PROFESSIONAL PRACTICE STANDARD. The first standard holds that adequate disclosure is determined by the traditional disclosure practices of a professional community—such as a community of physicians or psychologists. The custom in a profession establishes the amount and kinds of information to be disclosed. Only expert testimony from members of such professional groups could count as evidence that there has been a violation of a right to information. As one commentator correctly notes,

The view accepted by the majority of American jurisdictions bases the duty to disclose on a community standard; it requires only such disclosures of risks as is consistent with the practice of the local medical community. Expert medical testimony is required to show a breach of local medical standards.[13]

This standard was devised under the conviction that the doctor's proper role is to act in the patient's best medical interest. The obligation to disclose information is in effect subservient to a medical judgment of the patient's best interest. Medical care standards, rather than patients' rights, thus determine the operative guidelines for disclosure.

Several difficulties accompany the professional practice standard. It is unclear that a customary standard exists for particular situations in the medical profession, and if custom alone is taken as conclusive, then pervasively negligent care can be perpetuated with impunity. The majority of professionals can in principle offer the same inferior level of information. However, the chief objection to the professional practice standard is that this standard undermines patient autonomy, the promotion of which many—including the present authors—hold to be the primary function and justification of rules of informed consent. The weighing of risks against a person's subjective beliefs, fears, and hopes is not an expert skill to be measured through a professional standard and is perhaps better within the comprehension of an average juror than an average physician. Medical custom often expresses the values and goals of the medical profession, but information provided to patients and subjects should be as free as possible of the personal values and goals of medical professionals, especially those doing research. Physicians and investigators may well see risks and benefits in quite a different perspective than would others.

(B). THE REASONABLE PERSON STANDARD. Because of several recent cases, the reasonable person standard has gradually emerged as a substantial legal criterion, although approximately seventy-five percent of the legal jurisdictions in the United States cling to the more traditional professional practice standard. According to this newer standard, information to be disclosed is determined by reference to a hypothetical reasonable person, and the pertinence of a piece of information is measured by the significance a reasonable person would attach to a risk in deciding whether to submit to a procedure. Most proponents of the reasonable person standard believe that considerations of autonomy generally outweigh those of beneficence and that, on balance, the reasonable person standard better serves autonomy than does the professional practice standard. The purest autonomy-based argument holds that risk evaluation always belongs to the individual affected, not to the professional(s) involved, regardless of the latter's expert knowledge and ability to protect the individual from harm.

The best available resource for understanding this standard is recent case law, which has gradually assembled a set of considerations that explicate the concept of a reasonable person, such as the following:

1. All material information necessary for a decision must be given, as judged by persons who would compose a jury rather than by expert testimony or by a medical body.[14]
2. Known risks of significant bodily harm and death must be disclosed.[15]
3. The reasonable person is a composite or ideal of reasonable persons in society, and the individual subject is not in question.[16]
4. Standards of disclosure in medicine are not different from those of other professions where there is a similar fiduciary relationship.[17]

Differences between the reasonable person standard and the professional practice standard are clearly reflected in Case #8. In this case, a patient was told in general terms of the risks of undergoing a general anesthetic and the nature of ulcer surgery, but the physicians failed to disclose the inherent risks of the surgery itself. An apparently successful operation was performed, but injuries to the spleen were subsequently discovered and a gastric ulcer developed—both risks inherent in the original surgery. The patient sued the physician on grounds of a failure to disclose these inherent risks. The physician argued that disclosures of such low probability are uncommon in medicine and that he should be held only to the standards of disclosure accepted by surgeons—a clear invocation of the professional practice standard. The court, however, concluded that "the patient's right of self-decision is the measure of the physician's duty to reveal." A physician is therefore required by the reasonable person standard to disclose "all information relevant to a meaningful decisional process," with respect both to the proposed therapy and its inherent risks.

Judge Robinson argued in *Canterbury* v. *Spence*, a precedent on which this court relied, that medical duties to disclose are themselves ultimately based on moral considerations of autonomy. The judge calls these considerations "the patient's right of self-decision" and the patient's "prerogative to decide."[18] His point is that duties of disclosure are at their root moral rather than legal or medical ones, and these moral duties inform both law and medicine as to the appropriate standards. Such case law, when combined with the moral standards of autonomy we have proposed, suggests the following standard of disclosure: The patient or subject should be provided with information that a reasonable person in the patient's or subject's circumstances would find relevant and could reasonably be expected to assimilate. In this way the moral requirement to respect autonomy is translated into a reasonable person standard.

Unfortunately, this reasonable person standard is still plagued by conceptual, moral, and practical difficulties. First, "material information" and the central concept of "the reasonable person" are not clearly defined. A pressing conceptual problem is how to understand the information the reasonable person would want under circumstances *similar* to those of the patient. If, for example, a patient argues that a physician failed to disclose the risk of cancer associated with a therapy, how broadly should we construe that element of the standard that points to the patient's circumstances or position?

Second, there are problems about how the reasonable person standard can be employed in practice in some areas of biomedical research and clinical medicine. One such problem has been suggested on the basis of recent empirical studies that attempt to discover whether information disclosed to patients is actually used by these patients in reaching their decisions. For example, data collected in a study by Ruth Faden indicate, among other things, that although 93% of the patients surveyed believed they benefited from the information disclosed, only 12% actually used the information in their decision to consent.[19] This study, involving family-planning patients, reaches conclusions similar to an earlier study by Fellner and Marshall of persons consenting to be kidney donors.[20] In both studies data indicate that patients make their decisions largely prior to and independent of the actual process of disclosing information. Other studies indicate that patients generally accept a physician's recommendation without weighing risks and benefits carefully[21] and that as many as 86% of patients would agree without any discussion of risks to a procedure (upper gastro-intestinal endoscopy in one particular study).[22] These data do not in any way show that patient decisions were uninformed or that disclosed information was irrelevant, for the patients may have believed only that the additional information was not such as to shake their prior commitment to a particular course of action. For example, a kidney donor could reasonably decide that the eventual death of his brother far outweighs any information disclosed by a physician. Nonetheless, the above empirical findings do throw into question what should count as material facts for the *individual* patient, as contrasted to the *reasonable* patient. This problem leads to a discussion of the third standard.

(C). THE SUBJECTIVE STANDARD. In the reasonable person model, sufficiency of information is judged by reference to the informational needs of the "objective" reasonable person, and *not* by reference to the specific informational needs of the individual subject—as proposed by the subjective stand-ard. Individual informational needs can differ, because a person may have highly personal or unorthodox beliefs, unusual health problems, or unique family histories requiring a different informational base than most other persons. For example, a female employee with a family history of reproduc-tive problems might need information that other persons would not wish to obtain before becoming involved in research on sexual and familial relations or accepting employment in certain industries. If a physician knows or has reason to believe that a person needs and wants such information, then withholding it may deprive the patient of the opportunity to make an informed choice, and thus may undermine autonomy.

At issue here is the extent to which the reasonable person standard should be tailored to the individual patient—i.e., made "subjective." There is a continuum of possible interpretations: At the conservative end, the phrase "in the patient's or subject's position" could be taken to include only the person's medical condition and related physical characteristics. Under this interpretation, the physician would be obligated to disclose only medical information that would be needed by the reasonable patient with these conditions and characteristics. At the liberal end of the continuum, the patient's position could be construed to include any factor particular to the patient's need or desire for information that a physician could reasonably be expected to know (or even to discover). Under this construal the reasonable person standard perhaps becomes indistinguishable from the subjective standard. The physician is obligated to disclose information a particular patient wants or needs to know, so long as there is a reasonable connection between these informational needs and what the physician should know about the patient's position. This construal suggests that the *moral* question is not whether the information necessarily, probably, or possibly would have led the patient to forego therapy—a critical *legal* question—but rather whether the information was necessary for an informed decision regardless of the outcome.

Despite the problems of using the subjective standard as a legal standard, it is a proper standard of disclosure from a moral point of view, based on respect for autonomy. We therefore suggest that the average reasonable person standard presently operative in *law* should be supplemented by some standard that takes account of the independent informational needs of actual reasonable persons in the process of making a difficult decision. Nevertheless, an *entirely* subjective standard—c above—seems inappropri-ate, because patients often do not know what information would be relevant for their deliberations, and a doctor cannot reasonably be expected to do an exhaustive background and character analysis of each patient to determine relevant information.

Perhaps the best solution is a compromise standard, combining B and C: Whatever a reasonable person would judge material to the decisionmaking process should be disclosed, and, in addition, any other information material to an individual patient should be provided through a process of asking a patient what else he or she wishes to know and providing truthful answers to any questions asked. Autonomy is not adequately protected unless some more rigorous criterion of this sort is adopted. If subjects do not have an adequate idea, given their concerns and needs, of what they are deciding, then there is no *informed* consent, even if they do possess all the information a disembodied "reasonable person" would possess. Because protection of autonomy is the central justification of rules of informed consent in morals and law, this modified, more stringent version of the reasonable person standard seems morally required.

Intentional nondisclosure

This proposed standard involves practical difficulties, however, especially for clinical medicine. According to the legal doctrine of "therapeutic privilege," a physician may intentionally and validly not disclose or may underdisclose information, based on a "sound medical judgment" that to divulge the information would be potentially harmful to a depressed, emotionally drained, or unstable patient.[23] Courts have increasingly curtailed physician latitude in the use of this therapeutic privilege, just as they have increasingly adopted the reasonable person standard instead of standards operative in the medical profession. (The courts have thus far described the physician's duty in such circumstances only in extremely general terms, and the proper formulation of this privilege is widely discussed.)

However, discretion by physicians must be permitted in many delicate cases, and this indisputable need has led courts to hold that the patient's right to information, based on autonomy, must on occasion yield to a professional judgment of welfare, based on beneficence and nonmaleficence. What may be doubted, as psychiatrist Jay Katz has illuminatingly argued, is that there can be "consistency" between physician discretion in disclosing information and the full disclosure of facts demanded by some courts. Physicians risk a malpractice charge by not providing sufficient information for an intelligent choice; and, yet, courts have often noted that the duty to disclose can be validly qualified by the physician's professional discretion.

"Only in dreams or fairy tales," Katz contends, "can 'discretion' to withhold crucial information so easily and magically be reconciled with 'full disclosure.' . . . Clearly informed consent was born in confusion."[24]

There is of course no formal inconsistency between respecting autonomy and protecting from harm. Both purposes can be promoted through informed choice. Yet, the history of informed consent has left a legal and medical legacy in which demands for patient autonomy are present in such cases as *Canterbury* and *Cobbs*, but with valid exceptions recognized in both law and medicine. This is an understandable complexity: Disclosures can harm some patients, and in many circumstances patients have a deep need to have a health professional in charge who assumes authority and, with reassuring confidence, issues orders that will restore the patient to health. Human needs for such authority are constant in the medical context, and they everywhere challenge the health professional's task of informing patients so that they can make decisions.

Problems of not harming or causing undue alarm to the patient are further complicated by remote risks. In Case #7 a woman had a fatal reaction during urography. The radiologist had intentionally not disclosed the slight chance of death (roughly 1/10,000) because of the unsettling effect such a discussion of possible death might have had on the patient. The radiologist justified the nondisclosure on grounds of beneficence: The disclosure could be "dangerous" and "not in the best interest of the patient." Although inherently threatening to autonomy, this argument is not implausible in all clinical contexts (a matter we take up in Chapter 5 while discussing paternalism). It can also be applied to the use of placebos, which are among the clearest examples of nondisclosure in clinical practice. (See Case #4 for an illustration.)

Two types of intentional nondisclosure have also raised important issues in *research* contexts. First, there is the use of randomized clinical trials— random assignment to one of several alternative treatment categories. Some subjects could receive placebos or an experimental therapy, such as a new drug, while others receive a standard or alternative therapy. Such procedures are blind, at least in that the subject does not know which treatment or placebo is received. Second, certain research, especially in psychology, methodologically requires deception for its successful completion without biasing its results. The major moral problem is how much information, if any, ought to be disclosed in either of these cases.

Consider randomized clinical trials further. It has been argued, on the one hand, that patients and subjects should not be informed that randomization is involved, because completion of the trial with adequate information would be rendered impossible,[25] and, on the other hand, that both the fact of randomization and the progress of the trial itself should be divulged to participants.[26] Case #28 is a widely discussed instance of this problem. In this case, a new drug (ara-A) was tested for the treatment and cure of herpes simplex encephalitis, a disease fatal to approximately seventy percent of those who contract it. Ten of the 28 patients treated received a placebo instead of the experimental drug. Of the 18 patients treated with ara-A, five died. Of the ten given the placebo, seven died. This very complicated case cannot be reduced to these simple terms, but these numbers alone indicate why some have found moral problems with randomized clinical trials.

At a minimum the following should be said about such practices: The procedures involved should be carefully scrutinized—by investigators and review committees—to insure that several possibilities are explored. For example, the probability of generating resentment on the part of subjects and of destroying relations of trust, the possibility of humiliation, and the benefits of the research should be considered. In order that autonomy not be violated, information that a subject would need in order to make a decision about participation—as judged by the revised standard of the reasonable person—would have to be provided. So long as a subject comprehends the procedures envisioned, as well as what is commonly done in such research, consent can be reasonably said to be informed. Thus, it is not enough simply to assert that "Where scientific or humane values justify delaying or with-holding information, the investigator acquires a special responsibility to assure that there are no damaging consequences for the participant," as the Code of Ethics of the American Psychological Association reads.[27] Nevertheless, general information provided to patients—such as the information that the procedure involves a randomized clinical trial and that the results will later be divulged to the subjects—should in many cases be sufficient.

This approach to incomplete disclosures in randomized clinical trials can be more sharply formulated. Such research is justified only if:

1. There is no satisfactory alternative methodology that avoids withholding information.
2. The subjects are informed that they are involved in a randomized clinical trial and might be receiving a placebo or a nonvalidated therapy.
3. The research is well designed, including provisions for the evaluation of alternative therapies.
4. All therapies to be included have no substantial disparity in their prior probabilities of benefit.
5. Risks to patients either are fully mentioned prior to their consent or are minimal (not beyond the risk involved in a standard physical examination) if there are risks that cannot be divulged.

6. Consent safeguards, such as a surrogate consent system, have been put in place wherever appropriate.

This list specifies only necessary conditions of justified randomized clinical trial procedure and consent. The conditions are not sufficient to justify all such research, for many subtle problems may require further conditions to be satisfied. Nonetheless, it seems precipitous to maintain that patients and subjects *can never* be adequately protected in such research. If principles of nonmaleficence, beneficence, and autonomy are not violated in carrying out the research, the procedures are not inherently morally objectionable. Nonmaleficence and beneficence can be observed by careful scrutiny of possible harms that might result, and autonomy can be protected by insuring that subjects have an adequate idea of what they are accepting even if they do not have information about all details.

Nevertheless, the six conditions listed above may not be met at present in a significant amount of biomedical and psychological research involving intentional deception. While much of this research presents minor risk and minor deception, the deception may engender resentment by subjects subsequent to their involvement. If the research is important, it might plausibly be argued that minor deception and minimal risks are outweighed by the substantial knowledge or benefits to be gained. This justification of the research would turn on a favorable risk/benefit analysis. However, as substantial deception or substantial risk is added, justification becomes progressively more difficult. Stanley Milgram's well-known experiments in which subjects were falsely informed that they would be supplying electroshock to other subjects provide examples of this sort.[28] Another, and perhaps more fascinating, case is #3 in the Appendix. In this case a social scientist using substantial deception placed homosexual subjects at risk of public disclosure and embarrassment and invaded their privacy. Also, a remarkably revealing sociological study of the practices of Italian priests in hearing confessions of sexual sins—published in English as *Sex and the Confessional*[29]—involved the deception of priests and the taping of their questions and advice. While these cases are social-scientific rather than biomedical, they illustrate how deception (and resulting risk) can and does occur during research.

Can such research be justified? We think not when significant risk is involved, unless subjects can be informed that they are being placed at risk and consent to this placement. The critical question is whether subjects accept the risk of involvement in deceptive practices. If they do not, it seems a fundamental violation of the principle of autonomy *both* to place them at risk and to deceive them. This conclusion is far from innocuous; much research of this description has been carried out in the past, and is still being considered and in some cases approved by research review committees. This conclusion does not imply, however, that research involving deception cannot justifiably be undertaken. Relatively risk-free and significant research —especially in behavioral psychology and sociology—could not in some cases be undertaken without deception or incomplete disclosure. Simple examples include studies of visual and other perceptual responses. Cases in which disclosure would invalidate the research should be distinguished from cases in which disclosure would be inconvenient, time consuming, or expensive. Generally, deception should be permitted only if essential to obtain important information, when there is insubstantial risk, and when no other moral principles are violated.

Comprehension of information

A sufficient quantity of information is needed for a consent to be informed, but so is adequate comprehension. Many conditions other than lack of sufficient information can limit comprehension.[30] Irrationality and immaturity can do so, for example. In Case #9, a woman suffering from chronic brain syndrome with arteriosclerosis has periods of confusion and mild loss of memory; she is sometimes, but not always, unable to understand her condition. But even if there were no such problems about general competence, problems about adequate comprehension would remain, for information could be so distorted or unsuitable that communication fails.

With the exception of a few studies of patient comprehension, most studies of informed consent have given little attention to information processing. Yet current knowledge about information processing raises many issues. For example, a major obstacle to adequate reception in the consent context may be information overload. Most standards for adequate disclosure require that subjects be provided with substantial amounts of information, much of which may be unfamiliar or conceptually alien. It is possible that "over" disclosure is as likely as "under" disclosure to produce an uninformed consent, although the implications of this phenomenon are not well understood. Practical constraints also generally require that subjects be given this information in a compressed presentation. Thus subjects are likely to rely on some modes of selective perception, and it will be difficult to determine when words have special meaning for patients, when preconceptions distort their processing of the information, and when other biases intrude.

Even if a subject adequately receives and comprehends disclosed information, his or her ability to give an informed consent may be compromised by a refusal to accept the information as true or untainted. The distinction between mere *comprehension* of information and *acceptance* of information often has been obscured by a reliance on paper-and-pencil and other recall tests. At best "correct" answers on such tests provide evidence of a subject's comprehension of what the investigator has disclosed. These answers do not indicate whether the subject *believed* the investigator. The status of a consent given by a comprehending subject who holds a pertinent false belief is clearly problematic. If, for example, a patient is asked to make a treatment decision and refuses on grounds that he or she is not ill (a false belief), further discussion to ensure adequate comprehension and acceptance would be called for.

An adequate *appreciation* of some information can be as important as its comprehension and acceptance. However, to educate or inform a patient not only to comprehend but to appreciate risks and benefits, without disastrously undercutting patient confidence, can be a formidable task. For example, coronary bypass surgery, orthopedic surgery, and many other forms of surgery are aimed at the relief of pain. Often there comes a point where ill patients no longer can balance the threat of pain against the risks of surgery with clear judgment. At this point the benefits of surgery are overwhelmingly obvious to patients, and risks recede into the distance of their awareness. Many common situations in medicine require the physician to confront this problem. In Case #25, a fourteen-year-old daughter wishes to donate a kidney to her mother. Although she has exhibited a perceptive and relatively unemotional grasp of the situation, many would doubt that a fourte-year-old child can either adequately appreciate the significance of future risks or skillfully balance risks and benefits in the present. These examples indicate how the professional must be skillful and persistent in balancing the risks against the benefits in order to enable the patient to decide based on an appropriate appreciation of the situation.

It is sometimes argued that most patients and subjects simply cannot comprehend enough information or appreciate its relevance sufficiently for an informed consent. Franz Ingelfinger argues, for example, that "the chances are remote that the subject really understands what he has consented to,"[31] and Robert Mulford similarly argues that "the subject is ordinarily not qualified to evaluate the true risks and expected benefits."[32] This position is partially based on unwarranted presuppositions about "full" disclosure. The ideal of complete disclosure of all possibly relevant knowledge promotes such claims about the limited capacity of subjects to comprehend. But if this ideal standard is replaced by an acceptable reasonable person standard, any temptation to succumb to an Ingelfinger-Mulford form of pessimism should vanish. Because we are never fully informed, voluntary, or autonomous persons, it does not follow that we are never *adequately* informed, free, and autonomous. Apprehending one's medical situation is not substantially different from apprehending one's financial situation when consulting with a CPA, or one's legal situation when consulting with a lawyer, or even one's marital situation when consulting with a marriage counselor. The shades of understanding are manifold, but various degrees of information processing may nonetheless be adequate for an informed choice. The goal of informed consent requirements is to prevent the decisions of patients and subjects from being less informed than similarly important decisions they make in life. The goal of a "professional choice" is improper from the outset.

A further problem about comprehension is whether we ought to recognize *waivers* of informed consent. What are we to say about those individuals who choose to have less information than a "reasonable" person? At least two courts have held that "a medical doctor need not make disclosure of risks when the patient requests that he not be so informed."[33] Some persons do not want to know anything about what will be done. Indeed, some studies claim to show that over sixty percent of patients want to know virtually nothing about procedures or the risks of the procedures,[34] and other studies, as we have seen, indicate both that 86% would consent without disclosures of risk and that only about 12% use the information provided in reaching their decisions.[35] Some physicians claim that more uninformed patients defer to physicians than seek pertinent information.[36]

There are two major ways of treating such patients. First, it might be maintained that if the reasonable person standard is not met, the contemplated procedure cannot be undertaken until sufficient information has been comprehended, notwithstanding the person's autonomously expressed desire not to be informed. According to this approach, persons should be coerced, even against their autonomous wishes, into receiving undesired information. Second, a contrasting view is that when a patient or subject is sufficiently informed to know whether to want further information, and when he or she waives the right to further information, the professional should not insist upon providing further information. In this second view, the person's informed waiver is sufficient to constitute a *valid* consent to therapy or research, even if it is not an *informed* consent.

Here we face a dilemma. On the one hand, forced information is a prima facie violation of autonomy, and many circumstances can be imagined in which information waivers would be justified. For example, if a deeply committed Jehovah's Witness were to inform a doctor that he wished to have everything possible done for him, but did not want to *know* if transfusions or similar procedures would be employed, it is hard to imagine a moral argument to the conclusion that he must be told. On the other hand, to consider the second alternative, patients commonly have an inordinate trust in physicians, and the general recognition of waivers of consent in research and therapeutic settings could make patients more vulnerable to those who would use abbreviated consent procedures merely because of convenience.

There probably cannot be any general theoretical solution to this dilemma about waivers. Each case of consent and the possibility of a waiver will have to be considered in its complexity. There may, however, be procedural ways to alleviate the problem. There could be rules against allowing waivers, but provisions so that these rules could be considered prima facie duties that could be relaxed after special consideration by deliberative bodies, such as institutional review committees and hospital ethics committees. Such rules could be developed to protect patients and subjects, but if protective bodies themselves determined that the person's interest in a particular case was adequately protected by a waiver, they could allow it. This procedural solution is no mere avoidance of the problem. It would be easy to violate autonomy and to fail to live up to our responsibilities by inflexible rules that either permit or prohibit waivers. This procedural suggestion at least provides a flexible arrangement for meeting such problems. (One might wish to distinguish conditions of waivers for therapy and for research.)

A similar and related problem arises when patients or subjects reach their decisions on irrelevant or misleading grounds, even though adequately informed. Such persons comprehend the relevant information but reach their decision because of emotional, irrational, or false views. For example, a person might falsely and irrationally believe that a doctor will not fill out his insurance forms unless he consents to a procedure the doctor has suggested; and he might persist in this belief even when informed of its falsity. Similarly, a sufficiently informed psychiatric patient capable of consent might consent to involvement in nonpsychiatric, nontherapeutic research under the false assumption that it is therapeutic. In these cases the adequate information that is both disclosed and apprehended plays no role in the decision to be involved in the research or to accept the therapy. The question then arises whether autonomous patients and subjects should be made to give up their false beliefs and irrational tendencies in order that they may reach a more informed decision.

In a general statement about the coercion of information, H. Tristram Engelhardt has argued that "One cannot try (nor should one) to force subjects who can be rational free agents to use that rationality and freedom to its fullest,"[37] because informed consent only entails that patients and subjects make their *own* free and reasoned assessments. Robert Veatch has similarly argued that where subjects specifically object to further information or persuasion, the information should not be imposed.[38] These statements do not imply that we should never coerce patients or subjects to further information. When a patient's or subject's autonomy is limited by his or her ignorance, as in the case of a false belief a patient refuses to surrender, it may be legitimate to promote autonomy by attempting to impose the information. In this respect these cases resemble the waiver cases just discussed. In both, unsatisfactory comprehension generates the problem, and, as with the waiver cases, the best general solution is probably a procedural one.

It might be argued that these conclusions about comprehension hold for therapeutic settings but do not fit research settings where persons would be involved in nontherapeutic research. In the therapeutic environment the physician acts to the end of a patient's best interests, but in research settings the subject serves as a means to the investigator's ends. Nonetheless, we believe this distinction between the two settings is largely irrelevant to problems of deficient apprehension. Factors such as the amount of risk involved and the person's identification with the purposes of research could make a decisive difference as to whether he or she should be involved, quite independent of whether it is a clinical or a research setting. Moreover, by participating in research, subjects might derive certain benefits that they could appreciate and that would be important to them, even though they consented on what the "reasonable person" would judge to be irrelevant grounds.

Finally, it deserves notice that, relative to the other elements of informed consent, there is substantial empirical literature on comprehension. The data reported in this literature point tentatively to the conclusion that consents to medical treatment or research display quite limited actual comprehension and limited ability to see data objectively. Evidence for this conclusion comes principally from three kinds of investigations—(1) studies of the readability of actual consent forms, (2) studies that use recognition tests or recall methods to assess patient knowledge, and (3) studies of how variation in the way information is presented affects choices between alternative therapies. Unfortunately, this somewhat erratic literature has severe methodological problems when applied to comprehension in a consent setting.[39]

Voluntariness

The nature of voluntariness

The primary meaning of "voluntariness" is exercising choice free of coercion or other forms of controlling influence by other persons. Voluntariness thus refs to the ability to choose one's goals, and to be able to choose among several goals if a wide choice is offered, without controlling constraints presented by other persons or institutions. The mere absence of controlling influences may not indicate that a patient or subject is acting voluntarily. On some occasions a person may have to be provided with the means to realize a chosen end, as well as be given freedom of choice. For example, information might have to be provided. It makes no sense to say that a person voluntarily chooses not to have therapy X and chooses instead to have therapy Y when only Y has been mentioned or made available and the person is ignorant of X. In contexts of decisionmaking by patients, voluntariness is optimal when there is adequate disclosure, adequate comprehension, and a patient capable of choice who in fact chooses a specific action. Disclosure, comprehension, and influence are in fact causally connected, because influence through information control directly affects freedom of choice. The voluntariness of a choice is equally affected by the information a person possesses, by the person's state of mind, and by the operative influences in a situation.[40]

How shall we analyze the concept of an "influence"? Coercion, which occurs when one person intentionally uses an actual threat of harm or force to influence another, is the most frequently mentioned form of controlling influence. However, coercion does not cover all forms of controlling influence; it is at one end of a continuum of influence and entirely compromises autonomy. At the other end of the continuum are weak forms of influence such as rational persuasion. Other points on the continuum include indoctrination, manipulation, seduction, and the like.[41] As this continuum indicates, voluntariness admits of degrees. Rarely, if ever, are we entirely free from various pressures, and "*fully* voluntary choice" is clearly an ideal.

Noncontrolling influences must also be distinguished from controlling influences. We almost always make decisions in a context of competing wants, needs, familial interests, legal obligations, persuasive arguments, and the like. Many inducements will thus be influential but not controlling— though no *sharp* boundary can be drawn in many cases between controlling and noncontrolling influences. What we most need to know about an influence is the point at which it ceases to be resistible, and becomes obstructive or irresistible for a substantially autonomous agent. Rational persuasion will generally pass the test of a noncontrolling influence, and some nonrational techniques such as emotion-laden appeals to family dependencies may also pass. In each case the powers of an individual patient or subject must be assessed, because resistibility to influence varies significantly from person to person. Some persons are careless and thoughtless, others thorough and reflective. The health professional thus should consider the particular patient's capacities for autonomous choice and resistance to influence, not the yardstick of the reasonable person. Again we see the moral importance of using a subjective standard rather than an objective reasonable person standard in communicating with patients and subjects.

The duty to abstain from controlling influence

A patient's choice can often be *adequately* voluntary, and this must be our goal in biomedicine. Thus patients and subjects must not be subjected to controlling influences that render a decision substantially nonvoluntary. By this criterion, the subject or patient must not be deceived, or forced, or manipulated. For example, if admission to a hospital of persons needing care is made contingent upon enrollment in a research protocol unrelated to their illness, a controlling influence has been exerted, and any "consent" is thereby invalidated. By contrast, if the only temptation inviting enrollment in a nontherapeutic research project is time off from one's work at no extra pay for the duration of the experiment, the influence is not inappropriate.

The grounds for claiming that an influence is not only *controlling* but also *unjustifiable* seem clear in the abstract, but dark in many concrete cases. By depriving a person of voluntariness, we infringe the person's autonomy. In Case #4, a patient's drug (Talwin) was modified without his knowledge after he had refused to allow the modification. This is a case of nondisclosure where the intent is to control choice and to manipulate the patient to the best medical outcome. This case exhibits a rather clear infringement of the patient's autonomy. However, such control may not be unjustifiable. The physicians in this case appealed to maximal benefit for the patient as the justification for their action, a beneficence-based justification. Their controlling influence is thus conceivably a justified influence.

These distinctions have significant bearing on practical contexts of informed consent. In clinical medicine patients are often abnormally weak, dependent, and surrender-prone. Influences that might ordinarily be resisted become controlling. A patient may be influenced to a conclusion even though the health professional has no intention of orchestrating the outcome. Compliance may be induced by influencing or contributing to the desperation, anxiety, boredom, hope, or other human emotions pervasive in the lives of patients. Even the hope of more attention and better care can be a significant factor for a bedridden individual. Thus, what a health professional regards as an attempt at rational persuasion may in fact irrationally persuade or manipulate by tearing at the patient's vulnerabilities. One of the most difficult determinations to make is when a person desperately needing an authority *willingly* submits to that authority and when the authority figure uses that commanding position for purposes of control. We are not implying that health professionals *do* routinely manipulate or exploit the patient's vulnerabilities, but only that patients are vulnerable to such influence.

Similar problems are also present in research. In Case #27 hepatitis research was being done on mentally retarded children in New York. An allegation surrounding this case has been that the parents were "coerced" into "volunteering" their children. Allegedly they were coerced, or, at least unjustifiably influenced, because there was a waiting list for admission to the school and parents were told that their children could be immediately admitted if they were "volunteered" for the hepatitis study. If this allegation is historically accurate, which is still in doubt, it would be a clear case of a controlling influence. However, there is nothing about admission to institutions or about institutions themselves that makes controlling influence inevitable. Even in generally coercive environments, such as prisons, it is sometimes possible that informed consent to medical and research procedures can occur. It may be especially important to insure that the right of autonomous determination is preserved in such institutions, since there will be a natural presumption that voluntary action is impossible, as in the case of research with prisoners. Yet in environments where many options are foreclosed, not all options need be so. There is no reason why prisoners could not validly consent to medical research if coercive tactics were not specifically involved, and if undue inducements, such as large amounts of money, were not allowed. Even a highly coercive environment does not by itself render a person incompetent or his or her choices involuntary. The person *may* be vulnerable and *may* act involuntarily, but this is a matter for careful investigation in each individual case.[42]

Refusal of treatment

The problem of informed consent in the broadest sense is the problem of informed decisionmaking. Patients and subjects with the capacity to consent may refuse instead, and we are equally concerned that these refusals be competent, informed, and voluntary. Although refusals can occur in non-life-threatening circumstances, the major controversies emerge from refusals of medical therapy necessary to sustain life. Examples include refusals to allow a blood transfusion, an amputation, or continued kidney dialysis. While patients have refused treatments such as blood transfusions because of their religious convictions, the ethical issues are broader than freedom of religious conscience. The rights of autonomy and privacy are often invoked to justify refusals for nonreligious and even highly esoteric reasons. There are also problems of second-party refusal in the case of children and certain classes of incompetent patients, which we treat in the chapter on non-maleficence. In this section we concentrate on refusals by competent adult patients, where the critical question is, "What are the implications and limits of the principle of autonomy?"

The "Patient's Bill of Rights" (See Appendix II) holds that "the patient has the right to refuse treatment to the extent permitted by law and to be informed of the medical consequences of his action." This right of refusal cannot be specified without a discussion of the law because the question of justified legal compulsion is at the center of the debate. However, we still must ask whether the law is morally sound (e.g., whether it adequately expresses the principle of autonomy). Despite all the general standards in statutory law, common law, constitutional law, and regulatory law applicable to questions of refusal, the core issue is moral.

A number of precedent legal cases suggest that the patient's informed refusal should be decisive. In *Erickson* v. *Dilgard*[43] a patient with intestinal bleeding deliberately refused on religious grounds a transfusion necessary for continued life. The court upheld the patient's decision by appealing to the protection of individual choice. Similarly, in *In re Estate of Brooks,*[44] it was held that free religious exercise is constitutionally sufficient to prevent physicians from compelling the therapy if there is a competent refusal, even when it is known by both patient and physician that death will ensue. In the first case, bodily *self-determination* was regarded as an inviolable right, while in the second, *free exercise of religion* was cited as the basic right. But patient refusal was decisive in both.[45] While the law is at present tentative and uncertain in this area, courts appear to be moving in the direction of greater latitude of patient choice, unless there is questionable competence or some compelling state interest outweighs the patient's autonomy.

By examining some cases, we can both illustrate the complexities involved and indicate some conditions under which patient choice may justifiably be restricted. In Case #13, a Jehovah's Witness refused to authorize blood transfusions for herself and her newborn daughter, and her husband also refused to authorize blood transfusions for either his wife or daughter. The judge declined to order transfusions for the woman, but did not accept the parents' proxy (second-party) refusal of therapy for the newborn daughter. In effect, he accepted a first-party refusal, but drew the line at that point and would not accept a second-party refusal for the incompetent child. As we have seen, the doctrine of informed consent is applied differently to competent and incompetent parties because of considerations of autonomy and nonmaleficence: Informed consent functions to protect the right of autonomous choice for competents but functions to protect incompetents from harm. This moral position perhaps underlies the judge's legal decision in this case.

In some cases a patient's refusal of livesaving therapy may impose unjustified burdens on or bring excessive harm to others. The *Georgetown College* case (#14) is an oft-cited example of a case where the seriousness of the consequences to others might override a patient's autonomous wishes. The court used the following reason, among others, to justify forcing a transfusion on an unwilling patient: "The patient, 25 years old, was the mother of a seven-month-old child. . . . The patient had a responsibility to the community to care for her infant. Thus, the people had an interest in preserving the life of this mother."[46]

This justification is certainly challengeable, but it captures one form of the "compelling interests" (here, protection from harms caused by others) that the state must assert in the law in order to outweigh an individual's fundamental interest (here, privacy or freedom of religion). In line with this theory, it has been argued that the child, even more than the community, is seriously damaged by the mother's decision, and thus that the state should not allow the patient to abandon her child.[47] While we are uncertain of the actual status of obligations in this dilemmatic case, the court's findings are dubious. The woman merely asserts a liberty parallel to that asserted in placing a child for adoption. The case nonetheless presents considerations of social need and individual rights that might be sufficient to override patient choice.[48]

It is easy to imagine circumstances in which a refusal of treatment would seriously harm another. The following line of argument might then be invoked: A refusal of treatment in life-threatening circumstances may be overridden if and only if nontreatment would produce or would be reasonably expected to produce significant harm to others or to violate the rights of others. This formulation says little more than that in circumstances of refusal, as elsewhere in law and morals, interests and rights must be balanced. It recognizes that refusals of treatment can violate rights or cause harms. Thus, one cannot safely pronounce in advance that rights of autonomous refusal can never be justifiably limited.

Other limitations of any unqualified endorsement of the patient's right to autonomous refusal must also be appreciated. First, the approach does not consider hard cases of second-party refusals, where someone other than the patient must accept the burden of the decision—e.g., cases where a family member consents to the withholding or cessation of treatment for someone in a vegetative state. (See Chapter 4.) Second, almost all court cases and many common situations in hospitals involve patients of questionable autonomy and thus of questionable capacity to consent. The conclusions we have reached do not apply to such patients. Only when there is an adequately informed refusal, as judged by our modified reasonable person standard, must a patient's decision be fully respected. In cases of doubtful competence, we should err on the side of preserving life. Of course, if persons are acting irresponsibly and thereby harming another person (usually a dependent), their decisions may be overridden, even if informed and voluntary.

Autonomous suicide

Refusal of therapy in life-threatening circumstances is not the only way to terminate one's life. Many seriously ill patients end their lives by carefully planned suicides. Not all such suicides are autonomous, but some are, and in this section we critically evaluate certain views about the morality of autonomous suicide.

In the history of philosophy and theology there is a rich literature on the morality of suicide. In addition, certain contemporary currents have revived interest in this topic. First, as with refusal of treatment cases, biomedical technology has made it possible for seriously ill and injured persons to prolong their lives beyond the point at which, in former times, they would have died. The suicide rate is substantial in some of these populations, and many people have come to think that some suicides can be justified and even justifiably assisted. Slogans such as "the right to die" and "death with dignity" have grown up around such cases. Second, while criminal laws prohibiting suicide have been repealed in most jurisdictions in the United States, repeal is still under debate in others. This lively debate focuses on the rightness and wrongness of taking one's own life. However, before we can assess this moral controversy, it is necessary to clarify the notion of "suicide" itself.

The definition of suicide

Ordinarily a death would be considered a suicide if it is an intentionally caused self-destruction and is not forced by the action of another person. However, the refusal of treatment cases that we have just studied make it difficult to accept such a simple definition. When persons suffer from a terminal illness or mortal injury and intentionally allow their own deaths to occur, we are reluctant to call the act "suicide." But if a patient with a terminal illness takes his or her life by an active means, such as a revolver, we generally do classify the act as a suicide. The more we have patent cases of actions that intentionally and actively cause one's own death, the more we are likely to classify them as suicide; but the more the context is one of merely allowing one's own death when a fatal condition is present, the less inclined we are to call the act a suicide. For example, if a seriously but not mortally wounded burn patient takes a weapon in hand and intentionally brings about his death, it is a suicide. But if a seriously burned patient is suffering terribly from a terminal wound and refuses yet another painful tubbing or blood transfusion, we are not likely to regard the death as a suicide (see Case #12). The passive nature of the death in the second case makes us reluctant to affix the label "suicide," whereas the active character of the act in the first case renders the death a suicide.

However, our concept of suicide is not quite as clear as these examples might suggest, for suicide does not always involve active steps. For example, a patient with a terminal condition might easily avoid dying for a long time but choose instead to end life immediately by not taking cheap and painless medication. We are not sure what to say in such cases, but at least it can be explained *why* our concept of suicide leaves us in this state of uncertainty.

Terms in their ordinary meaning often contain evaluative accretions from social attitudes that render them difficult to analyze. The meaning we have located for "suicide" appears to be a premier example. Self-caused deaths are often inexplicable; they may leave the living with a deep sense of loss, guilt, or even revulsion. An emotive meaning of disapproval has therefore been incorporated into our use of "suicide." Because of this already attached disapproval, we find it hard to view acts of which we approve, or at least do not disapprove, *as* suicides. For this reason we have been led to the semantic exclusion of such actions from the realm of suicide. For example, if coercion, refusal of treatment, or sacrifice is present, we are inclined not to attach the stigma of the label "suicide," and so *generally* (but not always) exclude deaths under these conditions. Because self-caused deaths under conditions of terminal illness or altruistic actions are commonly understandable, acceptable, and perhaps even laudable, semantic exclusion of them from the realm of the suicidal is tempting and is a *fait accompli* in the English language. We thus, by the very logic of the term, prejudice any pending moral analysis of the action of a suicide as being right or wrong, let alone praiseworthy or blameworthy.

Because this prejudicial feature infects our ordinary understanding of "suicide," it needs to be replaced for purposes of moral thinking by a more objective, though we admit *stipulative*, meaning. It will not be easy to employ a standard term in a nonstandard way in the discussions that follow, but this usage will enhance our investigations of the morality and autonomy of suicide. We propose, then, that suicide occurs if and only if one intentionally terminates one's own life—no matter what the conditions or precise nature of the intention or the causal route to death. If an autonomous refusal of treatment is made with the intention to terminate one's life, then it would be suicide. Death through an *act* of refusal is no mere *passive* natural death. There are problems about what the person's precise intention must be; but these problems plague virtually all definitions of suicide and cannot be further examined here.[49]

The morality of suicide

How are we to determine whether a particular act of suicide is or is not morally acceptable? As with other moral issues, this question should be answered by reference to those moral principles that permit us to take a consistent position on the issues. We believe that three moral considerations are directly relevant to discussions of suicide.

1. The first of these considerations derives from *the principle of autonomy* itself. As we have seen, to show a lack of respect for an autonomous agent is either to show disrespect for that person's deliberate choices or to deny that person the freedom to act on those choices. It would, therefore, show disrespect to deny autonomous persons the right to commit suicide if, in their considered judgment, they should do so. (If someone else is harmed by the action this would constitute moral grounds for opposing it.)

2. A second consideration often appealed to in discussions of suicide is the *sanctity of human life*. According to this criterion, human life has an intrinsic value that is irrevocably destroyed by suicide. Therefore, suicide is an act of killing that is (prima facie, at least) morally wrong. This action-guide can be qualified in a variety of ways—for example, by restricting it to the *direct* killing of *innocent* human life. As usually construed, it is permissible to *allow* someone to die instead of attempting heroic efforts to save him or her, but it is not acceptable to *kill*, because the agent then becomes morally responsible for an active destruction of life. From this view, the act of killing is wrong neither because it produces social disutility nor because it violates autonomy. It is wrong merely because it is an intentional, active termination of human life. The sanctity-of-life consideration is thus usually taken as independent of the four principles discussed in this book, but we believe it is most plausibly derived from *the principle of nonmaleficence*. (See the discussion of the killing/letting die distinction in Chapter 4.)

There is a continuum of stronger and weaker ways of formulating this

second consideration. In the strongest formulation, it is always wrong intentionally to terminate any human life, whatever the circumstances—whether
in capital punishment, in war, in self-defense, in abortion, or in suicide. A
markedly weak version is that the intrinsic value of life itself is always a
consideration, but also merely a consideration, and not necessarily the most
important or overriding one. This formulation is weak because any quality-
of-life consideration, for example, could compete with the principle in the
case of suicide.

Few people would now defend either the strongest or the weakest versions
of this principle. A middle position—perhaps the dominant one in the
literature—is that killing violates the principle of nonmaleficence and so is
prima facie wrong. Killing may be permissible if necessary to save the life of
other innocent persons, or if necessary to preserve a morally worthy society,
or if some similarly serious and fundamental moral reason justifies the
action.[50]

3. The final consideration relevant to discussing the morality of suicide is
the principle of utility, which we shall construe in Chapter 5 as part of *the
principle of beneficence*. As we have seen, utility requires that one examine
the consequences of actions to determine the impact on the interests and
welfare of all concerned. The interests of the person contemplating suicide,
the interests of dependents, the interests of relatives, and perhaps the interests
of others must all be considered in the calculation of positive values and
disvalues. The facts that people love the person contemplating suicide and
that they value the person's contribution to the community are relevant to a
moral assessment of the contemplated action. In many cases a utilitarian
calculation would show that the disvalue of the suicide, including grief, guilt,
and deprivation, would be greater than the value to be gained. Hence the
principle of utility would dictate that an act of suicide is unjustified in these
cases.

However, there are cases where the consequences would not automatically
fall on the side of disvalue. For example, imagine someone suffering from
both brain cancer and apparently untreatable tic douloureux (an excruci-
atingly painful condition of the trigeminal nerve). Suppose further that this
person has neither dependents nor debts, that the suffering of this person's
family has been protracted, and that everyone concerned believes death
would be a merciful release from agony. An intentional overdose taken by
the person could satisfy the utilitarian demand that the greatest possible
amount of value or at least the smallest possible amount of disvalue be
brought about by the person's action. (Case #5 presents a more complicated

case in which a suicidal man may take his life irrationally once he learns of an inoperable carcinoma.)

Under the assumption that each of the above three moral considerations is acceptable, each should be regarded as asserting a prima facie duty, in some cases binding a person contemplating suicide and in other cases affecting those who might intervene to prevent suicides. As discussed in Chapter 2, prima facie duties are more than rules of thumb, because they are always binding from the moral point of view unless in conflict with stronger duties. In the present context, this approach to morality may be applied as follows: To the extent the principle of autonomy or one of the other two general considerations mentioned in this section is relevant, and does not conflict with other principles, it determines our duty. Thus, if a suicide were genuinely autonomous and there were no powerful utilitarian reasons or reasons of nonmaleficence standing in the way, then we ought to allow the person to commit suicide. Otherwise we would violate the person's autonomy.

A ready example of the use of prima facie reasoning about suicide is found in a classic essay on the subject, by the eighteenth-century philosopher David Hume.[51] In this essay he combined the principle of autonomy with the principle of utility to provide a powerful justification of certain types of suicide—though by no means did Hume draw the radical conclusion that all suicides can be justified by these two principles. His strategy was to show that the more one's life is plagued by suffering, the more justifiable is suicide. In the end he advanced the largely utilitarian thesis that if the value of relieving one's misery by taking one's own life is greater than the value to the community of one's continued existence, then suicide is justified.

Hume's claim might be applied in biomedical contexts by reference again to the desperate circumstances that often surround refusal-of-treatment cases. If a person's life is utterly miserable and pain management is inefficacious while the person's dignity and ability to relate to others are slipping away, then autonomous suicide is not morally improper and should not be an object of moral condemnation. Whether it would be justified to encourage suicide or to assist a person in committing suicide presents further questions.

Case #11 features a suicide attempt by a 32-year-old lawyer with Huntington's chorea, a painful neurological disorder that becomes progressively worse over a several-year period and is uniformly fatal. His mother had a horrible death from the same (autosomal dominant) disorder, and he has often said that he would prefer to die than to live longer and die like his mother. He has thought seriously about the disorder and about his life circumstance. After a psychiatrist refuses to help him commit suicide, he attempts to take his life, leaving a note of explanation to his wife and child. It is reasonably clear that this case involves an *autonomous* suicide, but whether it is *justified* requires a difficult balancing of the considerations discussed above.

Our general analysis of the morality of suicide leads to the conclusion that there are good reasons for suicide in some circumstances, but that suicidal action may be morally wrong and even cowardly in other circumstances. In some cases one may have moral obligations not to commit suicide, while in other cases one may have a right or even an obligation to commit suicide (the last situation being extremely rare). Even if persons sometimes have obligations not to commit suicide, it does not follow that when all interests are considered the obligation will always be to abstain from suicide. Moreover, weak duties are sometimes overridden not only by stronger *moral* duties but also by stronger *prudential* interests. Even though a daughter might beg her terminally ill father to stay alive for his last remaining month, his agony may nonetheless be sufficient to override the daughter's interest in his remaining alive.

At the same time, in determining whether to commit suicide, it is easy to exaggerate the direness of one's situation. One's desires, sufferings, and hopes in the present moment tend to overwhelm consideration of what one's desires, sufferings, and joys may be at future times. The young lawyer (in Case #11) with Huntington's chorea may well be overreacting to the horrors of his mother's death. His anxiety, heavy drinking, and intermittent depression may lead him to undervalue the possibilities, at least for the next few years. In the case of illness that leads to certain death we have one of the strongest justifications of suicide, but an optimistic and objective view about life's possibilities is likely to be deeply inhibited by such an illness. Indeed, depression is likely to increase steadily. Even if no terminal illness is present it is easy to miscalculate by substituting present feelings for rational calculations of future possibilities. It is thus of the utmost importance to frame a realistic appraisal of the circumstances and the actual state of mind of persons who perform "autonomous" suicide. Ideally, a person contemplating suicide would take account of all relevant variables and future possibilities, but this approach will not always be taken and our obligations to prevent suicide will always be difficult because of uncertainty surrounding the quality of autonomy.

In any final assessment of an act of suicide that one believes to be wrong, it is also important to consider different judgments of excusability that might be reached. We might say that a suicide is seriously mistaken, and even wrong, but not blameworthy; or, alternatively, we might say that the suicide is both morally blameworthy and morally wrong. The first alternative derives from the moral view that some wrong suicides may be excused.[52] We can excuse some suicides if they act on false information, if they are temporarily of unsound mind, or if depression or some other psychological state overwhelms a person of an ordinarily even disposition. Perhaps the most compelling cases are those in which a person acts altruistically but on false information in committing suicide. For example, a person might falsely believe that he or she has a disease that will produce prolonged agony and leave his or her family in financial ruin. We can sometimes say not only that such a person acted wrongly though excusably, but even that the person acted *commendably* (though wrongly). Many who would absolutely condemn suicide fail to distinguish the objective wrongness of an action from the moral excusability and even praiseworthiness of that same action. One virtue of our analysis of both suicide and the principle of autonomy is that it permits us to make these important distinctions and to adjust our moral judgments about suicide accordingly.

Problems of suicide intervention

It follows from the discussion above that autonomous persons have a *right* to commit suicide—a prima facie right entailed by the principle of autonomy. Thus, if persons act autonomously and do not seriously affect the interests of others, we ought not to intervene. Yet we certainly do not always act as if the suicide has such a right, for we often do intervene to prevent suicide. In days past, for example, it was not uncommon for several persons to place themselves at risk of death in order to prevent a person from reclining on subway tracks in the path of an oncoming train. It is easy to understand why such interventions occur, as acts of humanity; and we may believe that we are justified in intervening in the lives of such individuals. But if they have a *right* to commit suicide, are we really justified?

In the case of almost any other similarly intrusive action, the person interfered with could correctly argue that his or her autonomy had been violated by the intervention. For example, physicians can be successfully sued for malpractice if they intervene in certain unauthorized ways in the life of a patient. Yet in the case of potential suicide, many believe that we have obligations to suicidal persons, even if they act autonomously. These obligations are thought to necessitate prevention of suicide by almost any means, including direct intervention. But can we morally justify this conviction that intervention in the name of saving a life is better than nonintervention in the name of autonomy?

One account of our obligations, based on the principle of autonomy, is offered by Glanville Williams:

If one suddenly comes upon another person attempting suicide, the natural and humane thing to do is to try to stop him, for the purpose of ascertaining the cause of his distress and attempting to remedy it, or else of attempting moral dissuasion if it seems that the act of suicide shows lack of consideration for others, or else again from the purpose of trying to persuade him to accept psychiatric help if this seems to be called for. Whatever the strict law may be (and authority is totally lacking), no one who intervened for such reasons would thereby be in danger of suffering a punitive judgment. But nothing longer than a temporary restraint could be defended. I would gravely doubt whether a suicide attempt should be a factor leading to a diagnosis of psychosis or to compulsory admission to a hospital. Psychiatrists are too ready to assume that an attempt to commit suicide is the act of a mentally sick person.[53]

Yet many do not agree with Williams's estimate, chiefly for two reasons. First, failure to intervene indicates a lack of concern about others and a diminished sense of moral responsibility in a community. Attempts to save a person from suicide in subways are now comparatively rare, and this seems to indicate how times have changed in large cities—and how undesirable the change has been. Second, many believe that most suicides are mentally ill or at least seriously disturbed, and therefore are not capable of autonomous action. Notoriously, suicidal persons are often under the strain of temporary crises, under the influence of drugs or alcohol, beset with considerable ambivalence, or simply wish to reduce or interrupt anxiety, while not wishing to die. Case #5 presents a psychiatric patient with typical problems of depression and irrational reactions to disturbing information.

Many psychiatric and legal authorities can be cited in support of the belief that suicides are almost always the result of maladaptive attitudes needing therapeutic attention. Their underlying conviction is that the suicidal person suffers from some form of disease or irrational drive toward self-caused death, and that it is the business of medicine or behavioral therapy to cure the illness and prevent the patient's self-destruction. Freudians even argue that suicide is created by a breakdown of ego defenses and a release of destructive forces. These forces are said to reflect the ambivalent relationship to love objects with whom a person strongly identifies. While no single theory presently suffices for understanding the motivation to suicide, many such accounts characterize suicide as substantially nonvoluntary and therefore as nonautonomous. Also, other suicidal persons who are not ill nonetheless may not be in a position to act autonomously, because they are immature, are unable to process information or deliberate, have false or quite unrealistic beliefs, or are in a vulnerable position in which they might be manipulated by others.[54]

Virtually everyone agrees that nonautonomous suicidal actions may be justifiably prevented. Furthermore, there are often good reasons to intervene temporarily to determine the competence and the actual wishes of persons attempting suicide. For example, in the aforementioned case of Huntington's chorea (#11), John K. attempted to commit suicide, and was found unconscious by his wife, who had him taken to the emergency room. Both his wife and the emergency room staff had good reasons to try to save him in order to determine whether his actions were autonomous. Even if there is widespread agreement about justifiably preventing nonautonomous suicides and temporarily intervening to determine the competence and wishes of persons attempting suicide, there is controversy about whether autonomous suicides may be justifiably prevented when they do not harm others. This question is properly situated under the topic of paternalism, which will be treated in Chapter 5. We shall, therefore, defer further discussion of these issues until certain analyses essential to any adequate resolution have been considered.

Conclusion

The intimate connection between autonomy and informed decisionmaking unifies the four sections of this chapter. Although we have justified the obligation to obtain informed consent and to respect informed refusals by the principle of autonomy, several issues about the proper limits of the principle remain unsettled. Important issues concern the exact demands the principle makes in decisionmaking contexts in biomedicine, and how the principle is connected to truthfulness and individual rights, such as the rights of confidentiality and privacy. Several of these issues will be treated later in this volume, especially in Chapter 7.

We shall also witness several conflicts between the principle of autonomy and the three moral principles featured in the next three chapters. The argument in these chapters shows how entrenched and difficult these conflicts can be in biomedicine, and how respect for autonomy requires a use of discretion in the balancing process. Many authors in biomedical ethics tend to assume that if a person is acting autonomously, then the person's choices morally ought not be overridden by such considerations as beneficence and proper care. We make no such assumption. In many cases in clinical settings the weight of autonomy is minimal, while the weight of nonmaleficence or beneficence is maximal. Similarly in public policy contexts, the demands of justice can outweigh those of respect for autonomy. There also are occasions on which decisions must be reached about substantially but not wholly nonautonomous patients. As we discussed briefly in treating suicide, one form of beneficent treatment for such patients is to intervene directly to protect them against harms resulting from their illness, immaturity, psychological incapacitation, and the like. These might be medical interventions, coercive institutionalizations, or some other method of prevention. To the extent these actions can be justified, the justification will be found in beneficence or nonmaleficence—the principles now to be explored in Chapters 4 and 5.

Notes

1. Mill, *Utilitarianism, On Liberty, and Essay on Mill,* ed. with an Introduction by Mary Warnock (New York: New American Library, 1974), pp. 136–38, 184–89.
2. Cf. Robert Paul Wolff, *In Defense of Anarchism* (New York: Harper and Row, 1970). See also Wolff's even stronger claims in his article "On Violence," *Journal of Philosophy* 66 (October 2, 1969).
3. Wolff, *In Defense of Anarchism,* pp. 4–6, 13f. In "On Violence" (p. 608), Wolff maintains that "obedience *is* heteronymy [sic]. The autonomous man is *of necessity* an anarchist" (our italics). We can only understand this necessity as logical necessity.
4. These reflections owe much to Gerald Dworkin, "Moral Autonomy," in *Morals, Science, and Sociality,* eds. H. Tristram Engelhardt, Jr. and Daniel Callahan (Hastings-on-Hudson, N.Y.: The Hastings Center, 1978), pp. 156–71.
5. "Informed Consent in Catastrophic Disease and Treatment," *University of Pennsylvania Law Review* 123 (December 1974): 364–76.
6. Cf. Charles Fried, *Medical Experimentation* (New York: American Elsevier, 1974), pp. 18ff.
7. Robert M. Veatch, "Three Theories of Informed Consent: Philosophical Foundations and Policy Implications," in National Commission for the Protection of Human Subjects of Biomedical and Behavioral Research, *Appendix to the Belmont Report: Ethical Guidelines for the Protection of Human Subjects of Research,* Volume 1 (Washington: DHEW Publication No. (OS) 78–0013, 1978).
8. *Schloendorff* v. *Society of New York Hospitals,* 211 N.Y. 125, 127, 129; 105 N.E. 92, 93 (1914).
9. *Natanson* v. *Kline,* 186 Kan. 393, 350 P.2d 1093 (1960), rehearing denied, 187 Kan. 186, 354 P.2d 670 (1960).
10. See Daniel Wikler, "Paternalism and the Mildly Retarded," *Philosophy and Public Affairs* 8 (Summer 1979): 377–92.
11. We are indebted to Donald Bersoff for this tripartite approach.
12. Jeffrie Murphy, "Incompetence and Paternalism," *Archiv für Rechts-und-Sozialphilosophie* 50 (1974): 465–86.
13. "Informed Consent and the Dying Patient," *Yale Law Journal* 83 (1974): 1637. Much the same point is made in *Canterbury* v. *Spence,* 464 F.2d 772 (1972), where the standards operative in the biomedical professions are analyzed as of two types: (1) good medical practice standards, and (2) what a reasonable practitioner would disclose under the circumstances.

14. *Wilkinson* v. *Vesey*, 295 A.2d 676, p. 688 (1972).
15. *Cobbs* v. *Grant*, 502 P.2d 1 (1972).
16. *Canterbury* v. *Spence*, 464 F.2d 772 (1972).
17. *Berkey* v. *Anderson*, 82 Cal. Reporter 67.
18. *Canterbury* v. *Spence*, 464 F.2d 772 (1972).
19. Ruth R. Faden, "Disclosure and Informed Consent: Does It Matter How We Tell It?" *Health Education Monographs* 5 (1977): 198–215; Ruth R. Faden and Tom L. Beauchamp, "Decision-Making and Informed Consent: A Study of the Impact of Disclosed Information," *Social Indicators Research* 7 (1980): 313–36; and, for an extension, Ruth R. Faden, et al., "Disclosure of Information to Patients in Medical Care," *Medical Care* 19 (July 1981): 718–33.
20. C. H. Fellner and J. R. Marshall, "Kidney Donors—The Myth of Informed Consent," *American Journal of Psychiatry* 126 (1970): 1245, and "Twelve Kidney Donors," *Journal of the American Medical Association* 206 (December 16, 1968): 2703–7.
21. See Alan Meisel and Loren Roth, "What We Do and Do Not Know About Informed Consent," *Journal of the American Medical Association* 246 (November 27, 1981): 2475.
22. Gerald T. Roling, et al., "An Appraisal of Patients' Reactions to 'Informed Consent'," *Gastrointestinal Endoscopy* 24 (1977): 69–70.
23. For a fuller description pertinent to clinical medicine, including a survey of recent court cases, see Leslie J. Miller, "Informed Consent: II," *Journal of the American Medical Association* 244 (November 21, 1980): 2348–49.
24. Jay Katz, "Informed Consent—A Fairy Tale?: Law's Vision," *University of Pittsburgh Law Review* 39 (Winter 1977): 138 (see also p. 150); and "Disclosure and Consent in Psychiatric Practice: Mission Impossible?" in *Law and Ethics in the Practice of Psychiatry*, ed. Charles Hofling (New York: Brunner-Mazel, Inc., 1981), p. 93. Katz is quoting the words of the court in *Salgo* v. *Stanford University Board of Trustees*, 154 Cal. App.2d 560 (1957).
25. See Thomas C. Chalmers, "The Ethics of Randomization as a Decision-Making Technique and the Problem of Informed Consent," as reprinted in *Contemporary Issues in Bioethics*, 2nd ed., eds. Tom L. Beauchamp and LeRoy Walters (Belmont, Calif.: Wadsworth Publishing Co., 1982), pp. 538–41.
26. See Fried, *Medical Experimentation*, pp. 25–36.
27. *Ethical Principles in the Conduct of Research with Human Participants* (Washington: American Psychological Association, 1973), p. 2, Principle 8.
28. Stanley Milgram, "Behavioral Study of Obedience," *Journal of Abnormal Psychology* 67 (1963): 371–78; "Some Conditions of Obedience and Disobedience to Authority," *Human Relations* 18 (1965): 57–76; *Obedience to Authority* (New York: Harper & Row, 1974). Milgram provides some evidence to show that his subjects did not resent involvement in the research.
29. Norberto Valenti and Clara di Meglio, *Sex and the Confessional* (New York: Stein and Day, 1974).
30. A sensible approach to several problems of comprehension other than those mentioned here is found in Alan W. Cross and Larry R. Churchill, "Ethical and Cultural Dimensions of Informed Consent," *Annals of Internal Medicine* 96 (1982): 110–13.

31. Franz J. Ingelfinger, "Informed (But Uneducated) Consent," *New England Journal of Medicine* 287 (August 31, 1972): 455–56, and "Arrogance," *New England Journal of Medicine* 303 (1980): 1507–11.
32. Robert D. Mulford, "Experimentation on Human Beings," *Stanford Law Review* 20 (November 1967): 106.
33. *Cobbs* v. *Grant*, 502 P.2d 1, p. 12 (Case #8 in the Appendix) and *Sard* v. *Hardy*, 379 A.2d, p. 1022.
34. Cf. Ralph J. Alfidi, "Controversy, Alternatives, and Decisions in Complying with the Legal Doctrine of Informed Consent," *Radiology* 114 (January 1975).
35. Cross and Churchill, "Ethical and Cultural Dimensions of Informed Consent," pp. 111–12.
36. See the articles mentioned in note 19 above.
37. "Basic Ethical Principles in the Conduct of Biomedical and Behavioral Research Involving Human Subjects," in National Commission for the Protection of Human Subjects of Biomedical and Behavioral Research, *Appendix to the Belmont Report*, Volume I (see note 7 above).
38. Veatch, "Three Theories of Informed Consent."
39. On these problems, again see Alan Meisel and Loren Roth, "What We Do and Do Not Know About Informed Consent." Important studies are Barbara J. McNeil, et al., "On the Elicitation of Preferences for Alternative Therapies," *New England Journal of Medicine* 306 (May 27, 1982): 1259–62, and Barrie R. Cassileth, et al., "Informed Consent—Why Are Its Goals Imperfectly Realized?" *New England Journal of Medicine* 302 (April 17, 1980): 896–900.
40. This point, suitably modified for our purposes, derives from Joel Feinberg, *Social Philosophy* (Englewood Cliffs, N.J.: Prentice-Hall, 1973), p. 48.
41. See the analysis of this continuum in Donald P. Warwick and Herbert C. Kelman, "Ethical Issues in Social Intervention," in *Processes and Phenomena of Social Change*, ed. G. Zaltman (New York: John Wiley and Sons, 1973), pp. 377–419. See also Ruth Macklin, *Man, Mind, and Morality: The Ethics of Behavior Control* (Englewood Cliffs, N.J.: Prentice-Hall, 1982), pp. 12–15 and 42ff, for applications to biomedical ethics.
42. The problems mentioned in this paragraph are examined in *Kaimowitz* v. *Department of Mental Health*, Civil No. 73-19434-AW (Circuit Court, Wayne County, Mich., July 10, 1973), pp. 31–32. Summarized at 42 U.S.L.W. 3062 (July 31, 1973); see also Paul Appelbaum and Loren H. Roth, "Competency to Consent to Research: A Psychiatric Overview," *Archives of General Psychiatry* 39 (August 1982): 951–58; Jeffrie G. Murphy, "Therapy and the Problem of Autonomous Consent," *International Journal of Law and Psychiatry* 2 (1970): 415–30.
43. 244 Misc. 2d 27, 252 N.Y.S. 2d 705 (Sup. Ct. 1962).
44. 205 N.E. 2d 435, 32 Ill.2d 361 (1965).
45. These and related cases are intelligently discussed in comprehensive articles on the subject by Robert M. Byrn, "Compulsory Lifesaving Treatment for the Competent Adult," *Fordham Law Review* 44 (1975): 1–36; and John J. Paris, "Compulsory Medical and Religious Freedom: Whole Law Shall Prevail?," *University of San Francisco Law Review* 10 (1975): 1–35.
46. *Application of the President and Directors of Georgetown College, Inc.*, 331 F. 2d 1000, p. 1008 (Case #14 in the Appendix). Cf. also Byrn, *op cit.*, p. 33.

On some interpretations of the decision in *Georgetown College*, the judge's verdict was reached as much on grounds of questionable competence as on the utilitarian grounds cited above.

47. Norman Cantor, "A Patient's Decision to Decline Life-Saving Medical Treatment: Bodily Integrity Versus the Preservation of Life," *Rutgers Law Review* 26 (1973): 228, 251–54.

48. A related case involving paternalistic intervention is *John F. Kennedy Hospital v. Heston* 58 N.J. 576, 279 A.2d 670 (1971). A completely different approach is found in the appellate court decision in *In re Estate of Brooks* 32 I11.2d 361, 205 N.E. 2d 435 (1965). In the former case, see esp. pp. 584f, and in the latter esp. pp. 440f.

49. For detailed analyses of this problem and others about the definition of suicide, see Tom L. Beauchamp, "Suicide," in *Matters of Life and Death*, ed. Tom Regan (New York: Random House, 1980), pp. 67–108, esp. Part I; and M. Pabst Battin and David J. Mayo, eds., *Suicide: The Philosophical Issues* (New York: St. Martin's Press, Inc., 1980), pp. 33–68.

50. For a sensible discussion of this principle and its possible modifications when applied to the problem of suicide, see Margaret Pabst Battin, *Ethical Issues in Suicide* (Englewood Cliffs, N.J.: Prentice-Hall, 1982), Chap. 3.

51. David Hume, "Of Suicide," *Essays: Moral, Political and Literary* (Oxford: Oxford University Press, 1963), pp. 585–96.

52. In this analysis we have benefited from R. B. Brandt's useful discussion of the subject in "The Morality and Rationality of Suicide," in *A Handbook for the Study of Suicide*, ed. S. Perlin (New York: Oxford University Press, 1975), p. 124.

53. "Euthanasia," *Medico-Legal Journal* 41 (1973): 27.

54. A useful discussion of "Criteria for Rational Suicide" is found in Battin, *Ethical Issues in Suicide*, pp. 132–53. A reply to the views we advance here about rational suicide is found in Stanley Hauerwas, "Rational Suicide and Reasons for Living," in *Rights and Responsibilities in Modern Medicine*, ed. Marc D. Basson (New York: Alan R. Liss, Inc., 1981), Vol. II, pp. 185–199.

4

The Principle of Nonmaleficence

The Hippocratic Oath expresses the duty of nonmaleficence together with the duty of beneficence: "I will use treatment to help the sick according to my ability and judgment, but I will never use it *to injure or wrong them.*" Generally, the concept of nonmaleficence is associated with the maxim *primum non nocere*—"above all, or first, do no harm"—which has wide currency in discussions of the responsibilities of health care professionals, particularly physicians. The origins of this maxim, however, are obscure. Scholars have been unable to locate it in the Hippocratic corpus, and a venerable statement often confused with it—"at least, do no harm"—may not be the most accurate translation of a passage appearing in the Hippocratic corpus.[1]

A duty of nonmaleficence is recognized in most rule-deontological and rule-utilitarian theories. Many such theories accept this duty as the foundation of social morality. For example, H. L. A. Hart presents a utilitarian argument that it is possible to formulate a minimum content of moral and legal systems by examining certain characteristics of human beings. One of these characteristics is "human vulnerability," which leads Hart to argue that

The common requirements of law and morality consist for the most part not of active services to be rendered but of forebearances, which are usually formulated in negative form as prohibitions. Of these the most important for social life are those that restrict the use of violence in killing or inflicting bodily harm. The basic character of such rules may be brought out in a question: If there were not these rules what point could there be for beings such as ourselves in having rules of *any* other kind? The force of this rhetorical question rests on the fact that men are both occasionally prone to, and normally vulnerable to, bodily attack.[2]

Other formulations of the duty of nonmaleficence appear in deontological writings, such as W. D. Ross's *The Right and the Good*, where it is distinguished from the duty of beneficence, and John Rawls's *A Theory of Justice*, where it is distinguished from a duty of "mutual aid."[3] However, not all philosophers identify nonmaleficence and beneficence as distinct or separate duties. For example, William Frankena holds that the principle of beneficence includes four elements:

1. One ought not to inflict evil or harm (what is bad).
2. One ought to prevent evil or harm.
3. One ought to remove evil.
4. One ought to do or promote good.[4]

He acknowledges that the fourth element may not be a strict duty at all, and that these elements appear in a serial arrangement so that the first takes precedence over the second, the second over the third, and so forth. When these elements come into conflict, he appeals to the principle of utility as a heuristic maxim: Maximize good or minimize evil.

It is difficult to separate nonmaleficence and beneficence in this volume because many issues of biomedical ethics involve both—e.g., risk-benefit analysis, which we will discuss in the next chapter. However, to conflate them into one principle is to obscure distinctions that we make in ordinary moral discourse. Our discourse expresses the defensible conviction that certain duties not to injure others are not only distinct from but very often (not always) more stringent than duties to take positive steps to benefit others. For example, our duty not to push someone who cannot swim into deep water seems stronger than our duty to rescue someone who has accidentally strayed into deep water. It is also morally imperative for us to take substantial risks with our safety in many cases in order not to endanger others, but it is less obvious that even moderate risks are morally required to benefit others. When a philosopher tries to encompass the ideas of benefiting others and not injuring them under the single principle of beneficence, he or she will still be forced to distinguish, as Frankena does, among the various requirements of this principle that correspond roughly to what we call nonmaleficence and beneficence. Therefore, it seems to be more satisfactory to consider them as distinct prima facie principles that may on occasion come into conflict, as the notion of risk-benefit analysis suggests. In such cases of conflict we can expect nonmaleficence to be overriding on most but not all occasions.

Thus, in contrast to Frankena, we distinguish the duties of nonmaleficence and beneficence in the following way:

Nonmaleficence
1. One ought *not to inflict* evil or harm (what is bad).

Beneficence
2. One ought to *prevent* evil or harm.
3. One ought to *remove* evil.
4. One ought to *do* or *promote* good.

All three modes of beneficence involve positive acts—preventing or removing harm or promoting good—while nonmaleficence requires noninfliction of harm. There may, of course, be considerable dispute about the characterization or description of any action. For example, in Case #26, Robert McFall was dying of aplastic anemia, and his physicians thought that a bone marrow transplant from a genetically compatible donor could increase his chances of surviving one year from 25 percent to 40–60 percent. The patient's cousin, David Shimp, agreed to undergo the tests to determine his suitability as a donor, but after completing the test for tissue compatibility, he refused to undergo the test for genetic compatibility. He had changed his mind. McFall's lawyer sought to have a court compel Shimp to undergo the second test and to donate his bone marrow if the test indicated that this was feasible. Public discussion focused on whether Shimp had a duty of beneficence toward McFall, i.e., a duty to prevent or remove evil or to promote McFall's welfare. In fact, McFall's lawyer tried (unsuccessfully) another tactic. He contended that even if Shimp did not have a legal duty of beneficence to try to rescue McFall, he had a legal duty of nonmaleficence, which required that he not make McFall's situation worse. Thus, the lawyer argued, when Shimp agreed to undergo the first test, and then backed out, he created a "delay of critical proportions" and violated the duty of nonmaleficence. The judge ruled in favor of Shimp, but held that Shimp's actions were "morally indefensible."[5] (In the next chapter we will consider this case from the standpoint of beneficence.)

The concept of nonmaleficence

Exactly what does "nonmaleficence" involve? First, it must be distinguished from nonmalevolence, which describes a moral attitude or virtue rather than a moral action. Second, nonmaleficence is frequently explicated by the terms "harm" and "injury." Both terms are somewhat ambiguous. "Injury" may refer to harm, disability, or death, on the one hand, or to injustice or wrong, on the other. Ross, for example, views "not injuring others" as a synonym of "nonmaleficence" and includes under the duty of nonmaleficence a number of prohibitions of harmful activities drawn from the Decalogue, such as the rules against killing, stealing, committing adultery, and bearing false witness.[6]

Some definitions of "harm" are so broad as to include injuries to reputation, property, and liberty. For example, if the object of harm is always an *interest*, it is possible to have various interests that could be violated or damaged, such as health, property, domestic relations, and privacy.[7] Then it would be possible to distinguish trivial from serious harms by the order and magnitude of the interests involved. Some philosophers, however, use a narrow definition of harm, distinguishing physical—and mental—harms from injuries to other interests such as property and liberty. Whether the broad or the narrow definition of harm is most satisfactory is not critical for our discussion. We will concentrate on physical harms, including pain, disability, and death, without denying the importance of mental harms and other injuries. In particular, we will emphasize intending, causing, or permitting death and creating the risk of death.

Because of the wide range of harms, the principle of nonmaleficence can give rise to several specific moral rules. According to Bernard Gert, rules prohibiting harmful actions form the core of morality and include the following: "Don't kill," "Don't cause pain," "Don't disable," "Don't deprive of freedom or opportunity," and "Don't deprive of pleasure."[8] Neither the principle of nonmaleficence nor these derivative moral rules can be absolute; at most they are prima facie. For instance, it is often appropriate—with the patient's consent—to inflict harm in order to prevent worse harms, e.g., to cause pain or even disability in order to prevent death. Furthermore, it is sometimes justifiable to inflict harm on one person in order to protect another; for example, a policeman may sometimes justifiably shoot a criminal in order to protect the criminal's intended victims or hostages. But these prima facie principles and rules of nonmaleficence identify actions that always stand in need of moral justification because they inflict harm. Overriding them requires that a heavy burden of proof be met. Some philosophers such as Ross even assign priority to principles and rules that prohibit infliction of harm; although this priority will be evident in many cases of conflict, it is not absolute.[9]

In addition to debate about the weight or strength of the principle of nonmaleficence, there is debate about the range of beings protected by the principle. Consider the controversy about when human or personal life begins and when it ends. Both boundaries are in dispute in part because of what they imply about the duty of nonmaleficence. For example, if the fetus is not a human being or a person, then causing its death may not be a violation of the principle of nonmaleficence or its derivative rules. But even if a being is not a human or a person, it may still be protected in some ways by the principle of nonmaleficence. For example, it is widely agreed that researchers should not inflict certain harms on animals even to generate scientific knowledge.[10]

The duty of nonmaleficence encompasses not only actual harms, but also risks of harm. Risks vary according to the probabilities and the amounts of harm. Agents not only take risks for themselves, they also impose risks on others. For example, both risk taking and risk imposition are evident in driving an automobile. The imposition of risks of harm on others is so common that it does not usually require explicit justification unless it is out of the ordinary or unexpected. In cases of risk imposition, law and morality recognize a standard of "due care." This standard can be met when the goals sought are weighty and important enough to justify the risks—both the magnitude of harm and the probability of harm—imposed on others. Grave risks require commensurately important goals for their justification, and emergencies may justify risks that calculations of good and evil in nonemergency situations will not justify. For example, saving lives after a major accident may justify the dangers created by speeding emergency vehicles. We will return to these themes when we discuss both the weight of beneficence and risk-benefit analysis in Chapter 5.

The duty of nonmaleficence also requires that agents be thoughtful and act carefully. Not all harms or even risks of harm are intentionally produced. It is possible to violate the duty of nonmaleficence without acting maliciously and even without being aware of or intending the harm or risk of harm. The violation may involve omission as well as commission. As Eric D'Arcy emphasizes, the moral requirement to be thoughtful and careful is not separate from other moral rules and principles, such as the duty of nonmaleficence. There is no moral rule against negligence as such. Rather, negligence "applies to certain types of failure to meet moral obligations" of many different kinds,[11] and includes the failure to guard against risks of harm to others. Negligence is "conduct which falls below a standard established by the law [or morality] for the protection of others against unreasonable harm."[12]

For health care professionals, the legal and moral standards of due care include knowledge, skills, and diligence. In making services available, the physician creates the expectation that he or she will observe these standards. If his or her conduct falls below these standards, the physician acts negligently. Even if the therapeutic relationship proves to be harmful or unhelpful, the patient cannot successfully charge malpractice unless certain standards of care were not met. In *Adkins* v. *Ropp*, the Supreme Court of Indiana dealt with the claim of a patient that the physician had been negligent in removing foreign matter from the patient's eye and that, as a result, the eye became infected and blinded. The court held as follows:

When a physician and surgeon assumes to treat and care for a patient, in the absence of a special agreement, he is held in law to have impliedly contracted that he possesses the reasonable and ordinary qualifications of his profession and that he will exercise at least reasonable skill, care and diligence in his treatment of him. This implied contract on the part of the physician does not include a promise to effect a cure and negligence cannot be imputed because a cure is not effected, but he does impliedly promise that he will use due diligence and ordinary skill in his treatment of the patient so that a cure may follow such care and skill, and this degree of care and skill is required of him, not only in performing an operation or administering first treatments, but he is held to the like degree of care and skill in the necessary subsequent treatments unless he is excused from further service by the patient himself, or the physician or surgeon upon due notice refuses to further treat the case. In determining whether the physician or surgeon has exercised the degree of skill and care which the law requires, regard must be had to the advanced state of the profession at the time of treatment and in the locality in which the physician or surgeon practices.[13]

With regard to "due care," legal standards and moral standards should be identical, though of course they often are not.

What constitutes due care will, of course, vary from time to time and place to place. The practices and policies of the medical profession also in part define the applicable standards. For example, the AMA Code requires that physicians provide "competent medical service" and "continue to study, apply and advance scientific knowledge." Furthermore, in some circumstances, "a physician shall . . . obtain consultation, and use the talents of other health professionals when indicated." These dicta establish standards. Nevertheless, these standards must acknowledge the inherent fallibility of clinical judgment. Due care cannot eliminate mistakes or prevent all harms; it can only reduce the probability of error in diagnosis and treatment.

Albert Jonsen has constructed a typology of uses of the principle "do no harm" in biomedical ethics.[14] This principle is used to refer to several aspects of medicine and health care: (1) medicine as a moral enterprise requiring that practitioners develop motives and intentions to serve the well-being of their patients, (2) due care, (3) risk-benefit assessments, and (4) detriment-benefit assessments. Interpretation (1) is very general and is implicit throughout this volume, especially in our discussion of professional-patient relationships and virtues and character (Chapters 7-8); (2) has already been mentioned in this chapter and pervades a number of issues; (3) will be emphasized in the next chapter; and (4) will be a major subject of this chapter, as well as the next. The major distinction between risk-benefit analysis and detriment-benefit analysis is that the former is concerned with risks of harm, whereas the latter is concerned with the harms that occur at the time of the procedure or benefit. For example, an amputation is subject not only to risk-benefit analysis in view of possible infection but also to detriment-benefit analysis, for the loss of the limb itself is a detriment. (Since both "detriments" and "risks" are "costs," both can be viewed as subsets of cost-benefit analysis, which will be examined in Chapter 5.)

The detriment-benefit analysis figures prominently in determining when actions that cause or permit death can be viewed either as nonviolations or as justified infringements of the principle of nonmaleficence (and its derivative rules, such as the prohibition of killing). Because death is recognized as a major, if not the major, harm, causing death is at least prima facie prohibited by the principle of nonmaleficence. When there is an apparent causal connection between our actions and another's death, we have several ways to defeat a charge of moral—if not legal—failure or culpability. First, we might specify the principle of nonmaleficence to prohibit the infliction of harm on an *innocent* person and then try to show that the person we harm or kill is not innocent, perhaps because he is an unjust aggressor. Second, we might contend that the being is not yet or no longer a person or a human being; e.g., the being is a four-week-old fetus, or an individual who has been declared dead, but kept breathing only by a respirator. Third, we might argue that the death is merely a foreseen consequence of our actions; it is not direct and intentional. As an indirect and unintentional side-effect of an action aimed at a significant good, it does not fall, one might argue, under the prohibitions that flow from the duty of nonmaleficence. Fourth, we might contend that we did not kill the person but only allowed the person to die and hence did no harm. Fifth, we might appeal to the person's voluntary and informed expression of a desire to die. Sixth, we might hold that death is in the "harmed" person's best interests, e.g., because he is suffering from uncontrollable and unmanageable pain. We might even claim that sustaining life under these conditions would violate the principle *primum non nocere*. We will explore some of these options to see if and when they might be morally acceptable responses. We will, however, generally avoid the term "euthanasia," which is commonly used in discussions of these ethical issues in death and dying. Its connotations would obscure rather than illuminate the issues that we encounter in applying the principle of nonmaleficence.

The principle of double effect

Through a long history, primarily but not exclusively in the Roman Catholic tradition, the principle of double effect has been invoked to support claims that an act having a harmful effect, such as death, does not always fall under moral prohibitions, such as murder, suicide, or abortion. The harmful effect is seen as an indirect, unintended, or merely foreseen effect, not as the direct and intended effect of the action.

The Roman Catholic position on abortion is a useful initial example of the use of the principle of double effect. Catholic opposition to abortion is based upon an acceptance of the prohibition against killing innocent human beings and the conviction that human life begins at conception. Thus, a moral principle is combined with a claim about the beginning of human life (a claim that is as metaphysical as empirical). Despite the prohibition of abortion, considered as the moral equivalent of murder, Catholic teaching acknowledges at least two situations in which the death of the fetus—as a result of the physician's actions—does not lead to the judgment that the physician performed an abortion and thus committed a moral wrong. Both situations involve conditions that threaten the pregnant woman—a cancerous uterus and an ectopic pregnancy. In both, the death of the fetus is held to be the indirect and unintended effect of a morally legitimate medical procedure. The Catholic position is not that "abortion" is justified in these cases, but that these deaths do not count as abortions because they are indirect and unintended.[15]

The principle of double effect involves four conditions: (1) The action in itself must be good or at least morally indifferent. (2) The agent must intend only the good effect and not the evil effect. The evil effect is foreseen, not intended; it is allowed, not sought. Some philosophers prefer to use Bentham's language of "obliquely intentional" for these foreseen effects. (3) The evil effect cannot be a *means* to the good effect. That is, the good and evil effects must follow immediately from the same action. In many cases, this element is the most decisive in determining whether the agent is morally responsible for the harm or death. (4) There must be a proportionality or favorable balance between the good and evil effects of the action.[16]

Let us see how Catholic moralists have applied these conditions to the problem of the removal of a cancerous uterus that results in the foreseen but not intended death of the fetus. The action of removing the cancerous uterus in this situation is a legitimate medical procedure that has good and bad effects, and the medical practitioner intends only the good effect (saving the mother's life), not the bad effect (the death of the fetus). This claim about the agent's intention can be made in part because the fetus's death is not a means to save the mother's life. If the fetus's death were a means, it would be intended along with the end. But saving the mother's life is only contingent upon the fetus's removal, not its death. Its death is an unintended though foreseen effect, and this is neither an end nor a means to an end. Finally, saving the mother's life is a sufficient reason for performing the medical procedure and for allowing the death of the fetus, because the good effect outweighs the evil one. Suppose, by contrast, that a physician determines that it is necessary to perform a fetal craniotomy—now rare—in order to save a woman in labor; the woman will die if the fetus's head is not crushed. Such a procedure could not be brought under the principle of double effect, because killing the fetus would be the means to the good end of saving the mother's life, and thus would be part of the intention. The fetus's death would be directly, even if regrettably, willed. (For an abortion procedure that can only be described as killing, see Case #23.)

Sometimes the principle of double effect is invoked to justify the deaths of civilians as the indirect result of an attack on a legitimate military target or to justify an agent's acceptance of the risk of death for a good cause. If the conditions of the principle of double effect are met, the former is not considered "murder" and the latter is not considered "suicide."

Appeals to the principle of double effect are especially prominent when there is conflict between obligations or values, and it is not possible to meet or realize all of them simultaneously. While these obligations are often to different parties, such as the pregnant woman and the fetus, two obligations to the same party may conflict. Such a situation may occur in the care of terminally ill patients when there is a duty of nonmaleficence, including a duty not to kill, and there is a duty to make the patient comfortable by inducing sleep and alleviating pain. If these duties conflict, it may be possible to make the patient comfortable only by using measures that may hasten the patient's death. When the conditions of the principle of double effect are met, hastening the patient's death does not count as homicide and is justified. According to the Ethical and Religious Directives for Catholic Health Facilities, "it is not euthanasia to give a dying person sedatives and analgesics for the alleviation of pain, when such a measure is judged necessary, even though they may deprive the patient of the use of reason, or shorten his life."

The principle of double effect has come under attack from many directions.[17] Often critics hold that the conclusions based on the principle are implausible, especially in the instances of abortion and euthanasia. Usually the conclusion is questioned because either the moral principles and rules or the factual premises of the argument are suspect. For example, at least one factual premise involved in the application of the principle of double effect to the deaths of fetuses is widely rejected: It is not clear to many people that the fetus should be considered a human being or person from conception, even if we have some obligations to it. According to such critics, there are instances of morally justified fetal deaths outside the scope of the restrictive principle of double effect. Regarding death and dying in general, few would dispute the conclusions reached about the justifiability of hastening death by relieving pain and inducing sleep. While these cases *can* be brought under the principle of double effect, the principle fails to resolve most of the difficult cases, as we shall see in the next section.

Utilitarians, joined by numerous deontologists, argue that the principle of double effect is not morally relevant. First, they contend that it makes no sense to distinguish moral judgments about the death of a fetus by craniotomy and the death of a fetus that results from the removal of a cancerous uterus when the consequences are identical: A woman's life is saved and a fetus's life is lost in both cases. It is not possible to draw the distinction in terms of the degree of probability of the bad result, for the probability of death in at least some removals of a cancerous uterus may be so high as to approach virtual certainty. Second, some critics of the principle of double effect contend that it is not possible to distinguish the above two cases of fetal death in terms of the agent's intention, for the physician may not want, desire, or intend the death of the fetus and may regret the death whether he or she removes a cancerous uterus or performs a craniotomy.

Two different attempts to retain elements of the principle deserve mention. First, some Roman Catholic moral theologians now emphasize the fourth element of the principle—proportionality between good and evil effects— almost to the exclusion of other elements. As a result, it is difficult to distinguish their position as a mode of reasoning from utilitarianism, although, of course, their more general conceptions of values and disvalues often differ. Second, some theologians and philosophers focus primarily on intention rather than on direct and indirect causation; they thus emphasize primary and secondary intentions rather than direct and indirect effects.[18]

Related to the distinctions between primary and secondary intentions and direct and indirect effects is the distinction between killing and letting die, which is equally controversial and deserves separate examination.

Killing and letting die

In Case #15, a sixty-eight-year-old doctor, who suffered severely from terminal carcinoma of the stomach, collapsed with a massive pulmonary embolism. He survived because one of his young colleagues performed a pulmonary embolectomy. Upon recovery the doctor-patient requested that no steps should be taken to prolong his life if he suffered another cardiovascular collapse. He even wrote an authorization to this effect for the hospital records. He reasoned that his pain was too much to bear given his dismal prospects. He thus asked to be *allowed to die* under certain conditions, but he did not ask to be *killed*. In Case #22, a defective infant needed an operation to correct a tracheoesophogeal fistula. The parents and physicians determined that survival was not in this infant's best interests and decided to allow the infant to die rather than to perform an operation. In both cases, we need to ask whether certain actions, such as intentionally not trying to overcome a cardiovascular collapse and not performing an operation, can legitimately be described as "allowing to die" rather than "killing," and whether such actions are justifiable.

For many people, it is important to distinguish killing and letting die, and to prohibit the former while authorizing the latter in some range of cases. For example, after prohibiting "mercy killing" or the "intentional termination of the life of one human being by another,"[19] the AMA House of Delegates held that cessation of treatment is morally justified when the patient and/or the patient's immediate family, with the advice and judgment of the physician, decide to withhold or stop the use of "extraordinary means to prolong life when there is irrefutable evidence that biological death is imminent." Although several terms in this statement—such as "extraordinary," "irrefutable," and "imminent"—need careful examination, it is clear that the statement authorizes some instances of allowing to die by withholding or stopping treatment, while it excludes killing. Whether letting particular patients die— such as the sixty-eight-year-old man suffering from terminal carcinoma of the stomach and the defective infant needing an operation—is morally acceptable would depend on several conditions. But if their deaths involve killing rather than being merely "allowed deaths," they are not justifiable according to the AMA House of Delegates' statement.

In recent years, the distinction between killing and letting die has come under frequent attack. Some critics focus on developments in biomedical technology that appear to make it difficult to classify acts as instances either of killing or of letting die. Unplugging the respirator is now a standard example of this problem. Other critics dismiss the distinction itself, holding that it is a "moral quibble" without any "moral bite." As we explore the arguments for and against this distinction, it is important to emphasize that acceptance or rejection of the *distinction* does not necessarily determine *moral conclusions* about particular cases. For instance, it is possible to reject the distinction and to hold that some cases of what have been called "killing" and "letting die" are morally permissible, or that all cases are morally prohibited; and it is also possible to affirm the distinction and yet to hold that most cases of letting die and all cases of killing are morally wrong. Even if the distinction is morally significant, the label "killing" or the label "letting die" should not dictate a conclusion about a particular case. For example, it would be absurd to affirm the moral significance of the distinction and then to accept *all* cases of letting die as morally fitting. Even instances of letting die must meet other criteria such as the detriment-benefit calculation, and some cases of allowed death involve egregious negligence.

In a widely discussed argument for rejecting both the distinction between active and passive euthanasia and the AMA's policy statement, James Rachels contends that killing is not, in itself, worse than letting die.[20] That is, the "bare difference" between acts of killing and acts of letting die is not in itself a morally relevant difference. Part of his strategy is to sketch two cases that differ only in that one involves killing, while the other involves allowing to die. He contends that if there is no morally relevant difference between these cases, the "bare difference" between killing and allowing to die is demonstrated to be morally irrelevant. In his two cases, two young men want their six-year-old cousins dead so that they can gain large inheritances. Smith drowns his cousin while the boy is taking a bath. Jones plans to drown his cousin, but as he enters the bathroom he sees the boy slip and hit his head; Jones stands by, doing nothing, while the boy drowns. Smith killed his cousin; Jones merely allowed his cousin to die.

While we agree with Rachels that both acts are equally reprehensible because of the motives, ends, and actions, we do not accept his conclusion that these examples show that the distinction between killing and letting die is morally irrelevant. Several rejoinders to Rachels are in order. First, Rachels's cases and the cessations of treatment envisioned by the AMA are so markedly disanalogous that it is not clear what Rachels's argument shows. In some cases of unjustified acts, including both of Rachels's examples, we are not interested in moral distinctions per se. As Richard Trammell points out, some examples have a "masking" or "sledgehammer" effect; the fact that "one cannot distinguish the taste of two wines when both are mixed with green persimmon juice, does not imply that there is no distinction between the wines."[21] Since Rachels's examples involve two morally unjustified acts by agents whose motives and intentions are despicable, it is not surprising that some *other* features of their situations, such as killing and letting die, do not strike us as morally compelling considerations.

Second, while Rachels's cases involve two *unjustified* actions, one of killing and the other of letting die, the AMA statement distinguishes cases of *unjustified killing* from cases of *justified letting die*. The AMA statement does not, however, claim that the moral difference is identical to the distinction between killing and letting die. It does not even imply that the "bare difference" between (passive) letting die and (active) killing is the only difference or even a morally sufficient difference between the justified and unjustified cases. Its point is rather that the justified actions in medicine are confined to (passive) letting die. While the AMA statement holds that "mercy killing" in medicine is unjustified in all circumstances, it does not hold that letting die is right in all circumstances or that killing outside medicine is always wrong. For an act that results in an earlier death for the patient to be justified, it is necessary that it be describable as an act of "letting die," but this description is not sufficient to justify the act; nor is the bare description of killing sufficient to make *all* acts of killing wrong. This AMA pronouncement is meant to hold only in the context of the physician-patient relationship.

Third, in Rachels's cases Smith and Jones are *morally* responsible and *morally* blameworthy for the deaths of their respective cousins, even if Jones, who allowed his cousin to drown, is not *causally* responsible. The law might find only Smith, who killed his cousin, guilty of homicide (because of the law's theory of proximate cause), but morality condemns both actions because of the agents' motives and their commissions and omissions. While we would not condemn a nonswimmer for failing to jump into deep water to try to rescue a drowning child, we find Jones's actions reprehensible because he (morally) should have rescued the child. Even if he had no other special duties to the child, the duty of beneficence—which we will examine in the next chapter—requires affirmative action. The point of the cases envisioned by the AMA is that the physician is always morally prohibited from killing patients but is not morally bound to preserve life in *all* cases. According to the AMA, the physician has a right—and perhaps a duty—to stop treatment if and only if three conditions are met: (1) the life of the body is being preserved by extraordinary means, (2) there is irrefutable evidence that biological death is imminent, and (3) the patient and/or the family consents.

Fourth, even if the distinction between killing and letting die is morally irrelevant in some contexts, it does not follow that it is always morally irrelevant. The fact that the distinction does not show up in every sort of case does not mean that it is morally unimportant under all circumstances. Rachels does effectively undermine any attempt to rest judgments about ending life on the "bare difference" between killing and letting die, but his target may be a straw man. Many philosophers and theologians have argued that there are *independent* moral, religious, and other reasons for defending the distinction and for prohibiting killing while authorizing allowing to die in some circumstances.

One theologian has argued, for example, that we can discern the moral significance of the distinction between killing and letting die only by "placing it in the religious context out of which it grew."[22] That context is the Biblical story of God's actions toward his creatures. In that context it makes *sense* to talk about "placing patients in God's hands," just as it is important not to usurp God's prerogatives by desperately struggling to prolong life when the patient is irreversibly dying. But even if the distinction between killing and letting die originated within a religious context, and even if it makes more sense in that context than in some others, it can be defended on nontheological grounds without being reduced to a claim about a "bare difference." However important the religious context was for the origin of the distinction, religious doctrines are not presupposed by the distinction, and independent moral grounds are sufficient to support it.

Some nontheological arguments in favor of the distinction between killing and allowing to die invoke both moral and practical considerations. They hold that the distinction enables us to express and maintain certain principles such as nonmaleficence and to avoid certain harmful consequences. Probably no single reason by itself is sufficient to support the moral relevance of the distinction, and thus to prohibit killing while permitting some intentionally allowed deaths. But several reasons together indicate that the distinction is worth retaining or, in effect, that our current practices should be maintained with some clarifications and modifications. We now turn to this set of reasons.

The most important arguments for the distinction between killing and letting die depend on a distinction between *acts* and *practices*.[23] It is one thing to justify an act, i.e., to hold that it is right; it is another to justify a general practice. As we saw in our examination of rule utilitarianism and rule deontology, many beliefs about principles and consequences are applied to practices or rules rather than directly to acts. For example, we might justify a rule of confidentiality because it encourages people to seek therapy and because it promotes respect for persons and their privacy. Such a rule might, however, lead to undesirable results in *particular* cases. Likewise, a rule that prohibits "active killing," while permitting some "allowed deaths," may be justifiable, even though it excludes some acts of killing that in and of themselves might appear to be justifiable. Such a rule would not permit us to kill a patient who suffers from terrible pain, who rationally asks for "mercy," i.e., to be killed, and who will probably die within three weeks. According to the rule of double effect, we should, of course, use measures to alleviate the patient's pain even though these would hasten death; we should allow the patient to die, but not kill the patient. It may be necessary to prohibit by rule and policy some acts that do not appear to be wrong in some circumstances in order to maintain a viable practice that, for the most part, expresses our principles and avoids seriously undesirable consequences. Thus, although particular acts of killing may not violate the duty of nonmaleficence and may even be humane and compassionate, a policy of authorizing killing would probably violate the duty of nonmaleficence by creating a grave risk of harm in many cases.

According to one line of argument, the prohibition of killing even for "mercy" expresses principles and values that provide a basis of trust between patients and health care professionals. Trust involves the expectation that others will respect moral limits. When we trust medical practitioners, we expect them to promote our welfare and, at least, to do us no harm without a corresponding prospect of benefit. The prohibition of killing in medical contexts is a basic expression of the ethos of care for the patient's life and health as well as the duty of nonmaleficence. Some claim that it is instrumentally as well as symbolically important, for its removal could weaken a "climate, both moral and legal, which we are not able to do without."[24] David Louisell, for example, contends that "Euthanasia would threaten the patient-physician relationship: confidence might give way to suspicion. . . . Can the physician, historic battler for life, become an affirmative agent of death without jeopardizing the trust of his dependents?"[25]

While this argument has plausibility, it needs to be stated carefully. It is a wedge or slippery slope argument that may take at least two different forms. One type of wedge argument focuses on moral reasoning and the logic of distinctions between different acts. It holds that there will be no defensible line between acts leading to deaths that we consider legitimate and others that we consider illegitimate, unless we can draw a clear distinction supported by moral reasons. A justification offered for one sort of act that strikes us as right may have logical implications for the justification of another sort of act that strikes us as wrong. For example, a justification of abortion under some circumstances also logically may imply a justification of infanticide under relevantly similar circumstances.

This first version of the wedge argument derives its power from the principle of universalizability discussed in Chapter 1. That principle commits us to treating similar cases in a similar way. If we judge X to be right, and we can point to no relevant dissimilarities between X and Y, then we cannot judge Y to be wrong. Because of this principle of universalizability, Paul Ramsey argues, ethical and legal mistakes tend to replicate themselves:

It is quite clear that at the point of medical, legal, and ethical intersections at the edges of life . . . , the so-called wedge argument is an excellent one. This is true because legal principles and precedents are systematically designed to apply to other cases as well. This is the way the law 'works,' and . . . also the way moral reasoning 'works' from case to similar case.[26]

This first version of the wedge argument, then, focuses on the logical implications of decisions—i.e., how support for one sort of action logically implies support for another sort of action when it is not possible in principle to identify morally relevant dissimilarities.

While we morally justify killing aggressors in such circumstances as self-defense and war, these killings presumably do not threaten the following rule, derived from the principle of nonmaleficence: Do not directly kill *innocent* persons. These killings are justified because the persons killed are not innocent. If, however, we justify the killing of innocent persons in medical settings, there is no logical way, according to some arguments, to limit the killing to legitimate cases, for the principle of nonmaleficence and the rule against directly killing innocent life have been eroded. Such arguments are not, however, as compelling as they may seem at first. As Rachels correctly contends, "there obviously are good reasons for objecting to killing patients in order to get away for the weekend—or for even more respectable purposes, such as securing organs for transplantation—which do not apply to killing in order to put the patient out of extreme agony."[27] In other words, relevant distinctions can still be drawn.

This first version of the wedge argument thus does not assist supporters of the distinction between killing and letting die as much as they might suppose. Indeed, it can be used against them by critics of the distinction in the following way: If it is rational and morally defensible to allow patients to die under X, Y, and Z conditions, it is rational and morally defensible to kill them under those same conditions. If it is in their best interests to die, it is (prima facie) irrelevant how death is brought about. Rachels makes a similar point when he argues that reliance on the distinction between killing and letting die will lead to making decisions about life and death on *irrelevant grounds*—such as whether the patient will or will not die without certain forms of treatment—instead of being made in terms of the patient's best interests.[28] For example, in Case #22 a baby suffering from several defects needs an operation to correct a tracheoesophogeal fistula, for otherwise the baby will die. A baby suffering from those same defects but without the fistula may be kept alive, while the baby who needs the operation may be allowed to die. It is possible to argue that we need to determine the conditions under which death would be in the baby's best interests and then choose to kill or to let die by determining which means would be more humane and compassionate in the circumstances. In the now famous Johns Hopkins

Hospital case, an infant with Down's syndrome and duodenal atresia took two weeks to die; the dying process was extremely difficult for all the parties involved, particularly the nurses. If a physician and family legitimately determine that a patient would be better off dead, does an act of killing violate the patient's interests if the patient will not die when artificial treatment is discontinued? A morally irrelevant factor, so the argument goes, would then be allowed to dictate the outcome, and this would violate the principle of universalizability.

If the first version of the wedge argument focuses on the logic of moral reasoning—the hammer back of the wedge—the second version focuses on what the wedge is driven into. It examines the culture and society in order to determine the probable impact of changing rules or making exceptions: If certain restraints against killing are removed, a moral decline will probably result, because various psychological or social forces make it unlikely that people will draw distinctions that are, in principle, clear and defensible. For example, in some settings, it would be possible (1) to argue that to authorize killing patients for their own benefit when they are suffering excruciating pain or have a bleak future could easily open the door to a policy of killing patients for the sake of social benefits such as reducing financial burdens, or (2) to argue that voluntary euthanasia would probably open the door to involuntary euthanasia.

Such arguments do not depend on the first version of the wedge or slippery slope arguments, for there are clear and defensible distinctions, rooted in moral principles, between voluntary and involuntary euthanasia and between killing patients for their own benefit and killing them for social benefits. Nevertheless, where there are certain psychological and social forces—such as racism, an increasing number of defective newborns who survive at great expense, or aging persons with vast medical problems requiring an increasing amount of a society's financial resources—the second version of the wedge argument might be compelling. It all depends on sometimes speculative predictions of what will probably happen independent of what our principles and rules logically imply. We need to make these predictions as accurate as possible. Thus, debates about the second version of the wedge argument concern empirical claims rather than the logical matters at issue in the first version.

If rules permitting active killing were introduced into a society, it is not implausible to suppose that the society over time would move increasingly in the direction of involuntary euthanasia—e.g., in the form of killing defective newborns for such reasons as the avoidance of social burdens. There could be a general reduction of respect for human life as a result of the official removal of some barriers to killing. Rules against killing in a moral code are not isolated; they are threads in a fabric of rules, based in part on nonmaleficence, that support respect for human life. The more threads we remove, the weaker the fabric becomes. If we focus on attitudes and not merely rules, the general attitude of respect for life may be eroded by shifts in particular areas. Determination of the probability of such an erosion depends not only on the connectedness of rules and attitudes, but also on various forces in the society.

When the second version of the wedge argument is combined with other considerations of consequences, the argument against the authorization of killing is strengthened. It is not a matter of combining several weak arguments in order to build a strong one—a ludicrous approach. However, when there are several good reasons to be suspicious of a proposed policy that offers only limited benefit, alterations in current practices may not be justified.[29]

In addition to fears of abuse, including abuse of the mentally disabled and others who cannot consent, there are other legitimate fears. First, easy resort to killing to relieve pain and suffering may divert attention and resources from other strategies that may be effective, such as the hospice movement. Second, consider the following two types of wrongly diagnosed patients:[30]

1. Patients wrongly diagnosed as hopeless, and who will survive even if a treatment *is* ceased (in order to allow a natural death).
2. Patients wrongly diagnosed as hopeless, and who will survive only if the treatment is *not ceased* (in order to allow a natural death).

If a social rule of allowing some patients to die were in effect, doctors and families who followed it would only lose patients in the second category. But if killing were permitted, at least some of the patients in the first category would be needlessly lost. Thus, a rule prohibiting killing would save some lives that would be lost if *both* killing and allowing to die were permitted. Of course, such a consequence is not a decisive reason for a policy of (only) allowing to die, for the numbers in categories (1) and (2) are likely to be small and other reasons for killing, such as extreme pain and autonomous choice, might be weighty. But it is certainly *a* morally relevant reason.

Proponents of the practice of killing some patients appeal to a range of exceptional cases to show the utility of the practice. Among the strongest reasons for killing some patients is to relieve unbearable and uncontrollable pain and suffering. No one would deny that pain and suffering can so ravage and dehumanize patients that death appears to be in their best interests. Prolonging life and refusing to kill in such circumstances may appear to be cruel and even to violate the duty of nonmaleficence. Often proponents of "mercy killing" appeal to nonmedical situations to show that killing may be more humane and compassionate than letting die—as, for example, in the case of a truck driver inextricably trapped in a burning wreck who cries out for "mercy" and asks to be killed. In such tragic situations we are reluctant to say that those who kill at the behest of the victim act wrongly. Furthermore, juries often find persons who have killed a suffering relative not guilty by reason of temporary insanity.

There are, nevertheless, serious objections to building into *medical practice* an explicit exception licensing physicians to kill their patients in order to relieve uncontrollable pain and suffering. One objection is that it is not clear that many, if any, cases in medical practice are really parallel to the person trapped in a burning wreck. The physician may be able to relieve pain and suffering short of killing—even if death is hastened—by means that are not available to a bystander at the scene of an accident. A second objection holds that we should not construct a social or professional ethic on borderline situations and emergency cases, even if medical practitioners confront some cases of unmanageable pain and suffering. It is dangerous to generalize from emergencies, for hard cases may make bad social and professional ethics as well as bad law. As Charles Fried writes,

The concept of emergency is only a tolerable moral concept if somehow we can truly think of it as exceptional, if we can truly think of it as a circumstance that, far from defying our usual moral universe, suspends it for a limited time and thus suspends usual moral principles. It is when emergencies become usual that we are threatened with moral disintegration, dehumanization.[31]

Third, there are ways to "accept" acts of killing in exceptional circumstances without altering the rules of practice in order to accommodate them. As mentioned earlier, juries often find those who kill their suffering relatives not guilty by reason of temporary insanity, as occurred in the Zygmaniak case in New Jersey.[32] In June 1973, George Zygmaniak was in a motorcycle accident that left him paralyzed from the neck down. The paralysis was considered to be irreversible, and Zygmaniak begged his brother, Lester, to kill him. Three days later, Lester brought a sawed-off shotgun to the hospital and shot his brother in the head, after having told him, "Close your eyes now, I'm going to shoot you." Verdicts like "not guilty by reason of temporary insanity" do not *justify* the act of killing a suffering relative. They differ from a verdict of not guilty on grounds of self-defense, for self-defense does justify killing, at least in some circumstances. Verdicts like not guilty by reason of temporary insanity thus function to *excuse* the agent by finding that he or she lacked the conditions of responsibility necessary to be legally guilty.

Others have proposed that we maintain the legal rule against killing even if physicians and others sometimes have to engage in justified conscientious or civil disobedience. Concurring with Robert Veatch, Paul Ramsey holds that "civil disobedience—the courage to go against the rule when morally warranted—may be better than to allow for exceptions in a rule of general practice."[33] But what conditions might justify conscientious refusals in medical practice to follow the rule against killing patients? According to Ramsey, when dying patients are totally inaccessible to our care, when our care is a matter of indifference to them because of intractable pain or a deep coma, "there is no longer any morally significant distinction between omission and commission, between standing aside and directly dispatching them."[34] "Total inaccessibility" is a limit of care itself; for care can become totally useless. It is not clear, however, that Ramsey's distinction between dying and nondying patients can carry his argument. Nor is it clear whether he considers someone in a deep and prolonged state of unconsciousness as dying and, if so, whether such a view is justifiable. In addition, it is necessary to ask whether Ramsey's exception can be limited to the cases that he endorses; it too may be the thin edge of the wedge. Nevertheless, even if pain and suffering of a certain magnitude can in principle justify active killing, as long as other conditions are met, they may only justify acts of conscientious refusal to follow the rule of practice, not basic changes in the rule itself.

Finally, which side in the debate has the burden of proof—the proponents or the opponents of a practice of selective killing? Antony Flew has argued that supporters of the current practice of prohibiting killing must bear the burden of proof because the prohibition of *voluntary* euthanasia violates the principle of liberty by refusing to respect individual autonomy.[35] However, a policy of voluntary euthanasia, based on either a negative right to die (a right to noninterference) or a positive right to die (a right to be killed), would involve such a change in society's vision of the medical profession and in medical attitudes that a shift in the burden of proof to the proponents of change is inevitable. The prohibition of killing is not arbitrary even when cases of voluntary request are factored in. It expresses some important moral principles, values, and attitudes whose loss, or serious alteration, could have major negative consequences. Because the current practice of prohibiting killing while accepting some "allowed deaths" has served us well, if not perfectly, it should be altered only with the utmost caution. Lines are not easy to draw and maintain, but in general we have been able to follow the line between killing and letting die in medical practice. Before we undertake any major changes, we need strong evidence that these changes are really needed in order to avoid important harms or secure important benefits, and that the good effects will outweigh the bad effects. Otherwise, we run the risk of undermining respect for the principle of nonmaleficence and its subsidiary rules.[36]

As mentioned previously, the distinction between killing and letting die does not suffice to decide all issues of life and death in medical practice, for not all "allowed deaths" are morally acceptable. There is considerable debate about when the description "letting die" can be applied and which instances of letting die are morally right. On the one hand, Ramsey clearly limits the application of "letting die" to the *dying*; only those who are irreversibly in the dying process may be allowed to die. On the other hand, Robert Veatch holds that we can justify allowed deaths when the treatments are unreasonable, even if the patient is not irreversibly dying.[37] What, then, are the conditions under which allowed deaths are justified? Serious consideration of this question requires that we examine the distinction between treatments that are obligatory and those that are optional.

Optional and obligatory means of treatment

Ordinary and extraordinary means

The language of "ordinary" and "extraordinary" means of treatment has a long history, especially in the Roman Catholic tradition, but this distinction has also played a prominent role in medical practice and in judicial decisions. The 1973 statement by the AMA House of Delegates holds that the patient and/or his immediate family can decide about the "cessation of *extraordinary means* to prolong the life of the body when there is irrefutable evidence that biological death is imminent." Even more recently, in the Quinlan case, the New Jersey Supreme Court implicitly invoked this distinction when it held that judgments about treatment should be based on the treatment's degree of invasiveness and its chance of success.

Like the distinctions between direct and indirect effects and killing and letting die, this distinction has been employed to determine whether an act that results in death counts as killing, and especially as culpable killing in violation of the duty of nonmaleficence. Historically, the distinction has been applied to decisions of patients, proxies, and physicians. As developed by Roman Catholics to deal with problems of surgery (prior to the discovery of antisepsis and anesthesia), the distinction was used to determine whether a patient's refusal of treatment should be classified as suicide. Refusal of "ordinary" means of treatment was considered suicide, while refusal of "extraordinary" means was not labeled suicide. Likewise, families and physicians did not commit homicide or violate obligations to patients if they only withheld or terminated "extraordinary" means of treatment.

Unfortunately, a long history does not guarantee clarity, and the distinction between ordinary and extraordinary means of treatment is vague and ambiguous. Several recent commentators have urged that the distinction be replaced by other categories. It is not always clear whether they intend to change only the vocabulary or also the substance of the distinction, but we at least agree that moral discourse would improve if the terms were replaced by such terms as "optional" and "obligatory." "Ordinary" would then be reconstructed to mean morally obligatory, mandatory, required, or imperative, while "extraordinary" would be reconstructed to mean morally optional, elective, or expendable.[38]

Such a translation is not alien to some traditional discussions of ordinary and extraordinary means of treatment, and it appears to be necessary because "ordinary" is often wrongly taken to mean "usual," while "extraordinary" is wrongly taken to mean "unusual." The "usual/unusual" distinction builds on what is *customary* in medical practice, which in turn is connected to the *professional practice* standard discussed in Chapter 3. But what is customary in medical practice is merely relevant to moral judgments and cannot always be construed as morally decisive. For example, it may be usual medical practice to treat disease X in manner Y, but whether this usual practice should be repeated for a particular patient depends on the patient's condition as a whole and not merely on what is usual treatment for disease X.[39] Ethics is not reducible to consensus or to traditional codes, oaths, and practices—as useful as these may be in many professional contexts.

It is possible to replace the misleading language of "ordinary" and "extraordinary," while retaining or only partially modifying the substance of the distinction. According to Gerald Kelly, S.J., the distinction can be understood in the following way:

Ordinary means are all medicines, treatments, and operations, which offer a reasonable hope of benefit and which can be obtained and used without excessive expense, pain, or other inconvenience. Extraordinary means are all medicines, treatments, and operations, which cannot be obtained or used without excessive expense, pain, or other inconvenience, or which, if used, would not offer a reasonable hope of benefit.[40]

Kelly's discussion of the distinction embodies two criteria: for a therapy to be obligatory or required, it must (a) offer a *reasonable prospect* of benefit, and (b) not involve *excessive* expense, pain, or other inconvenience. The substance of the distinction is a balance between benefit and detriment, if we assume that "excessive" is to be determined by the probability and magnitude of the benefit. If there is no reasonable hope of benefit, then any expense, pain, or other inconvenience is excessive. But if there is a reasonable hope of benefit, the amount of expense, pain, or other inconvenience may be significant without being excessive. Therefore, the point of the distinction and its application turns on a balance between benefits and costs, including immediate detriment, inconvenience, and risk of harm.

We will reserve a systematic treatment of such cost-benefit judgments for the next chapter. It is important now to consider substantive standards that distinguish obligatory treatment and optional treatment. These standards may vary for competent patients making choices about their own treatment and for second parties making decisions for incompetent patients. Competent and informed patients should have more latitude than second parties in balancing benefits and burdens and in accepting and refusing treatment. As noted throughout this chapter, the incompetent patient's vulnerability to harm may require uses of the principle of nonmaleficence that would violate respect for autonomy in a competent patient. We concentrated on competent patients in our discussion of autonomy in Chapter 3 and shall return to this class of patients in our discussion of paternalism in Chapter 5. Therefore, we shall here consider substantive criteria of optional and mandatory treatments mainly for incompetent patients. These substantive criteria specify the conditions under which it is possible to rebut the presumption, based on the principle of nonmaleficence, that the means to prolong life are obligatory. (In the last section of this chapter we shall also consider proxy decision-makers for incompetent patients.)

Conditions for overriding the obligation to treat

Pointless treatment
First, treatment is not obligatory when it offers no prospect of benefit to the patient because it is pointless. There are several classes of patients for whom treatment will not be efficacious. (a) Patients who are dead. It is unfortunate that a major impetus for refining criteria for determining death has come from the need for organs for transplantation. There are sufficient reasons for updating the criteria for determining death without considering the interests of potential recipients of organs. If the patient is dead, he or she can no longer be harmed by the cessation of treatment, and a standard of best interests does not dictate treatment. Of course, refined criteria of death will not help in most cases.[41] For example, few people argued seriously that Karen Ann Quinlan was dead. Yet among those holding that she was alive, there were moral and legal disagreements about what ought to be done.

(b) Patients whose death is imminent and who are irreversibly dying. The AMA statement, as we have seen, holds that some treatments may be discontinued when death is "imminent." It is not clear whether this statement holds that all means can be considered "extraordinary" when death is imminent, except those that are palliative, or that only "extraordinary" means can be discontinued when death is imminent. Whatever the intention of the AMA statement, the first interpretation is more defensible. When it can be determined, largely as a matter of medical judgment, that a patient's death is imminent and that a patient is irreversibly dying, such modes of treatment as resuscitation and respiration become optional. Because "ought" implies "can," there is no medical indication for starting or continuing curative treatment if the patient is irreversibly dying and death is imminent. Optimal care does not mean maximal treatment, and prolonging life is not the same as prolonging dying. Indeed, the paradigm of care for the dying needs to be dramatically revised so that technological interventions do not overwhelm human responses of care.

In cases involving (a) those who are dead and (b) those who are irreversibly dying, objective medical factors are primary, and the role of expert judgment is central. Expert judgment about objective medical factors is not, of course, infallible. The possibility of error should lead to efforts to prolong life in cases of serious doubt about whether patients are irretrievably in categories (a) or (b)—unless other conditions to be discussed below are met. Another problem is specifying central terms such as "imminence" of death. While "imminent" allows physicians latitude of judgment, it suffers from vagueness. It could mean, for example, "any second now" or "in less than a year." This lack of specificity also plagues attempts to classify patients as "terminally ill" and as "dying."

As important as medical judgments are in decisions about the treatment of dying patients, they should not always be decisive. Patient and family values are also important and sometimes decisive. For example, in Case #12, two elderly women were severely burned in an accident, and the burn team agreed that survival was unprecedented in their cases—they were irreversibly dying. According to the burn team, both women were competent and rational after the accident before they began to experience serious problems from the burns. The burn team asked both women if they wanted to choose between maximal treatment, which had never been efficacious in such cases at their burn center, and palliative care. Both women chose palliative care. But in Case #16, Mr. C., a patient irreversibly dying from emphysema, insisted on having his life prolonged as long as possible by all available means. He demanded aggressive treatment, even though the staff considered his condition hopeless. When Mr. C. became unconscious, his family and the staff had to decide whether to respect their earlier agreement with him or let him die. If this case did not involve a prior, clear statement of Mr. C.'s wishes, there would be no moral difficulty in terminating treatment on the grounds that it was only prolonging his dying. Following Mr. C.'s previous wishes might not be required or even justified if treatment under these conditions violated standards of justice in the distribution of health care resources—e.g., if other patients, who were not irreversibly dying, needed the ventilator and space in the intensive care unit.

Burdens outweighing benefits

Second, if the patient is not dead or dying, medical treatment is not obligatory when its burdens outweigh its benefits to the patient. (For now we will focus on the benefits and burdens to the patient, reserving for later an examination of the relevance and weight of benefits and burdens to the family and others.) We have already seen that objective medical factors are not always conclusive in cases of type (b), where considerations of value are frequently important. In other cases, where patients are not irreversibly dying and their deaths are not imminent, medical treatment may be optional even though it could possibly or probably prolong life for an indefinite period. Unless the principle of non-maleficence implies the sanctity of biological life, regardless of the patient's pain, suffering, discomfort, and other problems—which may be caused by medical conditions or by treatment—it does not mandate beginning or continuing maximum treatment for all nondying patients. For example, in Case #19, seventy-eight-year-old Earle Spring developed numerous medical problems, including chronic organic brain syndrome and kidney failure. The latter problem was controlled by hemodialysis. Although several aspects of the case are in dispute—e.g., whether Earle Spring was able to express his own wishes—there is at least a plausible argument that the family and health care professionals were not morally obligated to continue hemodialysis, which was necessary to sustain his life, because of the balance of benefits and burdens to the patient himself.

Few decisions are more important than those to withhold or stop a therapeutic procedure that in turn ends a life. But in some cases it is unjustified to begin or to continue therapy knowing that it will produce a greater balance of suffering for someone incapable of choosing for or against such therapy. As the Supreme Judicial Court of Massachusetts held in the Saikewicz case, "the 'best interests' of an incompetent person are not necessarily served by imposing on such persons results not mandated as to competent persons similarly situated."[42] An interesting example occurred in the case of In re Nemser, where a judge refused to require the amputation of the foot and ankle (a transmalleolar amputation) of an eighty-year-old woman. Her competency was doubtful, and her children sought to consent to the operation for her, although it was medically unclear how much benefit could be expected and clear that substantial suffering would be involved. While the operation did have a low probability of curing her, Judge Markowitz held that the substantial hazards and suffering involved outweighed the possible beneficial outcome—though he referred to his decision as "an example of a grave dilemma."[43]

Applications to defective newborns

Some of the most difficult questions about the treatment of incompetents involve the other end of the continuum of age: seriously defective newborns. Some societies have circumvented the duty of nonmaleficence in such cases by purely definitional ploys. For example, the Nuer tribe viewed defective newborns as nonhuman "hippopotamuses" who were mistakenly born to human parents and who should be put in the river, which was viewed as their natural habitat. Such definitional maneuvers are generally excluded in our society as far as newborns are concerned. But it remains important to consider the interests of these newborn human beings and to ask whether maximal treatment is always in their best interests. Some commentators even argue that intensive care for neonates may be "harmful," i.e., may violate the duty of nonmaleficence, if one or more of three conditions is present: "inability to survive infancy, inability to live without severe pain, and inability to participate, at least minimally, in human experience."[44]

Another commentator has drawn on the duty of nonmaleficence to develop a concept of the "injury of continued existence." Although he rejects active euthanasia on prudential grounds, H. Tristram Engelhardt, Jr., has argued that the duty of nonmaleficence may require that death be allowed under some conditions: "The concept of injury for continuance of existence, the proposed analogue of the concept of tort for wrongful life, presupposes that life can be of a negative value such that the medical maxim *primum non nocere* ('first do no harm') *would require not sustaining life*."[45] Engelhardt may be correct in suggesting that there is a moral *duty* not to sustain life in some circumstances where the burdens seriously outweigh the benefits. However, our conclusion is less severe. Our intention is merely to show that under some conditions allowing seriously defective newborns to die is morally *permissible* because it does not violate the duty of nonmaleficence (and satisfies other relevant justifying conditions).

Consider some candidate cases. It would be justifiable under the conditions mentioned thus far to withhold or to withdraw treatment from some who suffer Tay-Sachs disease—which involves increasing spasticity and dementia and usually results in death by age three or four—and from some who suffer Lesch-Nyhan disease—which involves uncontrollable spasms, mental retardation, compulsive self-mutilation, and early death. Children born with meningomyelocele (protrusion of part of the covering and substance of the spinal cord through a defect in the vertebral column), by contrast, are more problematic. It is difficult to know whether to treat vigorously all cases or to treat vigorously only selected cases. The difficulty stems from the fact that some children with meningomyelocele can have a meaningful life, while the chances are slim for others. Having argued at one point for vigorous and comprehensive treatment for all spina bifida babies (that is, babies who have a defective closure of the bony encasement of the spinal cord), Dr. John Lorber later concluded that such treatment results in only a marginal gain in survival rate and preserves life with severe disabilities and handicaps. He has proposed specific criteria, such as the site of the spinal lesion and the degree of paralysis, for determining the level of treatment on the first day after birth. When the decision is made to omit treatment for the disorder, normal custodial care and feeding are provided. But some of the babies who are not treated for spina bifida survive; however, their overall condition is not as good as it would have been had they been vigorously treated from the outset.[46]

In these and other cases, we should have a presumption in favor of the prolongation of life. Decision makers should then try to determine the patient's actual interests and should act accordingly. For an adult patient who has previously expressed a certain life plan, it may be possible for decision makers to balance benefits and burdens in terms of that life plan. It might be possible to say that "John Doe would not want to live under those conditions." In some cases, we may even be able to appeal to the patient's "living will." However, judgments about the patient's "interests" in the case of defective newborns must be made by considering the prospective benefits and burdens as objectively as possible, in light of the patient's condition, without benefit of their previous declarations. The possibility of error is substantial, but potentially no greater than in other judgments in medicine. Because of the possibility of error in diagnosis, prognosis, and judgments about the patient's interests, the normal duty to preserve life dictates erring on the side of sustaining life, at least in cases of serious doubt about the evidence.

Quality of life

Debates about whether treatment is optional or obligatory often presuppose or otherwise rely upon standards of the "quality of life." In the Saikewicz case (see #18) a sixty-seven-year-old man, with an I.Q. of 10 and a mental age of approximately two years and eight months, suffered from acute myeloblastic monocytic leukemia. Chemotherapy would have produced considerable suffering and possibly serious side effects. Remission under chemotherapy occurs in only thirty to fifty percent of such cases and typically only for between two and thirteen months. If not given chemotherapy, Saikewicz could expect to live for a matter of weeks or, perhaps, several months, during which he would not experience great pain or suffering. In not ordering treatment, the lower court considered "the quality of life available to him [Saikewicz] even if the treatment does bring about remission." The Supreme Judicial Court, however, rejected this formulation if construed to equate the value of life with a measure of the quality of life—in particular, with Saikewicz's lower quality of life because of mental retardation. Thus, the Court construed "the vague, and perhaps ill-chosen, term 'quality of life' . . . as a reference to the continuing state of pain and disorientation precipitated by the chemotherapy treatment."[47] It thus balanced the prospective benefit against the pain and suffering, finally determining that the patient's actual interests supported a decision not to provide chemotherapy. From a moral as well as a legal standpoint, we would agree that the conclusion reached in this opinion was justified. However, we object to its procedural requirements and standards in the last section of this chapter.

Because such slogans as "quality of life" and "sanctity of life" mislead more often than they illuminate, they should be replaced by more careful statements of substantive positions, such as those attempted by Paul Ramsey and Richard McCormick. Ramsey opposes all judgments about quality of life; for him what is important in the ordinary/extraordinary distinction can be "reduced almost without significant remainder to a medical indications policy."[48] Thus, to determine which treatment is obligatory and optional for incompetent patients, it is only necessary to determine which treatment is medically indicated. For the *dying*, the relevant choices are between further palliative treatments and no treatments. For unconscious or incompetent *nondying* patients, there is an obligation to use the treatment medically indicated. Ramsey contends that we are gradually moving toward a policy of active, involuntary euthanasia for unconscious or incompetent nondying patients. Against such a policy, he asserts an "undiminished obligation first of all to save life and in the second instance, to use palliative treatments where possible."[49] Above all, quality-of-life judgments are to be avoided, he argues, because they violate the principle of *equality* of life.

Ramsey's approach concentrates on medical factors that are objective even though they cannot be infallibly determined, e.g., criteria used in the classification of patients as dying and nondying and in the determination of treatment as medically indicated. It is not clear, however, that these objective medical factors will carry the weight he intends. In particular, it is not clear that such factors can be free of values that inspire, control, and limit them. Richard McCormick contends that it is impossible to determine what will benefit a patient without *presupposing* some quality-of-life standard. He believes that even the language of "medically indicated" presupposes judgments about the patient's condition, and "among the objective conditions of the patient to be considered, one of the most crucial is the *kind of life* that will be preserved as a result of our interventions."[50] Any attempt to make "life"—understood as metabolism and vital processes—good in itself is "vitalism" and should be rejected in favor of a view that such life has only conditional value. While the person possesses "an incalculable value," the maintenance of physical life should not automatically be considered a benefit to the person. Although McCormick does not spell out his criteria of the quality of life, he offers a minimal condition: the capacity for experience or social interrelating. If this minimal condition is not met, as in anencephaly, treatment is not required.

Ramsey has objected that such a quality-of-life approach shifts from the question of whether *treatments* are beneficial to patients to the question of whether patients' *lives* are beneficial to them. The latter question, he again insists, opens the door to active, involuntary euthanasia.[51] He appeals to the wedge argument and contends that qualify-of-life criteria logically commit us to active, involuntary euthanasia. The critical question is whether the criteria for "quality of life"—or, as we prefer, the criteria for determining the patient's best interests—can be stated with sufficient precision and cogency to avoid the dangers stressed by both versions of the wedge argument. We think that they can, but the vagueness of terms such as "dignity" and "meaningful life" is a cause for concern; and the increasingly widespread practice of allowing defective newborn infants to die when their "allowed deaths" are not justified provides a good reason for caution. A good example of an unjustified "allowed death" is Case #22, in which "Infant Doe" was allowed to die six days after he was born with Down's syndrome and respiratory and digestive complications requiring major surgery, which his parents refused to authorize. In this controversial case, the Indiana Supreme Court declined to review a lower court decision not to override the parent's action.

Some factors should be excluded from consideration. Just as the Supreme Judicial Court found it inappropriate in the Saikewicz case to include mental retardation in a determination of the quality of life, we too contend that this factor is irrelevant in determining whether treatment would be in the patient's best interests. Jonsen and Garland correctly urge that "a baby with Down's syndrome, although sure to be mentally deficient, should be given life-sustaining therapy as a rule whenever needed; an anencephalic baby (born without a developed brain) should not be resuscitated or sustained."[52] Unfortunately, the "gray area" between these two extremes is less easily handled by such general pronouncements.

There is debate about the relevance of burdens to the family and to the society in determining whether treatment is mandatory or optional. Robert Veatch holds that when second parties make decisions for incompetent patients, only the incompetent patients' burdens are relevant, while competent patients may include any burdens they find valid. He says emphatically that treatments are reasonable only if they do not give rise to "patient-centered objections." His position is not as restrictive as it appears, however, for the category of "patient-centered objections" is broad enough to include "patient-centered objections based on physical or mental burden; familial, social or economic concern; or religious belief."[53] He may mean that only some "patient-centered objections" are relevant, but it is not clear how he would treat the "patient-centered objection" that the treatment would be so expensive as to exhaust all the uninsured patient's funds. Apparently he would permit the competent patient to refuse treatment for this reason. But it is uncertain whether he would allow this same objection to be used *by family members* in order to refuse treatment for a patient whose imminent loss of resources directly affects them. Our contention is that such an objection should not be decisive in determining whether treatment is optional or obligatory. Rather, the patient's best interests should be decisive, and these may conflict with the interests of the family. To allow familial and social burdens to be determinative would open the door to a dangerous practice. Still, in situations of scarcity, difficult allocation questions do emerge, as we consider in our discussion of justice in Chapter 6.

Two final points need to be made. First, the distinction between *withholding* treatment that was never started and *withdrawing* treatment already started should be considered morally irrelevant when determining whether treatment is obligatory or optional. In many cases, it is necessary to begin and vigorously pursue certain kinds of treatment in order to diagnose the patient's condition with precision. Diagnosis and prognosis often require time that can only be gained by such vigorous efforts as resuscitation and respiration. If it is determined that treatment is optional because of the patient's interests, as analyzed through a benefit-cost calculus, treatment may be discontinued. The moral grounds for withdrawing are identical to those for withholding treatment. The critical issue is not that of an act versus an omission, for the description "allowing to die" may be consistent with such acts as turning off the respirator. Second, no classes of treatment procedures can be classified as "obligatory" or "optional." These terms do not refer to the nature of the treatment procedures or to customary medical practice, but rather to the patient's condition and interests. Even treatments such as intravenous feeding may be optional in some cases, as perhaps in the Karen Ann Quinlan case. Whether a particular treatment is *obligatory* depends on whether it serves a patient's best interests, including interests in comfort and in having his or her autonomous wishes carried out.

Proxy decision makers: standards and procedures

In the previous section, we accepted the point of the distinction between "ordinary" and "extraordinary" means of treatment while replacing the language with "obligatory" and "optional." Whether treatment is obligatory or optional depends on its chances of success and its balance of benefits and costs for a patient. In short, the standard is the patient's best interests. While competent patients can apply this standard for themselves, proxy decision makers must apply it for incompetent patients. In this section, we consider different proxy decision makers, and we elaborate the standard of the patient's best interests by comparing it to another standard that has sometimes been defended—substituted judgment.

John Rawls has argued that there are at least three possible relationships between procedures and right results or decisions. (1) Perfect procedural justice: There is an independent standard of a right outcome or decision, and it is possible to devise a procedure to insure this outcome. An example is insuring a fair distribution of a birthday cake at a children's birthday party by having the child who cuts the cake take the last piece. (2) Imperfect procedural justice: There is an independent standard of a right outcome, but the procedures are imperfect in that they cannot insure the desired outcome. For example, in criminal trials, we have an independent standard of a right outcome—the guilty and only the guilty should be convicted—but we lack a procedure that will produce this outcome in all cases. (3) Pure procedural justice: There is no independent standard of right results, and any result of the procedure is correct if the procedure has been followed. Gambling is an example of pure procedural justice.[54]

If our earlier argument in this chapter is correct, the most we can hope for in life and death decisions in medical practice is imperfect procedural justice. There are, we have argued, some independent standards, but there is no procedure to guarantee that decisions or outcomes will match those standards. Consider two significantly different situations. First, consider situations in which sick or dying but competent patients make their own decisions. The principle of autonomy requires that we recognize the competent patient's right to make the decision even if he or she improperly exercises that right. Nonetheless, we should not view the patient's decision as correct simply because the patient exercised it under conditions of competence, understanding, and voluntariness. Nor should we view the patient's right to make the decision as absolute. Thus, this first type of situation cannot be viewed as simply one of pure procedural justice.

A second type of situation involves incompetent patients who cannot make their own decisions about withholding or withdrawing treatment. In such cases, the principle of nonmaleficence requires that we establish procedures to protect their interests, although no procedure will *guarantee* that their interests will always be adequately protected. At best, this state of affairs represents imperfect procedural justice. Some have argued, however, that some procedures are justified by principles and values other than or in addition to nonmaleficence and are preferable for that reason. For example, Dr. Raymond Duff and Dr. A. G. M. Campbell argue that the family, in consultation with the physician, should make the decisions about the treatment or nontreatment of defective newborns, not only because the family can be expected to act in the infant's best interests—which would express the principles of nonmaleficence and beneficence—but primarily because the family needs to gain a sense of control over its destiny in the face of this misfortune.[55] Nevertheless, judgments about decision makers and procedures for incompetents should be made first in terms of the principle of nonmaleficence: Specific criteria protecting the person's interests should be employed; if it can be determined that a decision maker cannot be counted on to seek the patient's interests, a replacement should be sought. Thus, it is important to determine guidelines for decision makers and also whether various decision makers can render rational and impartial judgments about the patient's interests without major conflicts of interest.

Standards for proxy decision makers

If the patient is not competent to choose or refuse treatment, a physician or family member often goes before a court to seek resolution of the issues before any treatment decision is made. Such cases involve formerly competent patients like Karen Ann Quinlan, Earle Spring (see Case #19) and Brother Fox, as well as patients like Joseph Saikewicz (see Case #18) and John Storar, who have never been competent. Courts have recently been split over

the use of two proxy decisionmaking standards—the *best interests* standard
and the *substituted judgment* standards. Paradoxically, the doctrine of
parens patriae, or the state as parent, which represents the underlying
authority for the state's power to act in an incompetent's behalf, is the basis
for *both* legal standards applied by courts in medical decisionmaking for
incompetents. The doctrine of *parens patriae* has traditionally been built on
the principle of nonmaleficence and the principle of beneficence: the state's
duty to protect persons under legal disability from harm they cannot themselves avoid.

The state traditionally has had the power to act in the best interests of
persons under legal disability, such as incompetents and children. Long
before autonomy and privacy were ever thought to apply to incompetents or
minors, the responsibility of parents toward their children was legally defined
as the responsibility to act in the best interests of the child. It was assumed in
the law that parents act in their children's best interests, and that the state
would not interfere until the state and the parents disagreed in extreme circumstances regarding some decision with potentially serious consequences for
the child. Such cases include those where Jehovah's Witness parents have
refused lifesaving blood transfusions for their minor children. (See Case #13.)
When the court rather than the family decides, the court has thus already
made a judgment about the unreasonableness of the family's proposed
course of action.

However, when the parent is the decision maker, the best interests test is
highly malleable and can take into account intangible factors of questionable
importance. For example, in cases where parents seek court permission for a
kidney transplant from an incompetent minor child to a competent sibling,
determinations of the best interests of the donor have on occasion taken into
account projected psychological trauma from the death of the sibling and the
psychological benefits of the unselfish act of donation. But the most common
application of the best interests standard mainly considers highly tangible
factors—physical and financial risks, benefits and harms—and makes use of
such generalizations as "Health is better than illness and life is preferable to
death."

The other legal standard, the substituted judgment standard, is radically
different. Substituted judgment begins with the premise that the decision
properly belongs to the incompetent patient by virtue of the rights of
autonomy and privacy. Nonetheless, another decision maker must be substituted because the patient is unable to decide. In legal terms, the patient has
the right to decide but is incompetent to exercise it. Thus the very premise of
the standard is a fiction—for an incompetent person cannot truly be said to

have the right to make medical decisions if the right can only be exercised by competent persons and does not exist apart from its exercise. This fictional quality makes substituted judgment highly controversial.

The substituted judgment standard requires the substituted decision maker to "don the mental mantle of the incompetent," as the *Saikewicz* court put it—that is, to make the decision the incompetent would have made if competent. In *Saikewicz* the court had to contend with evidence that most people with Saikewicz's illness choose treatment, but it invoked the doctrine of substituted judgment to decide that Saikewicz, if competent, would not have chosen treatment. The court defined its task as determining "how the right of an incompetent person to decline treatment might best be exercised so as to give the fullest possible expression to the character and circumstances of that individual." The court recognized that what the majority of reasonable people would choose could differ from what this particular incompetent person would choose, and proposed the following test:

[T]he decision in many cases such as this should be that which would be made by the incompetent person, if that person were competent, but taking into account the present and future incompetency of the individual as one of the factors which would necessarily enter into the decision-making process of the competent person.[56]

Both the *Quinlan* and the *Saikewicz* courts apply the substituted judgment standard—first determining the subjective wants and needs of the individual, and then determining how a reasonable person with those wants and needs would decide. However, these two cases involve different applications of this standard. In *Quinlan*, Karen's father could draw on her life as a *competent* person to determine her wants and needs. The court then found that "if Karen herself were miraculously lucid for an interval . . . and perceptive of her irreversible condition she could effectively decide upon discontinuance of the life-support apparatus, even if it meant the prospect of natural death."[57] In *Saikewicz*, the lack of evidence as to the *incompetent's* own likely choice forced the court to look to what is known about other people in his particular circumstances, not only to determine whether his right of privacy could protect both possible choices, but also to help determine what a reasonable person in his circumstances, with his needs and desires insofar as they are ascertainable, would actually decide.

The substituted judgment standard, whether formulated by the *Quinlan* or *Saikewicz* courts, contains questionable uses of the principle of autonomy. The object of the standard is to give effect to what a reasonable person, with the needs and desires of the incompetent patient and taking into account the patient's present and future incompetence, would decide. The New York

Court of Appeals, in its recent decision consolidating *Eichner* v. *Dillon* (the Brother Fox case, a *Quinlan*-type case) and *In re Storar* (a *Saikewicz*-type case), held that trying to determine what a never-competent patient would have decided if competent was like asking "If it snowed all summer, would it then be winter?"[58] Paul Ramsey points out (correctly we think) that formulating the problem, as the *Saikewicz* court does, as that of how to afford an incompetent person the status in law of a competent person with respect to the right to refuse treatment is "question-begging."[59] George Annas has also correctly argued that in the *Quinlan* and *Saikewicz* cases "use of the more objective 'best interests' tests would have been more logical,"[60] because of the difficulty of ascertaining the actual (subjective) wishes of the incompetents. Annas is questioning the basis of the substituted judgment doctrine—the ascription of autonomy to incompetent persons.

We agree that this ascription involves a purely fictional autonomy and that the doctrine can be questioned in two ways. First, it is conceptually dubious to treat the nonautonomous as if autonomous; and second, the actual desires and preferences of incompetents are generally unknowable. It is John Robertson's position, however, that it is *desirable* to treat incompetent persons as fictionally autonomous, despite the superficial absurdity of treating the incompetent in a way that "diverges" from his "actual situation," because "it is precisely such a divergence that respect for persons requires and which generally confers benefits on the incompetent. Eliminating this divergence would mean that we treat the incompetent in all respects as a nonthinking, nonchoosing, irrational being—in short, as a nonperson."[61]

The *Quinlan* and *Saikewicz* courts, in echoing Robertson, add the further dimension of ascription to the incompetent of the right of privacy—an extension that may provide even greater formal protection of the incompetent's interests and desires. The application of the privacy right makes clear that a choice of either treatment or nontreatment is potentially acceptable, thus freeing the decision maker to consider carefully all the individual and subjective features of each case, including those cases in which the incompetent has not expressed a relevant preference, without feeling bound by the best interests standard or even the reasonable person standard.

If it is desirable to treat incompetent persons as fictionally autonomous, a means of doing so must be devised that is not totally without meaning and is superior to those thus far developed. If the preferences of persons are competently expressed, then the persons are competent for all immediately relevant purposes; if their preferences are incompetently expressed, they cannot be given effect without destroying the notion of autonomy; and if patients cannot express preferences at all, it is not possible to determine directly whether they have any preferences and what they might be. Because of these confusions and unresolved problems, it is best to rely most heavily, and perhaps exclusively, on the nonmaleficence-based, best-interests standard rather than on the allegedly autonomy-based substituted judgment standard.

Classes of proxy decision makers

Four major classes of decision makers have been proposed and actually used in cases of withholding and ceasing treatment of incompetent patients: families, physicians, committees, and courts. We believe that families of patients should be given first priority as decision makers—subject to the aforementioned qualifications. They should receive the advice and counsel of physicians, who should appeal to the hospital committee or to the courts to protect the patient's interests if the patient might be harmed by a family decision. We are proposing a structure of serial decisionmaking, with the family as the presumptive agent when the patient cannot make the decision. The family's role should be primary because of the presumed identity of interests with the patient, and intimate knowledge of his or her wishes and wants. Nevertheless, that role should not be final or ultimate. If families do not know or seek the best interests of their members, the physician(s) should attempt to persuade the family to reach a different decision. Should their attempts fail, they should invoke institutional procedures established to resolve such conflicts—perhaps by appealing to the ethics committee in the hospital, or, if appropriate, to the courts.

Arguments for giving primacy to some decision maker other than the family usually appeal to the importance of fair and impartial decisions. Such arguments frequently hold that families cannot be fair and impartial, because prolonged extensions of a relative's life may put a serious strain on financial, emotional, and other familial resources. Thus, so these arguments go, fair and impartial judgments about the patient's interests, and actions in accord with the principle of nonmaleficence, require independent decision makers. Such arguments also depend on empirical determinations. Is it true, for example, that patients' interests will likely be disregarded by allowing family members to make decisions? In the absence of convincing evidence that the principles of nonmaleficence and beneficence will be more closely approximated by decision makers other than family members, there are good reasons for allowing family members to make the decisions.

The consultative role assigned to physicians and other health care professionals cannot, however, be reduced to the mere provision of information. In Robert Veatch's analysis, the physician should only present information for the patient's or family's consideration and then should withdraw if he or she cannot comply with their request. Underlying his recommendation is a worry about societal acceptance of the fallacy of the "generalization of expertise"—the view that those who have technical knowledge also have moral insight. While it is true, as Veatch argues, that technical knowledge does not entail moral insight, it does not preclude moral insight.[62] Physicians and other health care professionals should engage in moral discussions of the options with patients and their families, and they should have the right to withdraw from cases when they cannot in good conscience act on a second party's decisions for treatment or nontreatment. We will discuss such cases of conscientious refusal by physicians and other professionals in Chapter 8. It is important, however, to emphasize here that mere withdrawal is not always morally adequate if there is a high probability of consequences seriously detrimental to the patient's interests. The duty of nonmaleficence and the duty of beneficence require that physicians and other health care professionals actively pursue measures to prevent such consequences.

In the Quinlan case, the New Jersey Supreme Court recognized Joseph Quinlan as Karen Ann Quinlan's guardian and thus acknowledged his right to make decisions about her treatment, after consultation with physicians of his choice.[63] And yet the Court held that even when the guardian and attending physicians concur that life-support systems should be discontinued because there is no reasonable possibility that the patient will return to a cognitive, sapient state, they must consult the hospital "ethics committee." Because its designated function is merely to assess the patient's medical prognosis, the "ethics committee" is surely misnamed. More importantly, it is not clear why this additional layer of decisionmaking is required, unless there is either uncertainty about the prognosis or disagreement between family and physicians.

Expressly departing from the *Quinlan* decision, the Supreme Judicial Court of Massachusetts held in *Saikewicz* (see Case #18) that questions of life and death require the "process of detached but passionate investigation and decision that forms the ideal on which the judicial branch of government was created."[64] Achieving this ideal is the courts' responsibility and is "not to be entrusted to any other group." The Massachusetts court held that probate courts should make these decisions after considering all viewpoints and alternatives, including those of an ethics committee. Saikewicz, as noted above, was sixty-seven and had an I.Q. of 10 and a mental age of approximately two years and eight months. He had lived in state institutions since 1923. Only two members of his family could be located—two sisters who did not want to become involved.

In such cases, where there is no family, or when the family is not interested, it is necessary to find some other decision maker—either physicians, a committee, or the courts—although there may also be other alternatives. There is nothing inherently objectionable about an appeal to probate courts as decision makers in such cases, although there is no evidence to suppose that physicians and hospital committees, including laypersons, would be inadequate for most cases of this sort. The Massachusetts court may, however, have mandated a procedure for other sorts of cases even where the families are involved and where there is no evidence of prejudicial decision-making. If so, the outcome is unfortunate. The decision may have also established a procedural presumption in favor of treatment until the probate judge specifically authorizes cessation. As we have seen, there should be a substantive presumption in favor of treatment until it no longer serves the patient's best interests. However, a procedural requirement of treatment unless and until the probate judge decides otherwise may not serve the patient's best interests. Such a procedural requirement is not needed unless there are conflicts of interest or reason to suspect abuse, which might occur in the case of wards of the state and other vulnerable parties.[65]

Who, in conclusion, should make final decisions in life and death matters in cases where there is reason to think that the patient is in some important respect incompetent, uninformed, or acting involuntarily? The principles of nonmaleficence and beneficence require that incompetent patients be protected against various harms—just as the principle of autonomy requires that competent patients be allowed to make their own decisions. Procedures and processes should be designed to protect the incompetent's interests, although at best we can only expect imperfect procedural justice. Apart from evidence to the contrary, families may be presumed to have the patient's best interests at heart and to have a firmer grasp of those interests. Thus, they should be the primary decision makers for incompetent patients. Physicians and other health care professionals, however, remain morally responsible in these settings, not only to provide information, but to engage in moral counseling, to withdraw when they cannot satisfy their consciences, and to take active measures to prevent abuses of patients' interests. Health care professionals, hospital committees, and courts should function to protect the patient's best interests when there are conflicting judgments or evidence of abuse.

Notes

1. W. H. S. Jones, *Hippocrates I* (Cambridge, Mass.: Harvard University Press, 1923), p. 165. See also Ludwig Edelstein, *Ancient Medicine* (Baltimore: The Johns Hopkins University Press, 1967) and Albert R. Jonsen, "Do No Harm: Axiom of Medical Ethics," in *Philosophical Medical Ethics: Its Nature and*

Significance, eds. Stuart F. Spicker and H. Tristram Engelhardt, Jr. (Dordrecht, Holland: D. Reidel Publishing Co., 1977).

2. Hart, *The Concept of Law* (Oxford: Clarendon Press, 1961), p. 190.
3. Ross, *The Right and the Good* (Oxford: Clarendon Press, 1930), pp. 21–26, and Rawls, *A Theory of Justice* (Cambridge, Mass.: Harvard University Press, 1971), p. 114.
4. Frankena, *Ethics*, 2nd ed. (Englewood Cliffs, N.J.: Prentice-Hall, 1973), p. 47.
5. Alan Meisel and Loren H. Roth, "Must a Man Be His Cousin's Keeper?" *Hastings Center Report* 8 (October 1978): 5–6.
6. Ross, *The Right and the Good*, pp. 21–22.
7. See Joel Feinberg, *Social Philosophy* (Englewood Cliffs, N.J.: Prentice-Hall, 1973), pp. 25ff.
8. Bernard Gert, *The Moral Rules* (New York: Harper and Row, 1973), p. 125.
9. For a careful criticism of the priority of avoiding harm, see Nancy Davis, "The Priority of Avoiding Harm," in *Killing and Letting Die*, ed. Bonnie Steinbock (Englewood Cliffs, N.J.: Prentice-Hall, 1980), pp. 172–214.
10. See, for example, David Sperlinger, ed., *Animals in Research* (London: John Wiley and Sons, 1981).
11. Eric D'Arcy, *Human Acts* (Oxford: Clarendon Press, 1963), p. 121.
12. William L. Prosser, *Handbook of the Law of Torts*, 4th ed. (St. Paul, Minn.: West Publishing Co., 1971), pp. 145–46.
13. Quoted in Angela Roddy Holder, *Medical Malpractice Law* (New York: John Wiley and Sons, 1975), p. 42.
14. Albert R. Jonsen, "Do No Harm," pp. 27–41.
15. See David Granfield, *The Abortion Decision* (Garden City, N.Y.: Doubleday, 1969).
16. For some of the literature on double effect, see Joseph T. Mangan, S. J., "An Historical Analysis of the Principle of Double Effect," *Theological Studies* 10 (1949): 41–61; Richard A. McCormick, S. J., *Ambiguity in Moral Choice* (Milwaukee: Marquette University, 1973); Paul Ramsey and Richard A. McCormick, S. J., eds., *Doing Evil to Achieve Good: Moral Choice in Conflict Situations* (Chicago: Loyola University Press, 1978); Joseph M. Boyle, Jr., "Toward Understanding the Principle of Double Effect," *Ethics* 90 (July 1980): 527–38. For criticisms see Jonathan Bennett, "Whatever the Consequences," *Analysis* 26 (1966): 83–102; Philippa Foot, "The Problem of Abortion and the Doctrine of Double Effect," *Oxford Review* 5 (1967): 5–15; and Susan Nicholson, *Abortion and the Roman Catholic Church, JRE Studies in Religious Ethics*, II (Knoxville, Tennessee: Religious Ethics, Inc., 1978).
17. See critical literature mentioned in note 16.
18. For the emphasis on proportionality, see McCormick, *Ambiguity in Moral Choice*; for the emphasis on intention, see Charles Fried, *Right and Wrong* (Cambridge, Mass.: Harvard University Press, 1978).
19. It is a mistake to view these expressions as synonymous, though the present statement appears to.
20. James Rachels, "Active and Passive Euthanasia," *New England Journal of Medicine* 292 (January 9, 1975): 78–80. For valuable discussions of the distinction between killing and letting die, see Bonnie Steinbock, ed., *Killing and*

Letting Die; and John Ladd, ed. *Ethical Issues Relating to Life and Death* (New York: Oxford University Press, 1979).

21. Richard L. Trammell, "Saving Life and Taking Life," *Journal of Philosophy* 72 (1975): 131–37.
22. Gilbert Meilaender, "The Distinction Between Killing and Allowing to Die," *Theological Studies* 37 (1976): 467–70.
23. See John Rawls, "Two Concepts of Rules," *Philosophical Review* 64 (1955): 3–32.
24. G. J. Hughes, S. J., "Killing and Letting Die," *The Month* 236 (1975): 42–45.
25. David Louisell, "Euthanasia and Biothanasia: On Dying and Killing," *Linacre Quarterly* 40 (1973): 234–58.
26. Paul Ramsey, *Ethics at the Edges of Life* (New Haven: Yale University Press, 1978), pp. 306–7.
27. James Rachels, "Medical Ethics and the Rule Against Killing: Comments on Professor Hare's Paper," in *Philosophical Medical Ethics: Its Nature and Significance*, eds. S. F. Spicker and H. T. Engelhardt, Jr., p. 65.
28. Rachels, "Active and Passive Euthanasia," pp. 78–80.
29. For an important debate about these issues, see Yale Kamisar, "Some Non-religious Views Against Proposed 'Mercy-killing' Legislation," *Minnesota Law Review* 42 (1958), and Glanville Williams, "'Mercy-killing' Legislation—A Rejoinder," *Minnesota Law Review* 43 (1958), reprinted in *Contemporary Issues in Bioethics*, 2nd. ed., eds. Tom Beauchamp and LeRoy Walters (Belmont, Calif.: Wadsworth Publishing Co., 1982), pp. 324–37.
30. We owe most of this argument to James Rachels.
31. Charles Fried, "Rights and Health Care—Beyond Equity and Efficiency," *New England Journal of Medicine* 293 (July 31, 1975): 245.
32. For a discussion of this case, see Paige Mitchell, *Act of Love: The Killing of George Zygmaniak* (New York: Knopf, 1976).
33. See Paul Ramsey, *Ethics at the Edges of Life*, p. 217; Robert Veatch, *Death, Dying, and the Biological Revolution* (New Haven, Conn.: Yale University Press, 1976), p. 97.
34. Ramsey, *Ethics at the Edges of Life*, pp. 195, 214, 216; cf. Ramsey, *The Patient as Person*, pp. 161–64.
35. Antony Flew, "The Principle of Euthanasia," *Euthanasia and the Right to Death: The Case of Voluntary Euthanasia*, ed. A. B. Downing (London: Peter Owen, 1969), pp. 30–48.
36. For other discussions by the authors of the main ideas in this section on Killing and Letting Die, see Tom L. Beauchamp, "A Reply to Rachels on Active and Passive Euthanasia," in *Ethical Issues in Death and Dying*, eds. Tom L. Beauchamp and Seymour Perlin (Englewood Cliffs, N.J.: Prentice-Hall, 1978), pp. 246–48; James Childress, "To Kill or Let Die," in *Bioethics and Human Rights*, eds. Elsie Bandman and Bertram Bandman (Boston: Little, Brown, 1978), pp. 128–31; Childress, *Priorities in Biomedical Ethics* (Philadelphia: The Westminister Press, 1981), chap. 2.
37. See Ramsey, *Ethics at the Edges of Life*, and Veatch, *Death, Dying and the Biological Revolution*.
38. See Ramsey, *Ethics at the Edges of Life*, p. 153, and Veatch, *Death, Dying and the Biological Revolution*, Chapter 3. For an analysis of these books, as well as

some other recent literature, see James F. Childress, "Ethical Issues in Death and Dying," *Religious Studies Review* 4 (July 1978): 180–88.

39. See Ramsey, *The Patient as Person*, p. 120.
40. Gerald Kelly, S. J., "The Duty to Preserve Life," *Theological Studies* 12 (December 1951): 550.
41. For the best statement of the issues in determining death, see President's Commission for the Study of Ethical Problems in Medicine and Biomedical and Behavioral Research, *Defining Death: A Report on the Medical, Legal and Ethical Issues in the Determination of Death* (Washington, D.C.: U.S. Government Printing Office, 1981).
42. *Superintendent of Belchertown State School* v. *Saikewicz*, Mass. 370 N.E. 2d 417 (1977), at 428.
43. 51 Misc. 2d 616, 273 N. Y. S. 2d 624 (Sup. Ct. 1966).
44. Albert R. Jonsen and Michael J. Garland, "A Moral Policy for Life/Death Decisions in the Intensive Care Nursery," in *Ethics of Newborn Intensive Care*, eds. Albert R. Jonsen and Michael J. Garland (Berkeley: University of California, Institute of Governmental Studies, 1976), p. 148.
45. Engelhardt, "Ethical Issues in Aiding the Death of Young Children," in *Beneficent Euthanasia*, ed. Marvin Kohl (Buffalo, N.Y.: Prometheus Books, 1975), p. 187. Emphasis added.
46. See R. B. Zachary, "Ethical Social Aspects of Treatment of Spina Bifida," *Lancet* 2 (1968): 274–76; John M. Freeman, "To Treat or Not to Treat: Ethical Dilemmas of Treating the Infant with a Myelomeningocele," *Clinical Neurosurgery* 20 (1973): 134–46; John Lorber, "Selective Treatment of Myelomeningocele: To Treat or Not to Treat?" *Pediatrics* 53 (1974): 307–8; several articles in Chester Swinyard, ed., *Decision Making and the Defective Newborn* (Springfield, Ill.: Charles C Thomas, 1978); and articles on "Ethical Perspectives on the Care of Infants" and "Public Policy and Procedural Questions" in the *Encyclopedia of Bioethics*.
47. *Superintendent of Belchertown State School* v. *Saikewicz*, Mass. 370 N. E. 2d 417 (1977).
48. Ramsey, *Ethics at the Edges of Life*, p. 155.
49. *Ibid.*, p. 165.
50. McCormick, "The Quality of Life, the Sanctity of Life," *Hastings Center Report* 8 (February 1978): 32. See also "To Save or Let Die: The Dilemma of Modern Medicine," *Journal of the American Medical Association* 229 (1974): 172–76.
51. Ramsey, *Ethics at the Edges of Life*, p. 172.
52. Jonsen and Garland, "A Moral Policy for Life/Death Decisions," p. 148.
53. Veatch, *Death, Dying and the Biological Revolution*, p. 112.
54. John Rawls, *A Theory of Justice*, pp. 85–86.
55. See Duff, "On Deciding the Use of the Family Commons," *Developmental Disabilities: Psychologic and Social Implications*, eds. Daniel Bergsma and Ann E. Pulver (New York: Alan R. Liss, 1976), pp. 73–84.
56. *Superintendent of Belchertown State School* v. *Saikewicz*, Mass. 370 N. E. 2d 417 (1977).
57. *In the matter of Karen Quinlan* 70 N. J. 10, 355 A.2d 647 (1976), at 663.

58. George Annas, "Help from the Dead: The Cases of Brother Fox and John Storar," *Hastings Center Report* 11 (June 1981): 19–20.

59. Paul Ramsey, "The *Saikewicz* Precedent: What's Good for an Incompetent Patient?," *Hastings Center Report* 8 (December 1978): 39.

60. George Annas, "Reconciling *Quinlan* and *Saikewicz*: Decision Making for the Terminally Ill Incompetent," *American Journal of Law and Medicine* 4 (1979): 367.

61. John Robertson, "Organ Donations by Incompetents and the Substituted Judgment Doctrine," *Columbia Law Review* 76 (1976): 65.

62. Veatch, "Generalization of Expertise," *Hastings Center Studies* 1 (May 1973): 29–40.

63. *In the Matter of Quinlan* 70 N. J. 10 (1976).

64. *Superintendent of Belchertown State School* v. *Saikewicz*, Mass. 370 N.E. 2d 417 (1977).

65. See Richard A. McCormick and Andre E. Hellegers, "The Specter of Joseph Saikewicz: Mental Incompetence and the Law," *America* (1978): 257–60. Contrast George J. Annas, "The Incompetent's Right to Die: The Case of Joseph Saikewicz," *Hastings Center Report* 8 (February 1978): 21–23. Annas holds that the adversary proceeding the court recommends is the most likely way to get a correct resolution of the difficult questions about a patient's interests and will. For further debate about such issues, see Cynthia B. Wong and Judith P. Swazey, eds., *Dilemmas of Dying: Policies and Procedures for Decisions Not to Treat* (Boston: G.K. Hall, 1981).

5

The Principle of Beneficence

The concept of beneficence

Morality requires not only that we treat persons autonomously and that we refrain from harming them, but also that we contribute to their welfare, including their health. Such beneficial actions are commonly placed under the heading of beneficence. While there probably are no sharp breaks or transition points on the continuum from the noninfliction of harm to the production of benefit, the principle of beneficence is generally thought to be more far-reaching than the principle of nonmaleficence because it requires positive steps to help others. Nonmaleficence, as we saw in the previous chapter, refers to the *noninfliction* of harm on others. "Nonmaleficence" is sometimes used to refer more broadly to the *prevention* of harm and also to the *removal* of harmful conditions. However, because prevention and removal generally require positive acts to assist others, we reserve the term "beneficence" for actions involving prevention of harm, removal of harm, and provision of benefit, while "nonmaleficence" is restricted to the noninfliction of harm.

In ordinary English, the term "beneficence" includes among its meanings mercy, kindness, and charity. However, in this chapter, beneficence will be treated as a *duty*, and thus as distinct from mere mercy, kindness, or charity. In its most general form, the principle of beneficence asserts the duty to help others further their important and legitimate interests. The duty to *confer* benefits and actively to prevent and remove harms is important in biomedical and behavioral contexts, but equally important is the duty to *balance* possible goods against the possible harms of an action. It is thus appropriate to distinguish two principles under the general heading of beneficence: The first principle requires the *provision* of benefits (including the prevention and removal of harm), and the second requires a *balancing* of benefits and harms. The first may be called the principle of positive beneficence, while the second is already familiar to us as a version of the principle of utility.

The principle of positive beneficence

Firmly established in the histories of ethics, medicine, and public health is the belief that the failure to benefit others when in a position to do so—and not simply the failure to avoid harm—violates social or professional duties. The Hippocratic tradition requires that physicians benefit patients, as well as not inflict harm, and one major justification of biomedical research is the production of positive benefits for society. Preventive medicine and active public health interventions provide other obvious examples. For instance, once methods of preventing yellow fever and cowpox were discovered in early modern medicine, it was universally agreed that it would be immoral not to take positive steps to establish preventive programs. To use a more current example, research in gene therapy is said to be justified on the basis of its promise to provide a therapy more beneficial than its alternatives (a cure that is genotypic as well as phenotypic).

In the practice of medicine perhaps the clearest cases of acting on the duty of beneficence involve extremely dependent patients who need social assistance. Case #30 in the Appendix provides an example. Here a bill has been introduced in a state legislature that would establish community-based homes for the care and education of the mentally retarded. The bill is intended to provide medical facilities for thousands of persons who live in unpleasant, impoverished, and medically unsatisfactory facilities. The problem of beneficence in this case reduces to the problem of how, in a situation of scarcity, goods and services should be distributed in society, if they should be distributed at all. Controversies thus arise concerning how beneficent society can *afford* to be. Here allocation rules and decisions quite properly function to restrain or at least to place limits on beneficence. Such problems should be situated under the umbrella of distributive justice—a topic considered in Chapter 6.

Because beneficence potentially demands extensive positive acts, such as generosity, some moral philosophers have argued that it is *virtuous* and morally *ideal* to act beneficently, but not a moral *duty* to do so. They have treated beneficent actions as akin to acts of charity and acts of conscience that exceed duty: Beneficent acts are laudable, but persons are not morally deficient if they fail to produce benefits, and therefore we do not have even a prima facie duty of positive beneficence. From this perspective, the positive benefiting of others is based on personal ideals beyond the call of duty and thus is supererogatory rather than obligatory. There is merit in this view, since we are not *always* morally required to benefit persons, even if we are in a position to do so. For example, we are not morally required to perform all possible acts of charity. However, the line between a duty and a moral ideal is not always easy to establish, and beneficence has proven to be the most troublesome moral principle to place firmly in one of these two categories (see Chapter 8). In what respects and within what limits, then, is beneficence correctly described as a duty?

Public support of biomedical research shows that we think some beneficent actions are demanded by social arrangements and the duties that flow from those arrangements. The obligation to benefit members of society, including future generations, is often cited as the primary justification for scientific research. For example, children who serve as research subjects often will not benefit individually from the research. Yet many believe that some research involving children, at least that which presents minimal or only slightly more than minimal risk, is justified. Children are often the only subjects who can be used to study childhood disorders and development in order to help other children, and research on infants has proven highly beneficial in learning about correct levels of fluids, nutriments, and oxygen in the treatment of newborns. This knowledge is generally of benefit only to succeeding generations.

In the Willowbrook case (see Case #27), we find precisely this justification of beneficence to future generations. It was advanced by those who conducted hepatitis research involving institutionalized and mentally retarded children. Willowbrook administrators argued that successful research would eventuate in generalizable knowledge about hepatitis that could benefit all potential victims of the disease. While it is controversial whether these children should have been involved in the research at all, concerted social actions intended to benefit others are sometimes morally justified, even if they involve certain risks.

Still, it is one thing to maintain that actions or programs are morally *justified* and quite another to maintain that they are morally *required* on grounds of some prima facie duty. Thus, we have not yet demonstrated that the principle of positive beneficence establishes duties. Several moral philosophers have proposed ways to do so.

A first proposal gives only weak support for beneficence as a duty. Frankena has argued that, "Even if one holds that beneficence is not a *requirement* of morality but something supererogatory and morally *good*, one is still regarding beneficence as an important part of morality—as desirable if not required."[1] Although quite correct, this contention is of little assistance for our purposes. No one denies that beneficent acts, such as the donation of a kidney to a stranger, are morally praiseworthy when they *exceed* what is morally required. If a man gave more money to a charity than he had pledged, he would obviously have performed a morally praiseworthy and generous action. Little is added by noting that beneficence forms an important "part of morality" when the issue is whether some different "part of morality" makes beneficence a *duty*. Frankena's observation can, however, be reconstructed for our purposes as follows: To say we "ought to do" something in general may mean that we ought to do it because it is a *moral* duty, or it may mean that we ought to do it because of a *self-imposed* requirement, such as a rule of charity.[2] This schema leaves open whether beneficence is a strict moral duty, or supererogatory, or a strict duty in some cases while not in others.[3]

A second and more pertinent proposal, offered by Marcus Singer,[4] is consistent with but moves beyond Frankena's thesis. Singer argues that beneficent actions spring from a moral requirement to perform acts that avoid undesirable consequences—a requirement *not* so strong as to make it obligatory to produce good consequences. Thus, loss must be avoided, but there is no duty to produce positive benefit. This approach has been defended in a modified and more sweeping form by Peter Singer, who speaks of "the obligation to assist"[5] and relies heavily on a distinction between preventing evil and promoting good:

I begin with the assumption that suffering and death from lack of food, shelter, and medical care are bad. . . . I shall not argue for this view. People can hold all sorts of eccentric positions, and perhaps from some of them it would not follow that death by starvation is in itself bad. . . .

My next point is this: if it is in our power to prevent something bad from happening, without thereby sacrificing anything of comparable moral importance, we ought, morally, to do it. By "without sacrificing anything of comparable moral importance" I mean without causing anything else comparably bad to happen, or something that is wrong in itself, or failing to promote some moral good. . . . This principle seems almost as uncontroversial as the last one. It requires us only to prevent what is bad, and not to promote what is good. . . .[6]

This argument may at first appear to be an instance of the nonmaleficence-grounded thesis that society may not be able to impose affirmative duties to promote the good, but may legitimately impose negative injunctions not to cause harm. For example, we would generally agree that a corporation creating health hazards because of poor pollution-control devices has an obligation to cease such harmful activities and that this obligation is much stronger than any corporate obligation to promote social welfare—*if* the corporation has the latter obligation at all. But this distinction does not quite capture Singer's strategy. He argues that requirements of *positive* actions can be grounded in the "*prevention* of what is bad," without pre-supposing a broader duty to promote what is good, e.g., in the form of government-sponsored exercise programs to improve health.

While Peter Singer may be correct in maintaining that at least some moral duties rest on his principles, this argument leaves us unclear both as to the *scope* of the duty to be beneficent and as to the moral *justification* of this duty. Singer's conception of the scope of the obligation to be beneficent is captured by his contention that we must always prevent what is bad unless something of "comparable moral importance" must be given up by per-forming the action. In effect, Singer argues that we must always act to prevent harm, unless a stronger prima facie moral duty conflicts with and overrides an opportunity to provide such a benefit.

So construed, this argument is unrealistic and overly demanding. As Michael Slote has pointed out:

> It also seems probable that there are limits to our obligations to help others by preventing harms and evils. To me at least it sometimes seems mistaken to suppose that one has an obligation to go and spend one's life helping sick and starving people in India or elsewhere. Part of the reason for this may be that it can at times seem perfectly understandable, from a moral standpoint, that one should want to lead one's own life and develop one's own plans and potentialities independently of what may be going on, for better or worse, with others outside one's own family. In other words, it can sometimes seem somewhat unfair or morally arbitrary that one's moral freedom to choose one's own special kind of fulfillment in life should be abrogated by the existence of states of affairs for which one was in no way responsible and which would tend not to enter into one's life plans. . . .
>
> It is only when something like a basic life plan has to be sacrificed in order to prevent some evil that we feel any genuine hesitation to make such prevention obligatory. . . .
>
> And so I am saying that the following principle may be true:
>
>> It is not morally wrong to omit doing an act if (it is reasonably believed that) doing it would seriously interfere with one's basic life style or with the fulfillment of one's basic life plans—as long as the life style or plans themselves involve no wrongs of commission. . . .

[And we could] add a *principle of positive obligation* to the effect that:

> One has an obligation to prevent serious evil or harm when one can do so
> without seriously interfering with one's life plans or style and without doing
> any wrongs of commission.[7]

There may be ambiguities and even serious moral problems in Slote's
argument, but it is hard to imagine that moral rules demand more than his
principles suggest. Of course individuals might accept a moral *ideal* of the
sort proposed by Singer. Society might even be more advantaged by attempting to make Singer's proposals an obligatory part of morality, but this
outcome is far from obvious, given what we know about our actual abilities
to live up to such high ideals.

Since the publication of the first edition of our book, Singer has attempted
to take account of the objection that his principle of beneficence sets "too
high a standard." He has come to agree that in the abstract the principle may
well be too demanding. To the question "What level of assistance should we
advocate?," Singer now offers a more explicit answer:

> Any figure will be arbitrary, but there may be something to be said for a round
> percentage of one's income like, say, 10%—more than a token donation, yet not so
> high as to be beyond all but saints. . . . No figure should be advocated as a rigid
> minimum or maximum. . . . [But] by any reasonable ethical standards this is the
> minimum we ought to do, and we do wrong if we do less.[8]

It is difficult to assess a percentage of income as an expression of one's
obligation, especially in light of conditions we advocate below. But Singer's
revised thesis certainly attempts to set additional limits on the scope of the
duty of beneficence—limits that reduce required risk and impact on the
agent's life plans.

The duty of beneficence is not strong enough in our view to require that
the passerby who is a poor swimmer try to swim a hundred yards to rescue
someone who is drowning. If he does nothing—for example, fails even to run
several yards to alert a lifeguard—his omissions are morally culpable. From
this and many similar examples, we would argue that, apart from special
moral relationships such as contracts (which we consider later), X has a duty
of beneficence toward Y only if each of the following conditions is satisfied:
(1) Y is at risk of significant loss or damage, (2) X's action is needed to
prevent this loss, (3) X's action would probably prevent it, (4) X's action
would not present significant risk to X, and (5) the benefit that Y will
probably gain outweighs any harms that X is likely to suffer.[9] Such conditions indicate when X's general duty of beneficence becomes a specific duty
of beneficence toward Y.

While we seem clearly to have such a duty of beneficence, we also have some discretion about discharging it. The duty is indeterminate in that it rarely requires that we specifically benefit Y. As we saw in our discussion of rights in Chapter 2, Mill and Kant judged beneficence an imperfect obligation rather than a perfect obligation; we are usually free to practice it as we see fit. Nevertheless, if our argument is correct, under the five conditions identified above, a person has a specific duty of beneficence toward Y, even apart from special moral relationships such as promises or roles. Only if one accepts greater risks or disruption to one's life plans is the act beyond the call of duty (a supererogatory action, which we analyze in Chapter 8).

The fourth condition above is critical because it enables us to avoid the problems that Peter Singer encounters and to limit the scope of Slote's duty of beneficence. Although it is difficult to specify "significant risk," the point is clear. Even if X's action would probably save Y's life, and would meet all conditions except the fourth, the action would not be obligatory on grounds of beneficence. Let us now consider two cases that test these theses about the demands of beneficence. In Case #26, which we introduced in Chapter 4, Robert McFall was diagnosed as having aplastic anemia, which is usually fatal, but his physician believed that a bone marrow transplant from a genetically compatible donor could increase his chances of surviving one year from 25 percent to 40–60 percent. David Shimp, McFall's cousin, was the only relative willing to undergo the first test, which established tissue compatibility. However, Shimp then refused to undergo the second test to measure genetic compatibility. Clearly the first two conditions were met for a duty of beneficence, independent of special moral relationships. The third condition was not as clearly satisfied, because McFall's chance of surviving a year would have only increased from 25 percent to 40–60 percent. These are the kinds of contingencies that make it difficult to determine whether beneficence demands a particular course of action. Shimp himself was especially concerned about the fourth condition, although most medical commentators contended that the risks were minimal. The necessary 100–150 punctures of the pelvic bone can be painlessly performed under anesthesia, and the major risk is a 1-in-10,000 chance of death from anesthesia. Bone marrow regenerates itself. Shimp, however, believed that the risks were greater ("What if I become a cripple?") and that they outweighed the probability and magnitude of benefit to McFall, even though there was no medical evidence to support his fears.

By contrast, a *clear* example of a duty of beneficence can easily be created by slightly modifying the *Tarasoff* case (#1), with which we began Chapter 1. The psychiatrist in this case learned of his patient's intention to kill a woman, but maintained confidentiality and did not attempt to warn her. Suppose we modify the actual circumstances in this case in order to create the following hypothetical situation: A psychiatrist has told his patient that he does not believe in keeping any information confidential. The patient agrees to treatment under these conditions and subsequently reveals his intention to kill a woman. The psychiatrist may now either remain aloof or make some move to protect the woman (by calling her or the police). What does morality demand of the psychiatrist in this case? It seems to us that only a remarkably narrow view of moral duty would hold that the psychiatrist is not under *any* duty to contact the woman. The psychiatrist is not at risk (and, moreover, will suffer virtually no inconvenience or interference with his life plan). If morality does not demand this much beneficence, it is hard to see how morality creates any duties at all.

Moreover, even if there is a competing duty such as the protection of confidentiality, beneficence may outweigh it—a rather sure indication that beneficence is not purely a principle of supererogation. For example, epidemiologists often must use confidential hospital records in order to trace patterns of disease. The reason for delving into confidential material is to prevent the spread of the disease, thus protecting the public health. If our "duty" to protect the public health were merely supererogatory, we would be far more reluctant to override a duty of confidentiality.

Both the general duty of beneficence and specific duties of beneficence of the sort just described have been justified in several different ways. Utilitarians such as Mill recognize (at least) a limited duty of beneficence because it would produce the greatest good for the greatest number, and deontologists such as Kant and Ross also recognize a duty of beneficence—Kant because it is required by the categorical imperative, and Ross because it is a clear part of common morality. In a more complex interpretation of the foundation of beneficence, David Hume argued that the duty to benefit others arises from our social interactions:

All our obligations to do good to society seem to imply something reciprocal. I receive the benefits of society, and therefore ought to promote its interests. . . .[10]

This view, which might be called the reciprocity theory of moral obligations, implies that we incur obligations to help others because we have voluntarily received, or at least will voluntarily receive, beneficial assistance from them. If a person had not incurred such obligations, then presumably he or she would have *no* duty to act beneficently, as in the case of a hypothetical, isolated individual—"an island unto himself." The idea that we can actually be free of indebtedness to our parents, to researchers in medicine and public health, to educators, and to other benefactors, is as hopelessly removed from the reality of the moral life as the idea that we can always act autonomously without affecting others by our actions. One justification, then, for the claim that beneficence is a duty resides in an implicit contract underlying the necessary give-and-take of social life. Such a view might be restated in terms of John Rawls's duty of "fair play."[11] It might even be correct to say that Hume's account *reduces* the duty of beneficence to a duty of fair play. While this reductionist thesis is too narrow, reciprocity of fair play is one appropriate way to root beneficence in ethical theory.

If we think about the beneficence of health care professionals in terms of reciprocity and fair play, we can see both the possibilities and the limitations of this approach. Health care professionals are not "self-made." They are indebted to society in various ways, so much so that some have interpreted their indebtedness as a "covenant" with society. Codes of medical ethics traditionally have viewed physicians as independent, self-sufficient philanthropists whose beneficence appears almost a matter of giving gifts. Such codes have sometimes distinguished between physicians' duties to their patients and obligations to their teachers and colleagues. For example, according to the Hippocratic Oath, the physician's duties to patients represent philanthropy and service, while his or her obligations to teachers represent debts incurred in becoming a physician. But in the contemporary world, the professional is greatly indebted to society (e.g., for education and privileges) and to patients, past and present (e.g., for research and "practice"). Because of this indebtedness, the medical profession's duty of beneficence is misconstrued as mere philanthropy. It is rooted in what William May calls the "reciprocity of giving and receiving."[12] Following May, it may be more appropriate to call this a covenant than a contract, because the relationship does *not* have a specific *quid pro quo*. It certainly creates an obligation to patients and to society, but the terms of that obligation are rarely specific. The professional usually has some discretion about discharging the obligation, and it is possible to have an obligation to Y, without having specific obligations to do a, b, and c. Our obligations to our parents are often of this nature. That there is an obligation often cannot be doubted; however, the scope and content of that obligation may be disputed, particularly the specific actions it requires.

Even if our general duty of beneficence derives in part from reciprocity and fair play, our specific duties of beneficence often derive from special moral relationships with persons, frequently through institutional roles. These duties stem particularly from our implicit and explicit commitments—for instance, making promises and accepting roles and positions that require beneficent actions—as well as from our previous wrongful actions and reception of benefits. To focus on the most relevant categories, we often ought to act to benefit someone either because of our "station and its duties" or because our promises require such acts. Thus, the professional lifeguard on duty has a strong obligation to try to rescue a drowning swimmer, even at considerable personal risk, just as a physician has a strong duty to accept some health risks in meeting the needs of his or her patients. We might also believe that the father had a stronger obligation to donate a kidney to his dying daughter (in Case #2) than Shimp had to donate bone marrow to his dying cousin (Case #26). The claims that we make upon each other as parents, spouses, and friends similarly stem not only from interpersonal encounters but also from fixed rules, roles, and relations that constitute a matrix of obligations and duties. John Reeder even claims that "the benefi-cence which is proper to the therapeutic role is a duty of *justice*."[13]

The aim of the relationship between health care professionals and patients, for example, is to benefit the latter. In the Hippocratic Oath, the physician makes a commitment to "come for the benefit of the sick" and to "apply dietetic measures for the benefit of the sick according to my ability and judgment." In the Hippocratic work *Epidemics*, the fundamental injunction is "help, or at least do no harm."[14] According to the AMA, its "body of ethical statements" was developed "primarily for the benefit of the patient," and the first principle is that "a physician shall be dedicated to providing competent medical service with compassion and respect for human dignity." Human needs, actual or perceived, usually form the basis of this benefiting relationship. However, these actual or felt needs are not enough in most circumstances to impose either a legal or a moral duty of service on the health care professional. The AMA Code affirms that "A physician shall in the provision of appropriate patient care, except in emergencies, be free to choose whom to serve. . . ." From a legal standpoint, both the patient (or the patient's representative) and the health care professional must assent to the relationship; the former's need is not sufficient to establish a contract for service. (When we examine paternalism later in this chapter, we will see how the principle of autonomy limits and constrains beneficence.)

Of course, we must distinguish different roles a physician or other health care professional may occupy. If a physician is in private practice, he or she has no legal duty to see patients even in emergencies where no other physician is available. Thus, a physician has no legal duty to stop at the scene of an automobile accident or to answer affirmatively when the manager of a restaurant or theater asks "Is there a doctor in the house?" But a physician on duty in a hospital emergency room may not refuse to care for a patient.

From a moral standpoint, however, the principle of beneficence some-times creates a duty where the law is silent. A request for help or a need for help, as in the case of an automobile accident, imposes a moral responsi-bility on a health care professional to respond with his or her special knowledge and skills, as long as there is only negligible or minimal risk and no major interference in lifestyle.[15] This final clause restricts the scope of the obligation: The health care professional would not be expected to climb a dangerous mountain to provide aid for a stricken climber or to go several hundred miles to care for someone in need, although he or she would merit our praise for such voluntary actions. A physician is not morally obligated to be a "Good Samaritan," but only what Judith Thomson calls "a minimally decent Samaritan."[16]

Because of the uncertainties surrounding the principle of beneficence, we have examined its possible meanings and its possible sources. As a principle it applies to both society and individuals, but often what it requires, espe-cially in terms of individual risk-taking, hinges on other duties, such as fair play, promise-keeping, and role commitments. Even though the distinction between beneficence and nonmaleficence is not always clear, the importance of the distinction is evident. It is accurate to say that the duty of nonmale-ficence is more independent of roles and relations, allows less discretion, and, in general, requires greater risk-taking than the duty of beneficence, which requires positive actions. For example, our duty not to harm others must be observed in all roles, but some duties to benefit others depend strictly on our roles.

An example of the significant difference in perspective between the duties of nonmaleficence and beneficence is found in debates about abortion. Traditionally, as we noted in the previous chapter, the pregnant woman's duty of nonmaleficence toward the fetus implied that she could not kill the fetus if the fetus were viewed as a human being from the moment of conception. Furthermore, she might have to undertake serious risks in order to avoid harming the fetus. But thinking about abortion in terms of bene-ficence offers another perspective. Even if the fetus is viewed as a human being from the moment of conception, the extent of the pregnant woman's obligations of beneficence to the fetus may be unclear or controversial. For example, perhaps she does not have an obligation to assume great risks or even to support the fetus for nine months. She may even have a moral right to sever the relationship with the fetus, even though the fetus will probably die as a result.[17] Some of these conflicts emerge sharply in Case #24, in which a woman was compelled to undergo a caesarean section in order to protect the life and health of her baby.

The principle of utility

Those engaged in medical practice and research know that risks of harm constantly must be weighed against possible benefits. The requirement that there should be such a weighing assumes that risks of harm and possible benefits can be measured and balanced. The principle that requires us to bring about the greatest possible balance of value (benefit) over disvalue (harm) is one way of formulating the principle of utility, especially as it has been understood by act utilitarians. This principle assumes that we not only have an obligation to be positively beneficent as well as nonmaleficent, but that we also have a moral duty to weigh and balance possible benefits against possible harms in order to maximize benefits and minimize risks of harm. As we saw in Chapter 2, both utilitarians and deontologists need a principle of utility as a principle for balancing benefits and harms, balancing benefits against alternative benefits, and balancing harms against alternative harms. The moral life does not permit us simply to produce benefits and avoid harms, and thus a balancing principle is essential.

This principle of utility is obviously not identical to the principle of utility exalted to preeminence by utilitarians. It thus should not be construed as the only principle or as one that justifies or overrides all other principles. Rather, it is one principle among others; all four of the principles advanced in Chapters 3–6 specify prima facie obligations, and any principle can compete with any other for priority in a particular case. (As we noted in Chapter 2, all four principles *can* in theory be derived from the principle of utility, but can be derived from deontological sources as well. Because we rejected act utilitarianism, while finding rule utilitarianism congenial for the derivation of our four principles, the following clarification is in order: The principle of utility now under discussion can be derived from the principle of utility relied upon by rule utilitarians, but in our system it is only one prima facie principle among others.)

The principle of utility advanced in this chapter should not be construed so that it allows the interests of society as a whole to override individual interests and rights. In the context of medical research, for example, a balancing principle might seem to dictate that dangerous research on human subjects could be undertaken, and even *ought* to be undertaken, when the prospect of substantial benefit to society or other individuals outweighs the danger of the research to the individual. But in our system utility merely competes with considerations of autonomy, nonmaleficence, and justice; it does not always triumph.

Thus, if an act conforms to the requirements of the principle of beneficence, it does not follow that the act is morally justified. When a beneficent act entails risk, as is common, considerations of nonmaleficence are unavoidable. Actions such as research on diseases that provide major social benefits frequently transgress the limits suggested by nonmaleficence alone, for they present significant risks of harm. For this reason the principles of beneficence and nonmaleficence jointly suggest a moral requirement of risk-benefit analysis. If the risks of the procedure are reasonable in relation to the anticipated benefits (however precisely the determination of reasonableness is to be made), then the action is morally permissible. At least this is so with respect to the two principles of beneficence and nonmaleficence in isolation from other moral considerations. Moral problems could arise if a risk-benefit assessment were not supplemented by considerations of autonomy and just distribution of the harms and benefits. As we shall see in Chapter 6, the patterns by which risks and benefits are distributed establish independent limits on the use of risk-benefit calculations.

However, abstract disputes about the priority of principles tend to function in a vacuum far removed from the actual dilemmas of the moral life. On most occasions when we might question whether individual rights are being sacrificed to some larger public interest, we will be uncertain about the correct answer. There can be no definitive formulation as to appropriate risks and benefits of, for example, human subjects of research and of society; and so the application and implementation of the principle of utility calls for a sensitive and discriminating analysis of the issues raised in particular cases. For example, consider cases of defective newborns with diseases such as myelomeningocele. These cases involve issues about whether society's beneficence should extend to paying medical costs for such children and whether surgeons have an obligation to operate (rooted in beneficence) when there is a chance of a favorable outcome, but a greater likelihood either of nonsurvival or of survival with multiple defects, including severe mental retardation. Assessing costs and benefits is inescapable in each case.

Costs and benefits

The principles of positive beneficence and utility are applied to moral problems when questions arise about the comparison and relative weights of costs—including risks—and benefits. Questions about the most suitable medical treatment are commonly decided by reference to likely benefits and costs, including risks, and questions about the justification of research involving human subjects are resolved, in part, by showing that the risks are outweighed by the probable benefits. Members of institutional review committees, and certainly the investigators conducting the research, are expected to describe the risks and benefits for potential subjects prior to the subjects' consent to participation in the research. Investigators are customarily required not only to *array* the risks and benefits but also to determine whether the benefits *outweigh* the risks imposed on subjects.[18] All such applications of the principle of beneficence to research can, with only slight reformulation, be applied to the treatment of patients and to the delivery of health services.

The nature of costs, risks, and benefits

"Costs" are popularly conceived in financial terms, but in cost-benefit analysis a cost can be any negative value that detracts from human health and welfare. In biomedical contexts the specific costs most often mentioned are not quantifable and already ascertained financial costs; rather, they are risks to health or welfare. Accordingly, we shall often employ the term "risks" rather than "costs" when making a comparison to benefits. For such purposes, the term "risk" refers to a possible future harm, and statements of risk are estimates of the probability of such harms. However, the probability of a harm's occurrence is only one way of expressing a risk and should be distinguished from the magnitude of the potential harm. When expressions such as "minimal risk" or "high risk" are used, they usually refer to the chance of experiencing a harm—its probability—as well as the severity of the harm—its magnitude—in the event of occurrence. Of course uncertainty may be present in assessments of either the probability or the magnitude of harm.

The contrasting term "benefit" is sometimes used merely to refer to cost avoidance, but more commonly in biomedicine it refers to something of positive value that promotes health or welfare. Unlike "risk," "benefit" is not a probabilistic term; hence, "probability of benefit" is the proper contrast to risk, just as benefits are comparable to harms rather than to risks of harm. Accordingly, cost-benefit relations are more precisely expressed through the language of the probability and magnitude of an anticipated benefit and the probability and magnitude of an anticipated harm.

Obviously all three terms—"costs," "risks," and "benefits"—express evaluations. Values determine what will count as costs and benefits, and they also determine how much particular costs and benefits count, that is, how much weight they have in calculations. While the process of determining costs and benefits and assigning them weights is clearly value-laden, the process of determining probability is not so clearly evaluative. Certainly it is, or may be, more value-free than the determining and weighing of costs and benefits. However, as Harold Green has argued,

the values of those performing the analysis dictate the manner in which uncertainty as to potential adverse consequences will be resolved. To some, the absence of evidence that there will be injury connotes the belief that injury will not in fact result; to others, the absence of proof that injury will not result connotes the belief that injury may result. A basic question, therefore, is whether uncertainty will be resolved optimistically or pessimistically, and the manner in which the resolution is accomplished reflects the value judgments of those who perform the analysis.[19]

Later we will consider whose values are relevant to cost-benefit analyses.

There are many different kinds of risks and benefits. As we have seen, there are risks of physical and psychological harm, but also of damage to other interests such as reputation and property. Case #21 illustrates this range of risk. In this case a baby girl suffers from Seckel or "bird-headed" dwarfism, a recessive genetic disease, as well as multiple other medical complications. The child is at risk of starvation if an operation is not performed, but also is at risk of severe physical and mental suffering, as well as further serious medical complications, if the operation is performed. The family is at risk of psychological harm and perhaps of economic harm (because of the extremely low state per capita funding for institutions that house the retarded). Eventually, the parents decide against the surgery—a decision that in some states might place them at risk of legal harm.

Cost-benefit analysis

Cost-benefit analysis is a much discussed but as yet underdeveloped economic and evaluative tool for decisionmaking.[20] It is applied with some frequency to problems of health and safety. It is especially promising as a method for making explicit the overt and covert trade-offs that must be made as a matter of individual, institutional, or public policy. There are trade-offs, for example, between the possible benefits and risks of heart surgery, on the one hand, and a life of severely restricted activity without the surgery, on the other hand. Other trade-offs are between lives lost and money expended to save them, between the costs of research and the costs of treatment programs, and between the quality and cost of a product (such as gasoline) and the quality of the health of those who produce it.

The simple idea behind the cost-benefit approach is that costs and benefits should be measured by some acceptable device, while uncertainties and trade-offs are similarly outlined, in order to present decision makers with specific, relevant information that can serve as a rational basis for a decision.

Although such analysis usually proceeds by measuring different quantitative units—such as number of accidents, statistical deaths, dollars expended, and number of persons treated—it attempts in the end to convert and express these seemingly incommensurable units of measurement into a common one, such as money, or at least to bring as many units as possible to commensurate status. This goal of an ultimate reduction gives the method its appeal, because judgments about trade-offs can be made on the basis of perfectly comparable quantities. As it is often metaphorically put, risks and benefits can then be "weighed" and "balanced" and shown to be "in a favorable ratio." Some examples will make this point clearer.

First, consider a study by Klarman of the benefits of eradicating syphilis in the United States.[21] Benefits in this case are the reductions in the costs of, for example, medical care expenditures, economic deprivation from loss of employment, and pain and disability during and after the disease. In this study, the costs incurred in 1962 were measured at $117.5 million. The value of the disease's total eradication would be equivalent to this annual sum projected in perpetuity. By employing discount rates, Klarman argued that the present capital value of this eradication would be several billion dollars. Having arrived at these benefits (based on cost eradication), analysts could then figure the costs of treatment programs for purposes of comparison. Different but parallel studies could also be provided—such as cost-benefit calculations for a control program that reduced the *incidence* of the disease but did not eradicate it. Because of the rapid emergence of highly resistant strains, the latter kind of cost-benefit analysis would be the most useful, though Klarman unfortunately did not provide it.

Consider as a second example the proposed standards for occupational exposure to the carcinogen benzene, which was recently studied by OSHA (Occupational Safety and Health Administration) because of reports of excessive leukemia deaths related to benzene in industrial manufacturing plants. In his testimony in this case, Richard Wilson argues both that "an average level of benzene in the workplace of 10 parts per million (ppm) is much more acceptable than many other actions" and that the social benefits of the manufacture of benzene at these levels outweigh the risks associated with such production.[22] Wilson recognizes that benzene is a carcinogen and that we must be cautious about the level allowed. His point is that we have no choice except to settle for a conservative estimate of the risks, as determined largely by dose levels generalized from animal studies. If he is correct, our only rational policy option is to accept a dose level in the vicinity of that point at which we cannot scientifically demonstrate that benzene in such doses produces cancer in humans, even though it demonstrably is a carcinogen. This argument turns on a showing that the entire hazard cannot be banned because too many significant benefits (not directly related to health) would be lost. The manufacture of gasoline, for example, would have to be prohibited. Yet compliance costs at levels less than 10 ppm would be in the hundreds of millions of dollars and would potentially render manufacture nonprofitable—without any evidence that workers would be more, rather than less, protected when possible harms are taken into consideration. This general viewpoint was ultimately accepted by the United States Supreme Court in its 1980 ruling on benzene.[23]

Although in the benzene case risks beyond the testable level are not known, Wilson's reasoning is not remote from decision analysis required elsewhere in biomedicine—for example, in deciding whether to produce the implantable artificial heart, as reported in Case #32, and in deciding about proper health policies to control hypertension, as reported in Case #34. In both cases we must ask how much society should pay to reduce health-related risks. These risks are continually reducible to lower levels, but at geometrically increasing financial costs. Moreover, in both cases the risk of death itself cannot be eliminated. The ideal presumably is a level of risk that is socially acceptable, where acceptability is determined by what benefits must be given up elsewhere in order to achieve the appropriate level. In its most dramatic form, the level of acceptability is sometimes stated as "the value of life"—i.e., how much it is worth to reduce the risk of death.[24] Cost-benefit analyses promise to provide, or at least to help us determine, this level of acceptability. This promise should not be construed to mean either that all costs and benefits can be fully quantified or that all uncertainties about probabilities can be eliminated. Rather, it means that the principles and values operative in risk-benefit decisions often can be stated in considerable detail so that *unclarity in the judgmental process is reduced*. This reduction of intuitive weighing in policy formulation is the great promise of the cost-benefit approach.[25]

The need for this reduction of unclarity has been aptly illustrated in many recent decisions by federal regulatory and administrative agencies (such as the Environmental Protection Agency, the Occupational Safety and Health Administration, and the Food and Drug Administration), whose decisions directly affect the nation's health. An example is found in Case #31 in the Appendix, which recounts the difficulties in, but also the necessity of, a cost-benefit decision at the National Institutes of Health concerning how much to budget for cancer research and how much to budget for arthritis research. The frustration of the Director of the National Institute of Arthritis, Metabolism, and Digestive Diseases is directly due to the unavailability of an objective means of assessing the relative worth of funding arthritis research by comparison with cancer research. It is difficult if not impossible to measure and compare death, on the one hand, with pain, suffering, and disability, on the other.

Despite the promise held out by some of the examples mentioned above— and by cost-benefit methodology in general—it will only rarely be possible to use precise quantitative techniques in the ultimate assessment of whether a medical treatment or research protocol is justified, and we must candidly face the difficulties presented by a purely quantitative model of weighing risks and benefits. This problem is illustrated in debates about the use of CAT scanning for diagnostic purposes: Larger dollar costs of using CAT scans must be weighed against the greater value of the procedure as well as the lower risk presented to patients.

Instead of a purely quantitative ideal, then, the proper model for bio-medical evaluations is the systematic, nonarbitrary, and nonintuitive comparison of benefits and risks. Such a model demands that justifications of a mode of treatment or a research protocol be thorough in the assimilation and evaluation of information about all aspects of the procedures under consideration. It also requires that those assimilating the data be explicit in stating operative standards and values as well as quantitative measurements for considering and weighing alternative procedures. When carefully spelled out, cost-benefit analysis can render the entire process of evaluating clinical procedures, research protocols, and preventive measures more rigorous and precise, while at the same time enhancing the quality of information transmitted when informed consent is solicited.

In some cases the risks and benefits are well-known, yet determining whether the benefits *outweigh* the risks may prove impossibly difficult. For example, consider the case of a premature infant born by caesarean section after a 34-week gestation period. At birth the baby was "blue, limp, had no reflexes, and a very slow heart rate"—and also had excessive fluid and an enlarged liver and spleen. The parents wanted the child very much, and intense resuscitation measures were initiated. At 14 minutes of age the child was doing poorly and had no spontaneous activity. The doctors feared that "there is an extremely high risk" that a retarded baby (at best) would result from further medical efforts. Physicians and nurses expressed strong differences of opinion as to whether resuscitation efforts should continue, at least if the baby once stopped breathing. Such a dispute can be anchored in considerations other than an assessment of risks and benefits, of course. But how can we weigh the high risk of mental retardation and the probable disappointment of the parents against the low possibility of a healthy baby and the parents' known desire to have the child? This is a matter clearly subject to differences of opinion, even if the probability of harm and the probability of benefit were well established and agreed upon by all. Risk-benefit assessments thus will not function as a panacea for decision makers.

Finally, even if it were possible to measure all risks and benefits with precision, it would not follow that a favorable or positive net sum of benefits would justify a particular therapeutic intervention or research procedure or that an unfavorable comparison of risks and benefits would render the treatment or research unjustified. Some criteria of risk *acceptability* are independent of the analysis and comparison of risks and benefits themselves. In some cases the same level of risk may be acceptable if borne by those who will receive the benefits, but unacceptable if borne by those who will not receive the benefits. Thus, one major factor in determining the acceptability of risk is the presence or absence of an informed and consenting individual. In order to show respect for autonomy, consenting patients and subjects must often be allowed to assume risks that would be impermissible for persons incapable of consent.

Cost-benefit analysis, and the principle of beneficence generally, can be applied not only to the interests of individuals but also to the interests of society. To determine whether a medical practice is justified traditionally involves comparing risks and benefits only for individual patients, but determinations of justified research are more complicated and have an inherent social dimension. While patients and subjects should always be protected by the scrutiny of risks, it would not satisfy the principles discussed in this chapter (especially utility) if the need to protect individuals against harm were not balanced against possible benefits of an intervention— in many cases benefits for an entire population. For example, beneficent acts should not only protect subjects of research against risk of harm but also should protect society against the risk of losing the substantial benefits that might be gained from the research. When skillfully done, risk-benefit analysis shows that such complex balancing judgments are generally present in hard cases.

Several crucial ethical questions are raised by cost-benefit and risk-benefit analysis. First, whose values should enter into the determination of what will count as costs and benefits, and how much will various costs and benefits count or weigh in the calculation? As we will see in the next section, when a practitioner treats an individual patient, he or she must determine whether to respect the patient's values or to impose his or her own values. But when several parties may be affected by an action or policy, whose values are relevant? The complexity of this issue can be seen in controversies about the value of life. According to the discounted-future-earnings approach, the value of life can be determined by considering what people at risk of a certain disease or accident could be expected to earn if they survived; future income is discounted, because money earned now could be invested and thus has more worth than future income. One problem with this approach is that it tends to give priority to young adult white males, who can be expected to earn more. Thus, a program to encourage motorcyclists to wear helmets would be selected over a cervical cancer program.

Another, more defensible approach is willingness to pay. This approach considers how much we would be willing to pay to reduce the risk of death. It determines the value of life by finding out how much persons affected by the policy are willing to pay to reduce the risks of death (first by summing up the individual amounts, and then by dividing by the anticipated number of deaths that could be prevented). Obviously, this approach bears a distinct resemblance to preference utilitarianism. One way to determine such preferences is by observing behavior (e.g., in the workplace), while another approach uses opinion polls. For example, Jan Acton used the following question, among others, to determine how people value life:

They are thinking about putting ambulances and other devices in communities around the country, but only if people are willing to pay enough for them. This program would be for you and 10,000 people living around you. In your area, there are about 100 heart attacks per year. About 40 of these persons die. With the heart-attack program, only 20 of these people would die. How much would you be willing to pay in taxes per year for the ambulance so that 20 lives could be saved in your community?[26]

Obviously such questions are relevant in decisions about developing the totally implantable artificial heart (Case #32) and about funding heart transplants (Case #33). To the charge that putting a value on life is immoral, it is appropriate to respond that individuals and society frequently decide how much they are willing to spend in order to reduce risks to health and survival. Analysis simply transforms our implicit, informal, unsystematic processes into more explicit, formal, and systematic studies that can clarify the trade-offs.

Another crucial ethical question raised by cost-benefit analysis is distributive justice. Utilitarianism and cost-benefit analyses are commonly said to fail to take account of problems of justice because they focus on the net balance of benefits over costs, without considering the *distribution* of those benefits and costs. (Such criticisms may not work well against rule utilitarianism, but act utilitarianism does seem open to such objections.) For example, in Case #34, which we discussed earlier, Weinstein and Stason argued that the most cost-effective approach for control of hypertension would be to concentrate resources on known hypertensives, but they recognized that this approach might be criticized on grounds of equity. Many poor people and blacks (who have a higher rate of hypertension than whites) would not know of their hypertension because they would not be in the health care system. Similarly, a study of the costs and benefits of treating mental retardation might show that the costs outweigh the benefits, while justice might demand that special benefits be extended to mentally retarded persons. In both examples, justice may require a different distribution of resources than cost-benefit analysis would support. In Chapter 6 we will examine these problems of distributive justice in detail.

Cost-benefit analysis has been accused of several serious deficiencies. There are methodological problems in the measurement of values, and especially in rendering commensurable all the units of value that must be compared. This problem can itself lead to arbitrary decisionmaking, and cost-benefit methods as developed in economics have proven difficult to implement concretely. There are also problems concerning how to compute discount rates, psychological effects, and indirect effects of certain personal and social interventions. We have attempted to circumvent these problems in our presentation of cost-benefit analysis by treating such analysis as including nonquantitative considerations.

Some critics worry that the tool of cost-benefit analysis may come to dominate its users. They fear that economic language, already evident in discussions of "the health care industry," "providers," and "consumers," as well as "cost-benefit analysis," will replace the traditional language of the doctor-patient relationship, including humanity and decency.[27] Our view is that a number of moral principles and rules are relevant to research, medicine, and health care, including the principle of utility. The requirements of this principle often can be determined with greater precision through systematic cost-benefit studies. This approach is acceptable and indeed commendable if it encompasses a wide range of values, including some that are not easily quantifiable, and if it respects such constraining principles as autonomy and justice.

Paternalism

The nature of paternalism

The health care professional or bureaucrat sometimes has a conception of benefits, harms, and their balance that differs from that of the patient. Whose conception of the requirements of beneficence and nonmaleficence should prevail? This issue is complicated by the fact that depressed patients, patients on dialysis, and patients addicted to potentially harmful drugs may not be likely to reach adequately reasoned decisions. Even patients who are competent and deliberative can make poor choices about courses of action recommended by physicians. Some health care professionals are inclined to respect autonomy by not interfering beyond attempts at persuasion when patients choose harmful courses of action, while others are inclined to protect patients against the potentially harmful consequences of their choices. The problem of whether or not to intervene in the decisions and affairs of such persons is the problem of paternalism.[28]

Although the *Oxford English Dictionary* dates the term "paternalism" from the 1880s, the idea is much older and, indeed, appears very early in human thought. Its root meaning, according to the OED, is "the principle and practice of paternal administration; government as by a father; the claim or attempt to supply the needs or to regulate the life of a nation or community in the same way a father does those of his children." When the analogy with the father is used to illuminate the role of professionals or the state in health care, it presupposes two features of the paternal role: that the father is benevolent, i.e., that he has the interests of his children at heart, and that he makes all or at least some of the decisions relating to his children's welfare rather than letting them make the decisions. Paternalism poses moral questions precisely because it involves the claim that beneficence should take precedence over autonomy, at least in some cases.[29]

The problem of paternalism is implicit in our previous discussions of autonomy, particularly in our analysis of informed consent in Chapter 3. There we studied two alternative models of informed consent, both of which can influence one's perspective on paternalism. According to the first model, which may be called the autonomy model, consent is required because it respects autonomy by recognizing that individuals have the right to choose what shall be done to them. According to the second model, which may be called the protection model, consent in medical contexts functions to maximize benefits and minimize harms for individuals. The protection model, based on the duty of beneficence, tends to support paternalistic intervention, while the autonomy model generally opposes it. For the autonomy model, the individual's conception of good should control what is done; for the protection model, to fail to maximize benefits and minimize harms for individuals, even against their wishes, is to violate the principle of beneficence.

The principle of nonmaleficence has played a parallel role in the justification of medical paternalism. Physicians have traditionally taken the view that disclosing certain forms of information can be directly harmful to patients under their care. In a classic article, L. J. Henderson argued that "the best physicians" use the following as their primary guide: "So far as possible, 'Do No Harm.' You can do harm by the process that is quaintly called telling the truth. You can do harm by lying. . . . But try to do as little harm as possible, not only in treatment with drugs, or with the knife, but also in treatment with words."[30] Henderson and others in the medical community go on to argue that for the patient's good some information should be withheld or disclosed only to the family.

Case #7 illustrates these problems of informed consent and paternalism. A woman had a fatal reaction during urography (visualization of the urinary tract made after injection of an opaque medium). The radiologist had not informed her of a possible fatal reaction to urography on grounds that his duty was to do "what is best for our patients medically." He apparently thought it was best in this case not to inform the patient of risks of death because the information might actually have been "dangerous" instead of protective. In other words, he conceived the doctor's role in informed-consent situations as that of judging whether the presentation of information is more or less harmful to the patient. In this particular case, he determined that it was not in the best interest of the the patient to be informed because the risk of death was small, while the possibility of causing undue alarm was great. This paternalistic attitude is clearly grounded in nonmaleficence and beneficence, but is it justified to act on such an attitude?

The case just considered is only one of many different types of truth-telling cases involving paternalism. Other cases arise when unwelcome news might adversely affect someone's health or lead to suicide, as when a cancer victim is told the truth about his or her condition. If a patient sincerely asks to be told the truth, it is paternalistic under most understandings of paternalism to withhold that information. In Case #5 an inoperable, incurable carcinoma is discovered in a sixty-nine-year-old male. The physician had treated this patient for many years and knew that he was fragile in several respects. The man was quite neurotic, had an established history of psychiatric disease, and had recently suffered a severe depressive reaction, during which he had behaved irrationally and attempted suicide. When the patient blurted out, "Am I O.K.?" and "I don't have cancer, do I?", the physician answered, "You're as good as you were ten years ago," knowing that the response was a paternalistic lie, but also believing it justified. The physician was obviously worried that an indelicately worded response would seriously disrupt the man's life plans, and possibly cause mental instability or suicide.

Cases of paternalism involve overriding a person's wishes or actions in order to benefit or to prevent harm to that person. Paternalistic interventions usually restrict liberty, and they often are coercive. According to many definitions of "paternalism," a paternalistic action inherently involves a limitation of liberty. While this definition is not implausible, we here accept the broader definition suggested by the *Oxford English Dictionary*. We thus understand paternalism as the overriding of a person's wishes or actions for beneficent reasons. If these wishes or actions do not derive from an *autonomous choice*, but nonetheless express the person's *intention*, then overriding the person's wish or action would be paternalistic. For example, if a man wholly ignorant of his condition and sick with a raging fever expresses his wish to leave the hospital, it would be paternalistic to detain him even if we judged that his expressed wish did not derive from an autonomous choice. "Paternalistic interventions," in our usage, do not always straightforwardly override the principle of autonomy by appeal to the principle of beneficence.

Of course, there are reasons for overriding a person's wishes and actions. Most importantly, we generally believe that it is morally justified to restrict a person's liberty when the person's exercise of liberty would cause harm to other persons. This principle, sometimes called the harm principle, was articulated by John Stuart Mill in *On Liberty*, a classic text of antipaternalism:

The object of this Essay is to assert one very simple principle. . . . That principle is, that the sole end for which mankind are warranted, individually or collectively, in interfering with the liberty of action of any of their number, is self-protection. That the only purpose for which power can be rightfully exercised over any member of a civilized community, against his will, is to prevent harm to others. His own good, either physical or moral, is not a sufficient warrant. He cannot rightfully be compelled to do or forbear because it will be better for him to do so, because it will make him happier, because in the opinion of others, to do so would be wise, or even right. These are good reasons for remonstrating with him, or reasoning with him or persuading him, or entreating him, but not for compelling him, or visiting him with any evil in case he do otherwise. To justify that, the conduct from which it is desired to deter him must be calculated to produce evil to someone else. The only part of the conduct of anyone, for which he is amenable to society, is that which concerns others. In the part which merely concerns himself, his independence is of right, absolute.[31]

Both paternalism and Mill's harm principle arguably rest on some form of the principle of beneficence, because beneficence includes producing good, preventing harm, and removing harm. But in a system such as Mill's, which recognizes only the harm principle as valid, an individual must be allowed to make his or her decisions when others are not affected, i.e., when he or she alone is adversely affected. By contrast, the principle of paternalism authorizes interventions to protect the individual from the consequences of his or her choices, wishes, and actions. In many cases, such as debates about legislation requiring motorcycle helmets, paternalism and the harm principle are both invoked, but the fact that these and various other principles are relevant to debates about the same case should obscure neither their distinctiveness nor the importance of being clear when one principle by itself would be sufficient to justify overriding a person's choices, wishes, and actions.

Are paternalistic interventions justified?

In the literature on paternalism, two main positions have been adopted: (1) "Justified Paternalism" and (2) "Antipaternalism." The first of these views has been held by such recent moral philosophers as H. L. A. Hart and Gerald Dworkin, while Mill represents the latter view.

(1) The justification of paternalism

Any supporter of the paternalistic principle will specify with care precisely which goods, needs, and interests warrant paternalistic protection. In recent formulations, it has been said that the state is justified in interfering with a person's intended course if that interference protects the person against his or her extremely and unreasonably risky choices, wishes, or actions—such as dangerous self-administered medical experiments. Supporters of justified paternalism argue nonetheless that it takes a heavy burden of justification to intervene in such cases, especially when intervention limits free choices and actions by competent persons. According to this position, paternalism can be justified only if (1) the harms prevented from occurring or the benefit provided to the person outweighs the loss of independence or the sense of invasion suffered by the interference, (2) the person's condition seriously limits his or her ability to choose autonomously, and (3) it is universally justified under relevantly similar circumstances always to treat persons in this way. Roughly this position is defended by a number of recent writers, some of whom regard paternalism as a form of "social insurance policy" that fully rational persons would take out in order to protect themselves.[32] Such persons would know, for example, that they might be tempted at times to make decisions that are far-reaching, potentially dangerous, and irreversible, while at other times they might suffer extreme psychological or social pressures to do something they truly believe too risky to be worth performing, e.g., where one's honor is placed in question by a challenge to fight. In still other cases, persons might not sufficiently understand or appreciate dangers that are relevant to their conduct, such as the facts about research on smoking. Thus, some writers conclude that we ought to consent to a limited grant of power to others to control our actions by paternalistic policies and interventions.

Case #10 in the Appendix presents one kind of action that inclines one toward paternalism. An involuntarily committed mental patient wishes to leave the hospital, though his family is opposed to his release. The patient argues that his mental condition does not justify confinement, yet after one previous confinement he plucked out his right eye, and after another confinement he severed his right hand. The patient functions fairly normally in the state hospital, where he sells news materials to fellow patients and handles limited financial affairs. The source of his "problems" is apparently his religious beliefs. He regards himself as a true prophet of God and believes that "it is far better for one man to believe and accept an appropriate message from God to sacrifice an eye or a hand according to the sacred scriptures rather than for the present course of the world to cause even greater loss of human life." Acting on this belief, he engages in self-mutilation. According to the paternalist, this person generally functions normally, by usual behavioral or observational criteria, yet desperately needs help. His capacities are too diminished and his dangerousness to himself is too severe to leave him without confinement and custodial care.

(2) *Antipaternalistic individualism*
Some believe that paternalistic interventions cannot be justified. This position is basically the one supported by Mill: Paternalism is not a valid principle for restricting liberty because it violates individual rights and allows too much restriction of free choice. The serious adverse consequences of giving such power to the state, or to any class of individuals, such as physicians, motivates antipaternalists to reject the view that the fully rational person would accept paternalism. Antipaternalists believe that the autonomous person can ascertain his or her best interests more competently than someone who would substitute a judgment about that person's best interests.

Why, from this perspective, is paternalism an unacceptable moral principle? The dominant reason offered by antipaternalists is that paternalistic principles are too broad and hence justify too much. For example, Robert Harris has argued that paternalism would in principle "justify the imposition of a Spartan-like regimen requiring rigorous physical exercise and abstention from smoking, drinking, and hazardous pastimes."[33] The more thoughtful restrictions on paternalism proposed by some writers would disallow such extreme interventions, but, according to antipaternalists, would still leave unacceptable latitude of judgment in contexts where authoritative controls are likely to be abused and also would leave unresolved problems concerning the scope of the principle. On the latter point, suppose that a man risks his life for the advance of medicine by submitting to an unreasonably risky experiment, an act most would think not in his best interests. Are we to commend him, ignore him, or coercively restrain him? Paternalism suggests that it would be permissible and perhaps even obligatory to restrain such a person. Yet if so, antipaternalists argue, the state is permitted in principle coercively to restrain its morally heroic citizens, not to mention its martyrs, if they act—as such people frequently do—in a manner "harmful" to themselves. Physicians could be authorized by the principle of beneficence to treat patients in parallel paternalistic ways.

The medical example that has the most extensive antipaternalistic literature is the involuntary hospitalization of persons who have neither been harmed by others nor actually harmed themselves, but who are thought to be at risk of harm by others or by themselves. These cases involve what might be called double paternalism: a paternalistic justification for both therapy and commitment. A widely discussed case of this sort is that of Mrs. Catherine Lake, included in the Appendix as Case #9. Mrs. Lake suffered from arteriosclerosis causing temporary confusion and mild loss of memory, interspersed with periods of mental alertness and rationality. All parties agreed that Mrs. Lake had never harmed anyone or presented any threat of danger, yet she was committed to a mental institution because she often seemed confused and defenseless. At her trial, while apparently fully rational, she testified that she knew the risk of living outside the hospital and preferred to take that risk rather than be in the hospital environment. The Court of Appeals denied her petition, arguing that she is "mentally ill," "is of danger to herself . . . and is not competent to care for herself." The legal justification cited by the Court was a statute that "provides for involuntary hospitalization of a person who is 'mentally ill and, because of that illness, is likely to injure himself'. . . ."[34] Antipaternalists resist the reasoning of this court on grounds that such actions involve an unjustifiable restriction of human liberty. This objection is commonly based on Mill's view that the harm principle alone provides valid grounds for the restriction of liberty. Since Mrs. Lake is not causing harm to others and understands the dangers under which she is placing herself, she should be free to proceed as she wishes, according to antipaternalists.

Strong and weak paternalism

Supporters of limited paternalism and opponents of paternalism often disagree about people's actual capabilities for autonomous action. (Cf. the discussion of competence in Chapter 3.) Supporters of paternalism tend to cite examples of persons of at least slightly diminished capacity—for example, persons on kidney dialysis and those in depression. By contrast, opponents cite examples of persons who are capable of autonomous choice, at least in some contexts—for example, those involuntarily committed merely for eccentric behavior, prisoners not permitted to volunteer for research on drugs, and those who rationally elect to refuse treatment in life-threatening circumstances.

Joel Feinberg's[35] distinction between *strong* and *weak* paternalism illuminates this disagreement. Weak paternalism is explained as follows:

[One] has the right to prevent self-regarding conduct only when it is *substantially nonvoluntary* or when temporary intervention is necessary to establish whether it is voluntary or not.

To say that conduct is "substantially nonvoluntary" is to say, in our language, that the person's action is not fully autonomous, even if it is autonomous in some respects. For example, the class of nonvoluntary actions includes cases of consent that are not adequately informed and thus not autonomous. Strong paternalism, by contrast, holds that it is sometimes proper to protect a person by limiting his or her liberty even when that person's choices are informed and voluntary.

Virtually everyone acknowledges that some acts of weak paternalism are justified acts of beneficence, e.g., preventing a person under the influence of LSD from killing himself. But weak paternalism may not be paternalism in any very controversial sense; it may not be an intervention to which antipaternalists would object, since it does not involve a violation of autonomy. That is, if the justification of so-called "paternalistic" interventions *always* rests on preventing harm to seriously compromised, effectively nonautonomous persons, then "paternalism" of this sort will not violate the antipaternalist's principles of autonomy and liberty. Rather, the antipaternalist will view these interventions as justified by reference to the principle of beneficence, and as free of conflict with the principle of autonomy.

To the present writers it is difficult to justify strong paternalism;[36] however, many forms of weak paternalism may be justified, as may an antipaternalism of the sort described in the previous paragraph. For example, some cases of coercive transfusions of blood are instances of strong paternalism that involve a serious violation of autonomy—a violation that cannot be justified by appeals to beneficence and nonmaleficence. (Compare Cases #13 and #14 in the Appendix.) Perhaps the most plausible kind of case *favoring* strong paternalistic interventions would be the following: A psychiatrist is treating a patient like the patient in Case #10 who plucks out his eyes and cuts off his hands for religious reasons. Presume that this patient is not insane and acts conscientiously on his quite unique religious views. Suppose further that this patient asks the psychiatrist a question about his condition, a question that has a definite answer, but which, if answered, would lead the patient to engage in self-maiming behavior in order to satisfy the demands of his religious convictions. Many would be inclined to say that the doctor acts paternalistically but justifiably by concealing information from the patient. Those who believe the physician acts justifiably probably believe the patient is acting on false religious beliefs and so is uninformed. But suppose the patient was genuinely rational and relevantly informed. Would this case then be an instance of strong paternalism with a plausible claim to justifiability? Paternalism may seem justified in this case for another reason. We may be uncertain about the extent to which the person's actions are autonomous or voluntary. This uncertainty pervades cases of strong paternalism that appear to be justified, and provides one reason why some writers believe that all justified paternalistic interventions are instances of weak paternalism.

There are many examples of justified weak paternalism. Everyone familiar with the practice of medicine knows that some patients who are mentally alert nonetheless suffer from conditions that affect their behavior, such as depression, drug addiction, and abnormal EEG patterns. Such persons are capable of making judgments that affect their lives, but their limitations can have important and immediate effects on their decisions. For example, while most people would favor allowing children to be consulted about important decisions affecting their lives in medical contexts, almost everyone believes that even the wishes of fairly mature children are sometimes validly overridden in order to provide important therapeutic benefits. If a child bitten by a rabid dog were terrified at the thought of undergoing treatment and refused to submit to it, we would regard the youth's parents and physician as irresponsible if they failed to override the child's wishes and force the treatment. Cases involving adult patients on dialysis and suffering from uremia (retention in the blood of toxic urinary constituents) or suicidal patients suffering from serious depression likewise invite paternalistic treatment. To allow persons to die through their own decisions would be callous and uncaring where certain conditions reduce the informed or voluntary character of their actions.

In some of his writings on medical ethics, Robert Veatch has argued that a "priestly model" of medical practice should be set aside in favor of what he calls a "contractual model," which he bases on marriage contracts and religious covenants. For him, informed consent should entirely replace medical paternalism. He argues that "society has the right to intervene to protect the welfare of individuals who are substantially nonautonomous, whose actions are essentially nonvoluntary";[37] but he bemoans what he calls a "paternalism in the realm of values" that leads physicians to rely on the principle "benefit and do no harm to the patient" without considering truly autonomous expressions of patients.[38] While Veatch's ideal is admirable, it is unrealistic for much of medical practice. The physician is thrust into a paternalistic role on numerous occasions by the questionable condition of patients, by their enormous regard for his or her knowledge of their conditions, and perhaps by their unwillingness or inability to make hard decisions.

It can be argued that on some occasions the physician actually protects autonomy by overriding the immediate wishes of a patient. For example, in Case #5, referred to previously, a sixty-nine-year-old unaware that he has prostate cancer asks his physician for the results of recent tests. The physician tells him that he is as healthy as he was ten years ago. Few would say that the doctor made an utterly indefensible choice, yet his action is a paternalistic lie. Moreover, it is particularly interesting because it straddles the boundary between strong paternalism and weak paternalism. Although the patient does act autonomously in making the request for the information, he would only questionably be able to act autonomously if he were actually given the information.

Such cases illustrate how complex the interactions sometimes become in the attempt to balance considerations of autonomy, beneficence, nonmaleficence, and justice in the treatment of patients. A necessary condition of justified paternalistic actions has already been set forth in rough outline: The paternalistic intervention would have to provide benefits that outweigh associated costs. Whether it would also be necessary that a state of incompetency, substantial ignorance, or substantial nonvoluntariness be present (or at least necessary that we cannot ascertain whether such a condition is present) is an unresolved matter of vigorous contemporary debate. This issue is whether strong paternalism is ever justified by balancing an act of beneficence against an invasion of autonomy.

Mill's example of a person about to cross a dangerous bridge provides a promising approach to these problems. If we are unsure whether a person's actions are voluntary or whether the person's judgment is uninformed, it would be justifiable to intervene temporarily in order to ascertain whether the person's actions are voluntary and informed. Once adequately informed under conditions of voluntary choice, the decision should rest with the autonomous agent. Still, what should be done in those cases of partially voluntary and partially nonvoluntary actions, where it is impossible to satisfy the demands of Mill's proviso? These might be cases involving mental retardation, ongoing psychotic compulsion, or repeated tendencies toward suicide. In such cases, we suggest, persons ought to be protected against harms that might result directly from their limiting conditions. To the extent one protects a person from harms produced by causes beyond the person's knowledge and control, the intervention has plausible claim to being morally justified, for the choices are substantially nonvoluntary. While degrees of control and voluntariness—and, indeed, autonomous choice—rest on a multilevel continuum, we can make informed discriminations in most important cases as to the substantial voluntariness or nonvoluntariness of the action.

In conclusion, it should be noted that in some cases a justification for an action may appear to be paternalistic when in fact it is based on nonpaternalistic grounds. An example is found in research involving prisoners. In 1976 the National Commission for the Protection of Human Subjects of Biomedical and Behavioral Research issued a report on *Research Involving Prisoners.*[39] It argued that the closed nature of prison environments creates a strong potential for abuse of authority and therefore invites the exploitation and coercion of prisoners. However, a Commission study indicated that most prisoners do not regard their consent to research as obtained under coercion or undue influence. The Commission argued that the inherent coercive possibilities in prisons nonetheless justified regulations prohibiting many prisoners from engaging in research, even if they wish to do so.

This justification may appear overtly paternalistic, but closer analysis of the Commission report shows that it is not. The Commission explicitly maintained that if an environment were *not* exploitative or coercive (and if a few other standards were met), then prisoners should be free to choose to participate in research. The Commission's justifying ground was the factual claim that most prisons could not be made sufficiently free of coercion and exploitation by drug companies and prison officials, not the moral claim that prisoners should be protected from their wishes or choices. Hence, the justification is only apparently based on a paternalistic principle. The harm principle provides the real basis: It is unpredictable whether prisoners will be exploited in settings that render them vulnerable, but research to which they might appear to consent validly should nonetheless be prohibited because we cannot adequately monitor the consent process. Many judgments about the justification of actions in medical practice and research turn on whether the harm principle or some paternalistic principle actually applies in the circumstances.

We conclude that weak paternalism is a coherent and defensible moral position, though it applies only to a narrow range of cases where patients and subjects are clearly endangered. It may also be quite compatible with those forms of antipaternalism that leave room for a principle of beneficence. Strong paternalism, by contrast, is more difficult and perhaps impossible to justify. While some cases of strong paternalism do not seem inherently immoral, the possibilities for abuse inherent in a *policy* of strong paternalism seem to outweigh its possible benefits, unless the lines could be more carefully drawn than they have been in the past. This conclusion follows from the general line of moral argument found in previous chapters. We have argued for a pluralism of moral principles, equally weighted in advance of information about particular circumstances. It therefore cannot be assumed that even an autonomous choice can *never* be validly overridden on grounds of beneficence; and it is easy to imagine many cases where the weight of autonomy is minimal, while the weight of beneficence is maximal. However, because strong paternalism involves a direct conflict with autonomy, the individual affected, not some external authority, almost always should make the judgment of desirable forms of benefit. What makes weak paternalism an attractive thesis is that on many occasions persons are genuinely not capable of making autonomous judgments about their best interests, and an external authority's decisions may be perfectly in order in those cases. This judgment is in no way inconsistent with our strong defense of the principle of autonomy in Chapter 3.

Notes

1. William Frankena, *Ethics*, 2nd ed. (Englewood Cliffs, N.J.: Prentice-Hall, 1973), p. 47. Frankena includes moral ideals under the umbrella of "the ingredients of morality" (pp. 67f).
2. See Joel Feinberg, "The Nature and Value of Rights," *Journal of Value Inquiry* 4 (1970): 243–57, especially 244ff.
3. Frankena later does say (*Ethics*, p. 47) that principles of beneficence specify "prima facie duties," but it remains unclear whether this means that they are moral *requirements* (as Ross's theory of prima facie duties entails that they are), because Frankena allows for an extremely lengthy list of possible prima facie duties (pp. 48, 56). See also Frankena's subsequent essay, "Moral Philosophy and World Hunger," in *World Hunger and Moral Obligation*, eds. W. Aiken and H. LaFollette (Englewood Cliffs, N.J.: Prentice-Hall, 1977), pp. 66–84, especially pp. 70, 73.
4. Marcus G. Singer, *Generalization in Ethics* (New York: Alfred A. Knopf, Inc., 1961), pp. 180–89.
5. Peter Singer, *Practical Ethics* (Cambridge, England: Cambridge University Press, 1979), pp. 168ff.
6. Peter Singer, "Famine, Affluence, and Morality," *Philosophy and Public Affairs* 1 (1972), as reprinted in T. Mappes and J. Zembaty, eds., *Social Ethics* (New York: McGraw-Hill, 1977), p. 317. This article is updated in "Reconsidering

the Famine Relief Argument," in *Food Policy: The Responsibility of the United States in the Life and Death Choices*, eds. Peter Brown and Henry Shue (New York: The Free Press, 1977), and in *Practical Ethics*.

7. Michael A. Slote, "The Morality of Wealth," in *World Hunger and Moral Obligation*, pp. 125–27.

8. Singer, *Practical Ethics*, p. 181.

9. Our formulation of these conditions is indebted to Eric D'Arcy, *Human Acts: An Essay in their Moral Evaluation* (Oxford: Clarendon Press, 1963), pp. 56–57. We have modified them by adding the fourth condition.

10. "On Suicide," as reprinted in S. Gorovitz et al., *Moral Problems in Medicine* (Englewood Cliffs, N.J.: Prentice-Hall, 1976), p. 386.

11. John Rawls, "Legal Obligation and the Duty of Fair Play," in *Law and Philosophy*, ed. Sidney Hook (New York: New York University Press, 1964). See also *A Theory of Justice* (Cambridge, Mass.: Harvard University Press, 1971), p. 148. Rawls prefers his contract account behind the veil of ignorance to the language of "benevolence," no doubt because of his Kantian convictions. However, Rawls does recognize a natural duty of beneficence (see pp. 114–15).

12. William F. May, "Code and Covenant or Philanthropy and Contract?" in *Ethics in Medicine*, eds. Stanley Joel Reiser, Arthur J. Dyck, and William J. Curran (Cambridge, Mass.: MIT Press, 1977), pp. 65–76, has greatly influenced this paragraph.

13. Reeder, "Beneficence, Supererogation, and Role Duty," in *Beneficence and Health Care*, ed. Earl E. Shelp (Dordrecht, Holland: D. Reidel Publishing Co., 1982), p. 101 (italics added).

14. *Epidemics*, 1:11, from W. H. S. Jones, ed., *Hippocrates* (Cambridge, Mass.: Harvard University Press, 1923), Vol. I, p. 165.

15. The AMA Code grants discretion to the physician in determining whom he will serve: "A physician shall, in the provision of appropriate patient care, except in emergencies, be free to choose whom to serve, with whom to associate, and the environment in which to provide medical services." (Section VI; see Appendix II.)

16. Judith Jarvis Thomson, "A Defense of Abortion," *Philosophy and Public Affairs* 1 (1971), as reprinted in Tom L. Beauchamp and Terry Pinkard, eds., *Ethics and Public Policy* (Englewood Cliffs, N.J.: Prentice-Hall, 1983), pp. 268–83. (Slote acknowledges an indebtedness to this essay for part of his analysis of the duty of beneficence.)

17. *Ibid.*

18. The functions and moral obligations of such committees are analyzed in a report on the subject of the National Commission for the Protection of Human Subjects, *Report and Recommendations: Institutional Review Boards*, including a separate *Appendix* (Washington: DHEW Publication Nos. (OS) 78-0008 and (OS) 78-0009, 1978). This study includes considerations of cost-benefit analysis.

19. Harold P. Green, "The Risk-Benefit Calculus in Safety Determinations," *George Washington Law Review* 43 (1975): 799.

20. A comprehensive source for economists' accounts of cost-benefit analysis is E. J. Mishan, *Cost-Benefit Analysis* (New York: Praeger Publishers, 1976), expanded ed. On the nature of risk, cf. William W. Lowrance, *Of Acceptable Risk: Science and the Determination of Safety* (Los Altos, Calif.: William Kaufmann, 1976). For applied studies in the area of health and medicine, see John P. Bunker et al., *Costs, Risks and Benefits of Surgery* (New York: Oxford University Press, 1977); and a special issue of the *George Washington Law Review* 45 (August 1977) devoted to "Risk-Benefit Assessment in Governmental Decisionmaking." For a philosophical critique of cost-benefit reasoning, see Alasdair MacIntyre, "Utilitarianism and Cost/Benefit Analysis: An Essay on the Relevance of Moral Philosophy to Bureaucratic Theory," in *Values in the Electric Power Industry*, ed. K. Sayre (Notre Dame, Ind.: University of Notre Dame Press, 1977).

21. H. E. Klarman, "Syphilis Control Problems," in *Measuring Benefits of Government Investments*, ed. R. Dorfman (Washington: Brookings Institution, 1965).

22. Richard Wilson. Direct Testimony. *In re Proposed Standards for Occupational Exposure to Benzene* (Washington: OSHA Docket No. H-059, 1977), pp. 10ff.

23. *Industrial Union Dept., AFL-CIO* v. *American Petroleum Institute et al.*, 448, U.S. 607 (1980).

24. For controversy about valuing lives, see Steven E. Rhoads, ed., *Valuing Life: Public Policy Dilemmas* (Boulder, Colo.: Westview Press, 1980).

25. This point has been repeatedly stressed in cases of environmental law that deal with problems of risks to health as balanced against other economic and social benefits. Cf., e.g., Judge David Bazelon's decision in *Environmental Defense Fund* v. *William D. Ruckelshaus and the Environment Protection Agency*, 439 F.2d 584 (1971).

26. Quoted in Steven E. Rhoads, "How Much Should We Spend to Save a Life?" in *Valuing Life: Public Policy Dilemmas*, ed. Steven E. Rhoads, p. 293. Rhoads's analysis greatly influenced this paragraph.

27. See Rashi Fein, "What is Wrong with the Language of Medicine?" *New England Journal of Medicine* 306 (April 8, 1982): 863f.

28. The term "paternalism" is not wholly felicitous, especially because it is sex-linked. While it might be desirable to use another term, such as "parentalism," the term "paternalism" is established by usage and philosophical discussion.

29. It is important to note, as Frankena has suggested, that "beneficence requires us to respect the liberty of others." *Ethics*, p. 53. Thus we have a conflict of obligations generated by beneficence itself when we attempt both to protect persons *and* to respect their liberty.

30. L. J. Henderson, "Physician and Patient as a Social System," *New England Journal of Medicine* 212 (1935): 819–23.

31. John Stuart Mill, *Utilitarianism, On Liberty, Essay on Bentham* (New York: New American Library, 1974), p. 135.

32. See especially Gerald Dworkin, "Paternalism," *The Monist* (January 1972): 64–84; and John Rawls, *A Theory of Justice, op. cit.*, pp. 248–49. See also

Charles Culver and Bernard Gert, *Philosophy in Medicine* (New York: Oxford University Press, 1982), Chapters 7–9; Jeffrie Murphy, "Incompetence and Paternalism," *Archiv für Rechts und Sozial Philosophie* 60 (1974): 466, 485; and James F. Childress, *Priorities in Biomedical Ethics* (Philadelphia: The Westminster Press, 1981), pp. 26–27, and *Who Should Decide?: Paternalism in Health Care* (New York: Oxford University Press, 1982).

33. "Private Consensual Adult Behavior: The Requirement of Harm to Others in the Enforcement of Morality," *UCLA Law Review* 14 (1967): 585n. Similar complaints, situated in the context of political philosophy, are found in Isaiah Berlin, *Four Essays on Liberty* (Oxford: Oxford University Press, 1969), pp. lxi–lxii, 132–33, 137–38, 149–51, and 157.

34. Cf. Jay Katz, Joseph Goldstein, and Alan M. Dershowitz, eds., *Psychoanalysis, Psychiatry, and the Law* (New York: The Free Press, 1967), pp. 552–54, 710–13; and Robert A. Burt, *Taking Care of Strangers* (New York: The Free Press, 1979), Chapter 2.

35. Joel Feinberg, "Legal Paternalism," *Canadian Journal of Philosophy* 1 (1971): 105–24, especially 113, 116. Also, Feinberg, *Social Philosophy* (Englewood Cliffs, N.J.: Prentice-Hall, 1973), p. 33. (Italics added.)

36. This thesis is argued in Tom L. Beauchamp, "Paternalism and Biobehavioral Control," *The Monist* 60 (January 1977): 62–80. See also James Childress, "Paternalism and Health care," *Medical Responsibility: Paternalism, Informed Consent and Euthanasia*, eds. Wade Robison and Michael Pritchard (Clifton, N.J.: Humana Press, 1979), pp. 15–27.

37. Robert Veatch, *A Theory of Medical Ethics* (New York: Basic Books, 1982), p. 195. Veatch therefore accepts "weak paternalism," construed as an intervention in essentially nonvoluntary actions (pp. 196f, 199).

38. Robert Veatch, "Models for Ethical Medicine in a Revolutionary Age," *Hastings Center Report* 2 (June 1972): 5–7, especially p. 6. Cf. also his "Medical Ethics in a Revolutionary Age," *Journal of Current Social Issues* 12 (Fall 1975): especially pp. 14–19. See also James Childress, "A Masterful Tour: A Response to Robert Veatch," *ibid.*, pp. 20–25.

39. *Report and Recommendations: Research Involving Prisoners* (Washington: DHEW Publication No. (OS) 76-131, 1976). See also, Office of the Secretary, DHEW, "Additional Protections Pertaining to Biomedical and Behavioral Research Involving Prisoners as Subjects," *Federal Register* 43, Part IV: HEW 53652-53656, November 16, 1978 and DHHS, Food and Drug Administration, "Protection of Human Subjects; Prisoners Used as Subjects in Research," *Federal Register* 45: 36386-36391, May 30, 1980.

6

The Principle of Justice

In a short story entitled "The Lottery in Babylon,"[1] Jorge Borges depicts a society in which all social benefits and burdens are distributed solely on the basis of a periodic lottery. Any given person, at the end of any lottery event, could be a slave, a factory owner, a priest, an executioner, a prisoner, etc. The lottery takes no account of one's past achievements, one's training, or one's promise. It is a purely random selection system, without regard to contribution, need, or effort. The story is compelling because of the ethical and political oddity of such a "system." We regard it as capricious and unfair, for we think there are *valid principles* of justice that determine how social burdens and benefits ought to be allocated. These principles seem distinct from and independent of the principles of autonomy, nonmalefi- cence, and beneficence.

However, if we attempt to state those valid principles with precision, our own political and moral rules for distributing burdens and benefits may seem as perplexing as the lottery method described by Borges seems capricious. Intuitively we believe that it would be wrong to ask another person to accept an unfair share of the burdens society might impose, but this judgment is not informative unless accompanied by an account of an *unfair* share. This problem is generally thought to be resolvable only by a general moral theory of justice, and yet our many moral requirements that persons be treated justly have proven difficult to bring together in a single comprehensive theory. We shall begin work on this problem by analyzing the terms "justice" and "distributive justice." We can then pass on to more substantive problems about social justice, including problems of allocation in biomedicine.

The concept of justice

The meaning and types of justice

Some moral philosophers, most notably John Rawls, have argued that justice is best explicated in terms of fairness. Clearly there are close conceptual connections between these terms, as we shall occasionally have reason to note. However, perhaps the concept most closely linked to justice in its broadest sense is *desert* ("giving to each his right or due," as it was put in some ancient accounts of justice[2]). One acts justly toward a person when that person has been given what is due or owed, and thus what he or she deserves and can legitimately claim. If a person deserves to be awarded an M.D. degree, for example, justice has been done when that person receives the degree. What persons deserve or can legitimately claim is based on certain morally relevant properties they possess, such as being productive or being in need. Similarly, it is wrong, as a matter of justice, to burden or to reward someone if the person does *not* possess the relevant property. For example, it is unjust to reward a superior for the work of his or her subordinates when the superior contributed nothing to the rewardable productivity. In these examples, we can see how both fairness and desert form the foundation of our intuitive sense of justice.

The expression "distributive justice" refers to the justified distribution of benefits and burdens in society. This distribution is conceived as a cooperative enterprise structured by various moral, legal, and cultural rules and principles. Rules and principles of distribution may be called the terms of cooperation for that society; they are the implicit and explicit terms under which individuals are obligated to cooperate. Questions such as the following can be raised concerning the justice of the terms: What gives one person or group of people a right to expect cooperation from another person or group if only one person or group benefits? Is it just for some to have more freedom or opportunities than others? Is it right for one person to gain an economic advantage over another, if both are abiding by existing societal rules? These are all questions about fairness and desert.

Although most societies proclaim the equal worth of all persons and back that proclamation with various legal guarantees of equal justice and rights, economic and political disparities between individuals in those societies (and internationally between nations) are ubiquitous. These disparities are often labeled "inequities," and those who so conceive the situation question some aspects of domestic and international systems for distributing power and wealth. Recent literature on distributive justice features problems of fair *economic* distribution, especially inequalities of income between different classes of persons and unfair tax burdens on certain classes. However, there are many problems of distributive justice, including a large number of issues about liberty and about the distribution of health-care resources.

Comparative justice and the problem of scarce resources

Justice is *comparative* when what one person deserves can be determined only by balancing the competing claims of other persons against his or her claims. Here the condition of others in society affects how much an individual is due, e.g., whether a person qualifies to receive a cadaveric kidney transplant or a heart transplant. (See Case #33.) Justice is noncomparative, by contrast, when desert is judged by a standard independent of the claims of others, e.g., by the rule that an innocent person never deserves punishment. This chapter deals exclusively with comparative justice and social distributions of benefits and burdens.

Such problems of distributive justice arise only under conditions of scarcity and competition. If there were plenty of fresh water for industries to use in dumping their waste materials and no subsequent problems of disease, then patterns of restricted use would not need to be established. Only when we are worried that the supply of drinking water will be exhausted or that public health problems will be created by the pollutants are limits set on the amounts, if any, of permissible discharge. Trade-offs are inherently involved in such judgments. The goal of a pollution-free environment helps to safeguard the "right to health," but this goal also squeezes the economy. A trade-off is involved here no less than in circumstances where capital and labor are used to produce one commodity when they could have been used to produce another. Similarly, the use of more raw materials today risks causing shortages in the future—another trade-off. The point is that there is no need for principles of distributive justice until some measure of scarcity exists, and this feature of social life usually strikes us most forcefully when a trade-off is manifest. Many contemporary discussions of "just" benefits in prepaid health maintenance programs, the justice of programs of care for the mentally retarded, and the like inescapably involve such trade-offs.

David Hume pointed out that the concept of comparative justice has been developed in order to handle problems of conflicting claims or interests.[3] As he put it, rules of justice would have no point unless society were composed of persons with limited sympathy for others in the competition for scarce resources. The rules of justice serve to strike a balance between those conflicting interests and claims. Because law and morality are our explicit tools for balancing conflicting claims, there is a close link between the lawful society and the just society. Nonetheless, the law may be unjust; and not all rules of justice are connected to the law or to legal enforcement. Accordingly, parties with conflicting claims often attempt to justify their claims by appeal to basic moral rules.

A compelling example of distributive justice appears in Case #32 in the Appendix. An interdisciplinary panel of distinguished figures in medicine, ethics, and law was assembled in 1972 to consider the merits and demerits of using modern technology to produce an artificial heart—the so-called totally implantable artificial heart (TIAH). The alternatives quickly narrowed to three possibilities: (1) produce no heart because it is too expensive, (2) produce a heart powered by nuclear energy, or (3) produce a heart with an electric motor and rechargeable batteries. The panel eventually concluded that, on balance, the battery-powered heart would pose fewer risks to the recipient, his or her family, and other members of society than would the nuclear-powered heart. In assessing each alternative, the panel considered implications for the quality of life of recipients, the high cost to society, and even whether it would be too expensive by comparison with other medical needs that might be fulfilled instead. The panel concluded that (i) despite the substantial costs, it would be an injustice not to allocate money for the provision of the artificial heart to those in need of it (on grounds that comparative justice requires it), and (ii) the nuclear-powered heart would create too much risk to society.[4] Such a weighing of alternatives, especially of risks and benefits, is typical of problems of distributive justice. In this case decisions would eventually have to be made regarding two separate problems: *whether* to allocate money for the production of the heart, and *how* to allocate the hearts to individuals once technology makes the hearts available. These two problems of distributive justice are distinguished later in the chapter as the problems of macroallocation and microallocation.

Formal and material principles of justice

Justice in the sense of comparative desert has been analyzed in different ways in rival theories. But common to all theories of justice is a rather minimal principle traditionally attributed to Aristotle: Equals ought to be treated equally and unequals may be treated unequally. This elementary principle is referred to as the principle of formal justice, or sometimes as the principle of formal equality. It is *formal* because it states no particular respects in which equals ought to be treated the same. It only says that no matter which relevant respects are under consideration, persons equal in those respects should be treated equally. More fully stated in negative form, the principle says that no person should be treated unequally, despite all differences with other persons, until it has been shown that there is a difference between them relevant to the treatment at stake.

The problem with the formal principle is its lack of substance. That equals ought to be treated equally is not likely to stir disagreement. But who is equal and who unequal? What respects are relevant for purposes of comparing individuals? Presumably all citizens should be provided equal political rights, equal access to public services, and equal treatment under the law. One thesis common to virtually all accounts of justice is that delivery programs and services designed to assist persons of a certain class, such as the poor and the aged, should be made available to all members of that class. To deny access to some, when others receive the benefits, seems clearly unjust.

Any plausible theory of justice must specify the relevant differences between individuals, and not just any proposed criteria are morally acceptable. For example, it might be judged a good reason for not producing artificial hearts that heart failure victims are often unflatteringly obese. This judgment introduces a *proposed* relevant difference to distinguish persons who should receive technological advances in medicine from persons who should not. Yet this difference is unacceptable. It allows an injustice based on the morally irrelevant property of unflattering obesity. Some of the most difficult questions about justice arise over how to specify the relevant respects by which people are to be treated equally. Principles that specify these relevant respects are said to be *material* principles, because they put material content into a theory of justice. Examination of these material principles is therefore in order.

Material principles of justice

Each material principle of justice identifies a relevant property on the basis of which burdens and benefits should be distributed. Each principle is made a plausible candidate by the relevance of the property it isolates. The following is a fairly standard list of the major candidates for the position of valid principles of distributive justice (though longer lists have been proposed):[5]

1. To each person an equal share
2. To each person according to individual need
3. To each person according to individual effort
4. To each person according to societal contribution
5. To each person according to merit

There is no obvious barrier to acceptance of more than one of these principles, and some theories of justice accept all five as valid. We hold that these material principles all specify prima facie duties that—like respect for autonomy, nonmaleficence, and beneficence—cannot have their actual weight assessed independently of particular circumstances.

Most societies invoke each of these material principles for public policy purposes, applying different principles in different contexts. In the United States, for example, unemployment and welfare payments are distributed on the basis of need (and to some extent on the basis of either rights or previous length of employment); jobs and promotions in many sectors are awarded (distributed) on the basis of demonstrated achievement and merit; the higher incomes of wealthy professionals are allowed (distributed) on the grounds of superior effort, merit, or social contribution (or perhaps all three); and, at least theoretically, the opportunity for elementary and secondary education is distributed equally to all citizens. While it seems attractive to use all these principles, conflicts among them create a serious weighting or priority problem.

A particular case may help to indicate the variety and interrelation of different material principles of justice (as well as their status as prima facie principles). The case involves one Mark Dalton, a histology technician in the employ of a large chemical company.[6] Dalton was an excellent worker, but a week-long sick leave led a company nurse to discover that he had a chronic renal disease. Furthermore, it was discovered that the permissible chemical vapor exposure levels of Dalton's job might exacerbate his renal condition. The company management found another job, at the identical rate of pay, for which Dalton was qualified. However, it turned out that two other employees eligible for promotion were also interested in the job. Both of these employees had more seniority and better training than Dalton, and one was a woman. In this situation, each of the three employees can appeal to a different material principle of justice to substantiate his or her claim to the available position. Dalton can cite the material principle of need, arguing that his medical condition requires that he either be offered the new position or dismissed from the company. With their superior experience and training, each of the other two employees can invoke material principles of merit, societal contribution, and perhaps individual effort in support of their claims to the position. In addition, considerations of equal opportunity might give the woman valid grounds for claiming that justice gives her a right to the position.

While this case is meant to illustrate the near baffling complexity of appeals to justice, most *theories* of justice attempt to systematize and simplify moral intuitions by selecting and emphasizing one or more of the available material principles of distributive justice, perhaps calling upon other moral principles as well. *Egalitarian* theories emphasize equal access to the goods in life that every rational person desires; *Marxist* theories emphasize need; *Libertarian* theories emphasize rights to social and economic liberty (implicitly invoking criteria of contribution and merit); and *Utilitarian* theories emphasize a mixture of criteria so that public and private utility is maximized. The acceptability of any such theory of justice is determined by the quality of its moral argument that some one or more selected material principles ought to be given priority, or perhaps exclusive consideration, over the others.

Neither principles nor theories of distributive justice can be considered here in detail. Nonetheless, it is important to see how both relevant properties and public policies based on justice can be developed from such meager and abstract beginnings as "the principle of need." This principle declares that distribution is just (fair, deserved) when it is based on need. But how are we to understand the notion of a need? In general, to say that a person needs something is to say that *without it the person will be harmed* (or at least detrimentally affected). We can expand this basic idea about need by calling on the formal principle of justice. Conjointly the two principles require that people of equal need should be treated equally in regard to the satisfaction of their needs, while those who have unequal needs should be treated unequally. Some common sense examples of actions based on this principle show its relevance in contexts of distribution. In hospital wards patients should be given equal amounts of blood and medication when they need equal amounts, and unequal amounts when they need unequal amounts —by contrast, say, to quality and size of rooms, which are distributed largely according to the ability to pay. However, this analysis of needs does not take us far. We are not required to distribute all goods and services equally for all needs, such as needs for pets, athletic equipment, and nightgowns (unless a radical form of egalitarianism is defensible). Presumably we are interested only in *fundamental* needs.

To say that someone has a "fundamental need" for something is to say that the person will be harmed or detrimentally affected in a fundamental way if that thing is not obtained. Examples of fundamental harms would be malnutrition, serious bodily injury, and the withholding of critical information. Without nutrition, health care, and education, these harms would befall anyone; hence we say we have a fundamental need for such primary goods.

The more we refine the notion of need, the closer we move toward the relevant properties necessary for the formulation of a policy position. For example, if there exists a fundamental need for health care, then we would have to decide which needs are fundamental and which are not in order to develop a national health policy. Anyone who had such needs would have the relevant properties. While such theoretical refinement cannot be carried out here, it is important to notice the significance of the first step in the argument—the acceptance of the principle of need as a valid material principle of justice. If one rejects the principle of need while accepting, say, only contribution and merit, then one would be opposed in principle to these refinements and their applications to public policy. All public and institutional policies based on distributive justice derive ultimately from the acceptance of one or more material principles of distributive justice and from some procedure for refining them.

One of the more intense debates about distributive justice in recent years has focused on the issue of national health insurance. The United States has largely, though not exclusively, operated on the principle that distributions of health care services and goods are best left to the marketplace, where the implicit distributive principle is ability to pay. This marketplace principle relies upon some form of libertarian theory of justice for its justification. Libertarian theories of justice concentrate on the individual rights of persons to enter and withdraw freely from arrangements in accordance with their perceptions of their interests. A commitment to this model of individual freedom characterizes "libertarianism": People choose to contribute to economic arrangements as they wish, and because contributions are freely chosen they can be considered morally relevant bases on which to discriminate among individuals in distributing economic burdens and benefits. Government action, by contrast, is justified only when it protects the fundamental rights or entitlements of such citizens. This theory of justice has been developed in considerable detail in the work of Robert Nozick, who emphasizes rights not to be coerced rather than redistribution of economic benefits and burdens.

Some theories of justice challenge this approach. John Rawls's theory of justice, briefly mentioned in Chapter 2, presents a challenge that has immediate implications for a national health policy.[7] Rawls's account has as its central contention that we should distribute all vital economic goods and services equally, unless an unequal distribution would actually work to everyone's advantage. He presents his views through a hypothetical social contract procedure strongly indebted to what he calls the "Kantian conception of equality." According to this account, valid principles of justice are those principles to which we would all agree if we could freely consider the social situation from a standpoint that he calls the "original position": Equality is built into that hypothetical position in the form of a free and equal bargain among all parties, where there is equal ignorance of all individual characteristics and advantages that persons have or will have in their daily lives. According to one interpretation of his views,[8] Rawls is committed to the following perspective on a national health policy: Rational agents would choose principles of justice that maximize the minimum level of primary goods in order to protect vital interests in uncertain but perhaps disastrous contexts. Social allocations to protect everyone's future health and health needs would thus be elected by such agents (if health is a primary good). Such an approach would at least partially supplement the conventional marketplace system of distribution. It would probably also rule out *utilitarian* systems (in the form of attempts to produce the highest possible level of health care) and systems based on distributions of *equal* sums to be invested in any health commodity the individual wishes.

The implications of this interpretation of Rawls's theory for national health care are egalitarian. Each member of society, irrespective of wealth or position, would be provided with equal access to an adequate (though not maximal) level of health care for all available types of services. The distribution would proceed on the basis of need, and needs would be met by equal access to services. Better services, such as luxury hospital rooms and expensive but optional dental work, would be made available for purchase at personal expense by those who are able to and wish to do so. Yet *everyone's* health needs would be met at the level Charles Fried has described as a "decent minimum."[9] This system presents only one of many approaches that might be taken to the vexed problem of a national health policy.

Relevant properties

We have seen that material principles of justice specify relevant properties that one must possess in order to qualify under a particular distributive principle, thereby excluding other respects as irrelevant to the distribution under consideration. There are, however, theoretical difficulties in explicating the notion of relevant respects, as well as practical problems in the development of public policies aimed at justice. In some contexts relevant respects are firmly established, perhaps by tradition and perhaps by moral principle. It is sometimes—though not always—inappropriate to challenge these established relevant respects or to attempt to substitute others. For example, trophies are awarded (distributed) at the end of tennis tournaments on the basis of achievement; and how achievement is to be determined is firmly set by the tradition-bound rules of tournament tennis. Similarly, prison terms are not distributed to those who are not found guilty of crimes; as a firm matter of law and morality, guilt is relevant to conviction.

However, in controversial contexts it is morally appropriate either to institute a policy that establishes relevant respects where none previously were established or to develop a new policy that revises standard "relevant" respects. If a person is chosen to be an ambassador to a foreign nation merely on the basis of wealth, party affiliation, and loyalty to the chief executive, it is arguably the case that these operative (and perhaps even traditionally entrenched) "relevant" properties are arbitrary and irrelevant from the point of view of justice. Here it might be argued: "You ought to shift your *operative* set of 'relevant' properties to the *right* set of relevant properties, which would include facility with the language, knowledge of the country, administrative experience, and past service." The argument is that certain properties accepted as "relevant" are actually irrelevant and that certain properties presumed "irrelevant" are actually relevant.

A contemporary issue that illustrates this problem occurs in Case #25, which involves an incompetent organ donor. In this case a forty-year-old woman's life depends on a kidney transplant, which her fourteen-year-old daughter offers to supply. The kidney is a fairly good match. However, the woman has a thirty-five-year-old mentally retarded brother who is a some-what better match. (Some would say the brother is a *much* better match.) A survey of nurses, social workers, and physicians who work with such patients indicates that a majority would seek a court order to take the kidney from the thirty-five-year-old, institutionalized, mentally retarded brother.[10] Here we have a straightforward question about which criteria shall be used to select between these two potential donors—or to determine whether to wait for a cadaveric donor (an unlikely prospect). The closeness of the match does seem to be a relevant property favoring use of the brother, but the lack of consent from the brother and the apparently knowledgeable consent of the child (a minor) introduces a reason favoring use of the child. There are also reasons against using either potential donor. The child is powerfully and perhaps overwhelmingly influenced by the fact that the recipient of her gift is her mother. The closeness of the relation and the emotion-laden situation undoubtedly exert pressure on the child—so much pressure that we might call into question the quality of the consent. (Cf. the section on informed consent in Chapter 3.) This case shows that when rather concrete policies must be formulated, abstract principles of justice provide only rough guide-lines, and further moral argument is needed to fix the specific relevant properties on the basis of which an actual choice can be made.

The role of argument and decision

It is sometimes assumed that relevant properties are fixed independently of moral arguments and human decisions. There is *something* right, but something just as certainly misleading, about such an assumption. The basic moral principles outlined in previous chapters of this book are neither arbitrarily selected nor changeable merely by individual fiat, and they often control the relevance and irrelevance of properties. These principles lead us to *find* some material criteria acceptable in some contexts, and others in other contexts. Any properties that such principles determine to be relevant are therefore neither arbitrary nor mere matters of individual preference.

Consider the issue of research involving adult human subjects. How shall we decide who should become involved in research? If such participation is burdensome, how should this burden be distributed? The formal principle of justice declares that we must treat equally everyone who is alike in relevant respects. But which respects are relevant? Suppose the members of one class of adult persons have *consented* to participation, are *informed* regarding the experiments and their risks, and have *voluntarily* given their consent. Suppose, by contrast, that the members of another class of persons either have not consented, or are not informed, or have been coerced. Consent, understanding, and noncoercion are clear examples of nonarbitrary, relevant differences. Their relevance is nonarbitrarily fixed by the moral principles surveyed in previous chapters.

It is a matter of theoretical importance that material principles of distributive justice may be justified by appeal to moral principles *other than* some basic principle of justice rooted in fairness or desert ("justice itself," as some have put it). A tempting but dubious account of ethical theory is that nonmaleficence generates its own rules, autonomy its own rules, beneficence its own rules, and justice its own rules. Rules of privacy and confidentiality, for example, can perhaps be derived solely from the principle of autonomy. While there are many such direct connections between derivative and basic action-guides, material principles of distributive justice are seldom connected to only one basic principle of justice; material principles may be justified on the basis of other moral principles such as those discussed in Chapters 3–5. Thus, there might be utilitarian reasons for a certain distributive principle—e.g., for allocation patterns for certain medical supplies in war zones; and there might be reasons of autonomy for disallowing a particular distributive principle—such as a requirement of mandatory genetic screening.

On the other hand, there are occasions when moral principles do *not* unambiguously determine applicable distributive principles. Usually this indefiniteness occurs not because moral considerations are unimportant, but because there are conflicting moral demands where there is no clearly right course. In such cases a moral *decision* concerning the weight of competing moral claims is required, and this decision in turn fixes the acceptable relevant properties. The words "decision" and "fix" should not be taken to mean that such decisions to fix the properties are arbitrary and without a principled basis. The point is that sometimes there may be several conflicting *good* reasons for choosing different ways and no sufficient or determinative reason. Decisions will play a significant role in such contexts. This was discussed in Chapter 1 as the problem of moral dilemmas. Whether members of minority groups formerly discriminated against should be given preferential consideration in hiring is one such issue with important policy implications. Whether 18-year-olds should be allowed to vote is another.

A particularly striking example is found in a current controversy over self-created health problems. Poor diets, high alcoholic intake, and habitual smoking can contribute to high health insurance premiums. Perhaps persons with "clean lifestyles" should not have to pay the same health insurance premiums as do those who engage in hazardous activities. Presumably, the only relevant property governing qualification for most group insurance programs is that of being an employee eligible for enrollment in a group plan. However, heavy drug intake by some persons might raise questions as to the appropriate criteria for enrollment without penalty in such a plan. Perhaps we shall have to *decide* whether alcohol consumption, cigarette smoking, diet, or exercise programs are relevant to the determination of premium payments, for it scarcely seems a matter that has been determined.

This issue may appear to be either an empirical or a conceptual dispute concerning the conditions of being "healthy." More plausibly, it is a straightforward moral problem of justice: On the one hand, is it *fair* to persons who carefully exercise and eat proper foods to allow those with undisciplined habits to affect increases in insurance premiums (without attached penalties)? Do they *deserve* a system of equal contribution and equal protection without penalty? On the other hand, is it *fair* to those who know and care little about health maintenance that they be excluded, and do they *deserve* such a system? Such an issue will be decided by considering the weight of moral arguments on each side, and in the end the relevance or irrelevance of drug habits, diet, and exercise programs will be decided by reference to specific moral arguments premised on fairness.

Numerous moral and public policy problems take such a dilemmatic form. There are powerful moral reasons—some based in justice, some in other principles—for accepting two or more sets of different and competing properties as equally relevant, even though only one can be adopted. Recently a President's Commission debated the issue of whether injured research subjects must be compensated for injury if they voluntarily consented to participate in the research and the injury was not the result of negligence. The Commission cast the problem of an "ethical basis for compensation" as follows: If "one ought to respect the autonomy of the potential subject, it is at least initially difficult to understand why there is a moral requirement to compensate a subject who consents to participation without the expectation of compensation in case of injury." The Commission then debated how to handle this straightforward conflict between respect for autonomy and justice, noting that "Fairness argues for compensation, but the alternative argument from the consent of free agents denies this."[11] It would be convenient if relevant properties were always fixed in the way tennis rules are established, but as in this case often they are not. They must be fixed by moral deliberation and decision. Sometimes it is not unreasonable, unfair, or unjustified if the final decision favors *either* of two or more competing positions.

Classes of persons

Suppose a statute governing jury duty excuses all men but excuses no women, on grounds that there are many more men in the working population than women. Here justice requires us to say that an undue burden is placed on women and an undeserved privilege is granted to men. Being male or female is irrelevant, and so is the use of either sexual grouping. If the relevant property excusing jury duty is employment, then employed men and employed women should be excused without regard to sex. In general, rules and laws are unjust when they make distinctions between classes that are actually similar in relevant respects, or fail to make distinctions between classes that are actually different in relevant respects.

An important issue about justice and classes of persons has emerged from reflection on the selection of human subjects of biomedical research. Two questions are involved. First, should a particular class of subjects be used at all? For example, should prisoners, fetuses, children, and those institutionalized for reasons of mental disability be involved as subjects of research, and, if so, under what conditions? Second, if it is permissible to involve such subjects, should there be some order of selection of subjects within that class, based on different properties possessed by members of the class? For example, we have seen how it is morally relevant to distinguish within the class of children between older and younger children—or, better, between those who comprehend and report their feelings well and those who have diminished capacity to comprehend and report. Typically, these distinctions have policy implications. For example, we might establish a national policy that animals, adults, older children, and younger children be used *in that order* when doing biomedical research.

These considerations of justice are illustrated by the data included in Case #27 in the Appendix—a case popularly known as Willowbrook. It involves a state institution for mentally retarded children, some of whom were used as research subjects in order to develop an effective prophylactic agent against strains of hepatitis that were persistent and continuing in the institution. Some of the research involved exposing children to the resident strain of hepatitis infection. Studies were carried out in a special unit that isolated the children and protected them from other infectious diseases. These studies precipitated a series of debates in various journals about the moral permissibility of this use of mentally retarded children. At the heart of these discussions are problems about justice to classes of persons: It must first be decided whether it is morally permissible to use children, the retarded, or the institutionalized for research. Assuming that it is permissible to involve some members of at least one of these three classes, is it permissible to use the class of children who are institutionalized and retarded? If it is, under what conditions may they be used, and should there be an ordering, such as older members first, or those most severely retarded last?

These questions have been widely debated. The American Bar Association has taken the position that no research can be done on the mentally disabled unless it relates immediately to the etiology, pathogenesis, prevention, diagnosis, or treatment of mental disability itself. This position would not permit studies such as Willowbrook, probably because it is believed that the children involved are already overburdened by their condition and by the somewhat oppressive institutional environments in which they live. Other parties, including a former editor of *The New England Journal of Medicine*, have taken the position that such research is highly valuable for understanding hepatitis, was of potential value to the children in the institution, did not overburden children (because they probably would have contracted hepatitis anyway), and was carried out by exceptionally competent investigators. These debates again illustrate how the acceptability of rather concrete and specific principles of distributive justice turns on such moral issues as equal and unequal treatment, the minimal obligations owed by all persons to society, and the role of consent. Without a moral perspective on these matters, it would be difficult to know which distributive principle should be allowed or disallowed when dealing with classes of persons such as institutionalized, mentally retarded children.

Fair opportunity

The relevant properties and material principles that inform our judgments about distributive justice have thus far been our preoccupation. Consider those properties that might and often do serve as bases of distribution, but that *should not as a matter of justice* be considered relevant. Sex, race, religion, I.Q., and social status are the primary examples. In some unusual contexts we may appropriately appeal to these properties; for example, if a script calls for an actor in a male role, then females are properly excluded ("Peter Pan" being but a feeble exception). These cases are anomalous. But why do we not permit the use of rules such as "to each according to sex" or "to each according to I.Q." as valid principles of justice? The most widely accepted reason why we exclude such properties, and indeed regard them as discriminatory, is because to use such rules would be "to treat people differently in ways that profoundly affect their lives *because of differences for which they have no responsibility*."[12] This fairness-based reason for excluding some possible distributive rules has important implications because it demands that differences between persons should be considered relevant only if those persons can be held responsible for the differences. This rule states a norm of fairness.

The *fair opportunity rule*, as it may be called, says that no person should be granted benefits on the basis of such properties, because no person is responsible for having these advantageous properties. The rule also says that no persons should be denied benefits on the basis of such properties, because they also are not responsible for their disadvantageous properties. Such properties are never grounds for morally acceptable discrimination between persons, because they are not the sorts of properties that one has a fair chance to acquire or overcome. Of course in many societies properties such as religion and social status may be altered by individual action and can be overcome. But race, sex, and I.Q.—those properties that bedevil fair treatment more than any others known to the human species—are not easily altered.

The fair opportunity rule could be applied to the problems of the institutionalized mentally retarded examined in the previous section. If I.Q. is something for which a person is indeed not responsible, and if no one should be denied the benefits of the state (or other distributional system) on the basis of any such property, then it would be unjust not to distribute to retarded persons the benefits generally conferred upon all who share in the system of benefits. But this claim is still vague. (Several issues about this claim are raised in Case #30.) Consider the more familiar example of a basic education. This benefit is conferred on all citizens equally, and we consider a person deprived or harmed if it is not received. Imagine a community in which an efficient school system gives a uniform opportunity for a high-quality education to all students with basic skills, regardless of sex, race, or religion. Such a system, let us stipulate, does not offer an education to students with reading difficulties or mental deficiencies. These students would require special training in order to overcome their problems and to receive what for them is a minimally adequate education. If the students were responsible for their slowness, we might say that they *deserve* no special training and simply have to expend more effort. But, if they are not responsible, through any fault of their own, they *deserve* special considerations; fairness demands it. Hence we introduce different levels of education for different kinds of students, regardless of the differential in cost (but within limits of resources).

At stake is not the *equal* distribution of economic resources. The mentally retarded or slow learners with special reading problems need not receive the same amount of money, training, or resources as other pupils. Rather, they should receive what for them is a quality education, even if it costs more, because the fair opportunity rule *requires* that they receive it.

This argument provides both a justification of unequal distribution to many classes of handicapped and disadvantaged persons and a basis for numerous health policies. Criteria such as effort and merit should not be introduced in cases where a person is handicapped or disadvantaged through no fault of his own. To determine a person's due or desert exclusively on the basis of such principles would be morally wrong, because the fair opportunity rule functions systematically as an exclusionary criterion that prohibits the use of these material principles. As several current debates indicate, many matters of health policy could also turn on this thesis. If, for example, one believes that alcoholics are not responsible for their health problems, whereas smokers are, then one might argue that smokers should pay for their health care but that the state should pay for the care of alcoholics. Similarly, if persons *cannot* reciprocally return benefits they have received through state aid (through no fault of their own), we could make an exception to normal reciprocity requirements.

Earlier in this chapter we noted that the term "desert" may best capture the general meaning of justice. If this term reflects the basic meaning of justice, then how can the retarded and other handicapped persons *deserve* preferential treatment? What, after all, have they done to deserve it? To look at the matter in this way is to miss the point of the fair opportunity rule, which is rather clearly rooted in fairness rather than in a merit-based sense of desert. Rules of distributive justice such as merit, effort, and contribution are irrelevant in these contexts, because they are excluded as inappropriate by the fair opportunity principle. Of course we can still say that such persons "deserve" the treatment they receive. They deserve it because it is *fair*. This shows that *both* fairness and desert are deeply entrenched in our fundamental understanding of justice. (See the debate in Case #30.)

Despite our convictions about fair opportunity, there are limits to the goods and services that can be provided for the handicapped. Comparative justice demands a fair share, but not an unreasonable share. One of the major continuing controversies in biomedical ethics centers on what a "fair share" is. An illustration of this problem is found in children treated for myelomeningocele, a severe central nervous system anomaly. These children often receive partial treatment rather than total care, in the expectation that they will die. But some do not die, and over a period of years a series of expensive medical treatments for a variety of problems may be required. These children may be afflicted by blindness, very low intelligence, and many medical problems in need of constant attention. For such persons it is perplexingly difficult to say what the principle of fair opportunity demands. There can be little doubt that society does not now provide the exceptional medical care and training that such a child would need to receive a "fair opportunity" by comparison with other eight-year-olds. But the moral question remains: How much ought to be provided?

If one accepts the full implications of the fair opportunity rule for our sense of distributive justice, a revisionary perspective on common practices of distribution is a certain outcome. For the sake of moral consistency we would have to say that whenever a person is not responsible for certain "disadvantageous" properties, he or she should not be denied important benefits because of those properties. But suppose, momentarily, that almost all of our "abilities" and "disabilities" are a function of what Rawls has referred to as "the natural lottery."[13] That is, suppose that our talents and disabilities result from heredity and environment and that consequently we are not responsible for them. Even the ability to work long hours is environmentally produced. Advantageous properties, from this perspective, are not something one deserves any more than are disadvantageous, handicapping properties (though one may deserve certain consequences that result from having such properties[14]). It follows that both the advantageous and the disadvantageous properties are irrelevant for purposes of distributive justice. If this theory of the causal origins of advantageous and disadvantageous properties were accepted, along with the rule of fair opportunity previously outlined, then we would be led to radically different views about distributive justice than the ones we now generally acknowledge.

The full implications of this approach are uncertain, though it does seem that similar assumptions and conclusions are found in Rawls's *A Theory of Justice*, where he argues as follows:

[A free market arrangement] permits the distribution of wealth and income to be determined by the natural distribution of abilities and talents. Within the limits allowed by the background arrangements, distributive shares are decided by the outcome of the natural lottery; and this outcome is arbitrary from a moral perspective. There is no more reason to permit the distribution of income and wealth to be settled by the distribution of natural assets than by historical and social fortune. Furthermore, the principle of fair opportunity can be only imperfectly carried out, at least as long as the institution of the family exists. The extent to which natural capacities develop and reach fruition is affected by all kinds of social conditions and class attitudes. Even the willingness to make an effort, to try, and so to be deserving in the ordinary sense is itself dependent upon happy family and social circumstances.[15]

At a minimum we would look at our system of rewards and punishments in a revisionary manner if this approach were accepted. Rather than allowing broad inequalities based on effort, contribution, and merit, as practices in Western nations presently permit, we would tend to regard justice as done when radical inequalities are diminished, so long as "disadvantaged" persons can be advantaged by such a system of conferring benefits. Fairness, by this rule, demands this form of distribution. On the other hand, as Bernard Williams has correctly pointed out,[16] this process of reducing inequalities introduced by the natural lottery will have to stop somewhere; and, as Tristram Engelhardt has cogently argued, one is likely to call a halt to the demands of justice (at least in the area of health care) where one draws the distinction between the *unfair* (and therefore obligatory to correct) and the *merely unfortunate*:[17]

The sense of the duty to allocate resources to health care is different depending on which viewpoint one takes, for if the natural lottery is morally neutral, then providing inadequate health care is not *prima facie* unfair or unjust, though it may be indecent and unfeeling. However, if we view the world and the natural lottery's distribution of social goods as it should have been, were it to have been structured in order to support the moral order, such differences should, in justice and fairness, be obliterated as far as is reasonably possible. Where one draws the line between what is *unfair* and *unfortunate* will, as a result, have great consequences as to what allocations of health care resources are just or unfair as opposed to desirable or undesirable. If the natural lottery is neutral, in the sense of not creating an obligation to blunt its effects, one does not have [even] *prima facie* grounds for arguing for a right to health care on the basis of claims of fairness or justice.

It thus remains uncertain what the full implications of the approach Rawls has suggested would be, and also whether the fair opportunity rule has a major role in moral thinking. As Engelhardt rightly hints, one's general theory of justice—such as Rawls's or Nozick's discussed previously—may in the end be the decisive consideration.

It would be inappropriate to pursue these more theoretical problems of justice here. The point of exploring them this far is to show that *if* one accepts a justification of unequal treatment based on the fair opportunity rule, then many areas of moral reflection and social policy will inevitably be affected in significant ways.

Macroallocation and health policy

We have thus far encountered several problems about justice that are created by situations of limited resources. We have seen, for example, that debates over a national health insurance policy, over unequal distributions of educational advantages to the handicapped, and over whether to provide extensive therapies for those afflicted with myelomeningocele all turn on the question of who shall receive what share of society's resources. The same problem recurs for the distribution of expensive medical equipment, artificial organs, and blood for the treatment of hemophilia. The issues are, in part, *economic*: How are these scarce resources to be most efficiently provided? How can more people be helped and how can costs be reduced? But the issues are also *ethical*: By what principles, policies, and procedures can justice in the distribution of resources best be insured? Because these economic and ethical issues cannot be neatly separated, we should perhaps say that there is both an economic dimension and an ethical dimension to problems of allocation and health policy.

Problems of justice in the allocation of resources arise on two levels: macroallocation and microallocation. At the macroallocation level, decisions must be made as to how much of society's resources should be used for various goods, including health-related expenditures, as well as how priorities are to be established for the distribution of these resources. Such decisions are made by Congress, state legislatures, private foundations, etc. There are at least two aspects of such decisions: What quantity of our total available financial resources should be allotted to health-related enterprises (such as medical research, routine services, clinical practice, and health education), and of the total amount so allocated, what quantity should go to which specific projects (such as cancer research and dialysis programs)? At the microallocation level, health care professionals, hospitals, and other institutions determine which particular individuals shall obtain available resources.

Even though macroallocation and microallocation decisions are analytically distinct, they frequently overlap and interact. For example, macroallocation decisions obviously determine how much of a good, such as artificial organs or intensive care units, will be made available and hence the extent of scarcity for microallocation. Controversies about microallocation decisions may in turn lead a society to reconsider its implicit or explicit macroallocation policies. For example, the controversy about rationing scarce kidney dialysis and transplants, particularly by ability to pay and by judgments of social worth, contributed to the federal government's decision in 1972 to allocate funds to provide almost universal coverage for dialysis and transplantation.[18] We will discuss macroallocation problems in this section, reserving microallocation problems for the next section.

Macroallocation decisions have become increasingly important because of heavy federal and foundation involvement in research and treatment programs. While such expenditures of funds cannot be based solely on economic considerations untempered by principles of justice, it has proven difficult to implement principles of justice in public policy. Not only is it difficult to bring abstract principles to bear on practical realities, but those principles frequently come into conflict, as we have seen.[19] Because of these conflicts, public policies often move in cycles as society tries to reaffirm the principles or values it has previously compromised. As Guido Calabresi and Philip Bobbitt note, "A society may limit the destructive impact of tragic choices by choosing to mix approaches over time. Endangered values are reaffirmed. The ultimate cost to other values is not immediately borne."[20]

These conflicts and tragic choices can be seen in two cases in Appendix I: Case #32 on the totally implantable artificial heart, and Case #33 on heart transplants. In the latter, in June 1980, Patricia Harris, then Secretary of the Department of Health and Human Services, withdrew an earlier tentative authorization for Medicare to pay for heart transplants because of the need to evaluate the technology's "social consequences," including its costs, which average over $100,000 per transplant. There may be 30,000 victims of heart disease whose condition is now hopeless and who could possibly benefit from cardiac transplantation if enough hearts as well as funds were available. The cost would be over three billion dollars for 30,000 transplants. Many people are not sure that we can afford another program as expensive as the end-stage renal disease program, which now costs over 1.5 billion dollars each year.

Both Cases #32 and #33 present specific and limited questions about whether to provide federal funds to produce the totally implantable artificial heart and whether to subsidize cardiac transplantation. But these can be analyzed into several discrete questions, all of which potentially involve conflicts among moral principles, including principles of justice. These questions concern whether health care should be a matter for the government or for the marketplace, how much of the government's budget should go for health care, how much of the health care budget should go for prevention and how much for rescue intervention, which categories of illness or disease should have priority, and finally which technologies should be funded. As this list suggests, answering the specific questions about funding the development of the totally implantable artificial heart or cardiac transplantation presupposes an implicit or explicit answer to these other more general questions.

First, should the government be involved in health-care allocation and distribution at all, rather than leaving these matters to the marketplace? Society sometimes allows the principle of ability to pay to determine the distribution of health goods and services, and it frequently considers precisely which goods and services should be distributed in this manner and which should be distributed by different principles. Major arguments for governmental involvement in health-care allocation and distribution appeal either to a sense of compassion and benevolence toward sick people or to a right to health care based on justice.

It has been difficult to specify a right to medical care, but two major views are (1) that there is a right to *equal access* to medical care, and (2) that there is a right to a *decent minimum* of medical care.[21] Those who argue that all citizens have a right to equal access to health care sometimes contend that medical needs deserve special attention because they are unpredictable, randomly distributed, undeserved, and overridingly important when they appear. A primary problem in specifying a right to equal access to health care is setting limits, because health needs and desires are very expansive. The other major view proposes a right to a decent minimum of health care, which implies a government obligation to meet certain basic health needs of all citizens. This approach generally favors a two-tiered system of health care: governmental coverage for basic and catastrophic health needs, but private coverage for other health needs and desires. The proposal of a decent minimum has proven both theoretically and practically interesting because it raises problems of whether society can fairly, consistently, and unambiguously structure a public policy that recognizes a right to care for primary needs without creating a right to exotic and expensive forms of treatment, such as heart transplants.

A second question is also presupposed by the cases of the totally implantable artificial heart and cardiac transplantation: If government is involved in the allocation and distribution of health care, as our government is, how much of its budget should be allocated for health care and how much for other social goods, such as housing, education, culture, and recreation? Health is not our only value, and expenditures for other goods inevitably compete with health care for limited resources. Some commentators have argued that this second question is basically "political" rather than "moral." They hold that it should be resolved through the political process, which can reflect the values, preferences and priorities of the society.[22] According to such an argument, a citizen may not be able to complain of injustice if the society puts more money into space programs or defense than into health care. Nevertheless, there may be grounds for complaint if there are rights or basic needs that must be met for justice to be realized. Thus, if there is a right to a decent minimum of health care, then society would act unjustly (at least prima facie) if it did not allocate enough funds to meet that decent minimum. However, as we have seen, assertions of such a right remain controversial, and it is not even agreed what constitutes a decent minimum.

Additional complications emerge because health care, particularly medical care, may not be the most effective and efficient way to protect and promote health. Many social goods, such as improved sanitation programs, directly and indirectly reduce morbidity and premature mortality. Indeed, many improvements in health can be traced to improvements in the standard of living rather than to improvements in medical care or technology. Some even argue that to concentrate resources on *medical* care is to misallocate them. For example, Paul Starr contends that "If one wishes to equalize health, equalizing medical care is probably not the most effective strategy."[23] Studies from Britain indicate that the National Health Service itself has not greatly improved health indices or reduced the inequalities in health indices among the social classes.[24] But such studies may only indicate that medical care itself has less to do with health than other conditions in the society, such as the standard of living. Nevertheless, as long as medical care is important for some needs and increases our security, society may have an obligation to provide resources for a decent minimum, if not for equal access. At the very least, provision of a decent minimum, such as coverage of catastrophic illness, would reduce anxiety about payment for medical care.

Third, once the government has determined its budget *for* health care, it still has to allocate funds *within* health care: Should priority go to *prevention* or to *critical care*?[25] For example, the government might choose to concentrate on prevention of heart disease rather than on rescuing individuals by heart transplants or totally implantable artificial hearts. Prevention may in some cases be more effective and efficient than crisis medicine in saving lives and raising health levels. How society might mix preventive and rescue strategies will depend in part on knowledge of causal links, e.g., between environmental or behavioral factors and disease. Polio vaccine is an example of what can be done in some areas, but since end-stage kidney failure and heart failure are not the result of single diseases or factors, prevention is only a remote possibility. Even for illnesses where prevention is more effective and efficient than critical care, concentration on prevention would neglect needy persons who could directly benefit from critical care. Most prevention reduces morbidity and premature mortality for "statistical persons," but critical interventions concentrate on "identified persons."[26] Society is more likely to favor "identified persons" and to allocate resources for critical care, even if prevention would be more effective and efficient. It has been argued that such a social preference in part led society to provide funds for the treatment of end-stage renal disease, a program that now costs over 1.5 billion dollars each year for approximately 50,000 persons. Nevertheless, principles of justice do not require concentration on critical care of "identified persons," even though they do not preclude such an allocation.

Fourth, which categories of illness or disease should receive priority in the allocation of public resources if it is not possible to fund maximal research and therapy in all areas? For example, should heart disease have priority over cancer? It is clear that an answer to this question, as well as to other questions, is presupposed by a policy to fund or not to fund heart transplants or the totally implantable artificial heart. When we discuss equal access or a decent minimum of medical care, we most often consider need, in contrast to geography, finances, and the like, as the relevant property justifying similar treatment. But, from the standpoint of public policy, it may be necessary to give certain diseases priority in research and therapy. Gene Outka has argued that it is more "just to discriminate by virtue of categories of illness, for example, rather than rich ill and poor ill."[27] For purposes of justice, according to this line of argument, the relevant similarity between persons under conditions of scarcity is the *type* of medical need rather than medical need as such. In trying to determine priorities among diseases, policymakers could take into account such factors as the communicability, frequency, costs, pain and suffering, and prospects for rehabilitation of various diseases. It might be appropriate, for instance, to concentrate less on killer diseases, such as some forms of cancer, and more on disabling diseases, such as arthritis. (See Case #31 in the Appendix.) While certain forms of treatment would not be developed and distributed for some categories of illness, care would still be provided to all persons, and no one would be abandoned.

Fifth, within disease categories, which technologies or procedures should be funded? For example, within the category of heart disease, should cardiac transplantation be supported? In order to answer this question, Secretary Harris argued that it is essential to have a technology assessment—that is, an examination of all the direct and indirect impacts of cardiac transplantation. The probable cost of a technology is certainly one factor, but by no means the only one. The cost of the end-stage renal disease program, for example, is staggering and suggests caution about funding new technologies in other areas; but when the U.S. government provided equal access to costly medical treatment for victims of kidney disease, the composition of the patient population changed dramatically, as measured by such criteria as sex, race, age, education, marital status, and employment status. In the late sixties, the patients were largely white, married, male high school graduates, between twenty-five and forty-five; and over forty percent were employed. Ability to pay and judgments of social worth were factors in their selection. But by the late seventies, the patient population more closely reflected the actual incidence of end-stage renal failure among various groups. Equal access was apparently achieved.[28]

Nevertheless, various policy questions remain. Critics ask whether society is now treating too many patients at excessive costs and whether overtreatment stems in part from government financial incentives, especially to for-profit dialysis centers. Because patients have to pay more of their costs for home dialysis, critics also wonder whether the current structure of reimbursement encourages dialysis in centers rather than at home. Others respond that an older, less educated population with other complicating diseases would probably prefer in-center dialysis. Finally, difficulties in overcoming tissue rejection have prevented kidney transplantation from increasing rapidly (by contrast to the dialysis program), even though many patients would prefer transplantation to dialysis and even though transplantation is more cost-effective.[29] In addition to medical difficulties, society's policies may be inadequate to encourage organ donations. Before a dead person's organs can be transplanted, it is currently necessary to have that person's prior consent or the family's consent, but few people fill out donor cards. One possible policy is to educate the public about the importance of organ donation; another is to force people to make a decision (for example, people might be required to sign a card indicating whether they consent or refuse to allow their organs to be used after death); and still another possible policy is routine salvaging of organs unless people have explicitly denied permission.

As the examples of cardiac transplantation and kidney dialysis and transplantation indicate, public policies frequently involve conflicting moral considerations, including those of justice. Nowhere are these conflicts more evident than in debates about public policies to promote health and to reduce morbidity and premature death. When we considered the third question above, we indicated some of these conflicts; now we examine other conflicts in more detail.

Prevention, which has been defended in some literature as the best way to improve the nation's health, includes strengthening individuals (e.g., through vaccinations), changing lifestyles and behavioral patterns, and altering the environment. Effective and efficient preventive programs, especially those concentrating on lifestyles and behavioral patterns, soon encounter the limits set by the principle of autonomy.[30] Some public policies, laws, and regulations are designed specifically to protect and promote the health of individuals personally opposed to these restrictions. Examples of policies that are objectionable to some on grounds of autonomy include: laws requiring motorcyclists to wear safety helmets and motorists to wear seat belts; taxation, allocation, and scaled insurance schemes designed specifically to prevent smoking, obesity, and alcohol abuse; prohibition of dangerous recreational activities, such as hang gliding or stunt flying; and banning the purchase of possibly harmful or inefficacious drugs and chemicals.

One critical element in the controversy over such rules concerns the quality of the choices made by the persons whose liberty might be restricted. It has been argued that those whose health is affected by smoking, alcohol abuse, or obesity are engaging in what may be for them substantially nonautonomous behavior, even though they knowingly engage in the behavior and might oppose policies that penalize them for such behavior. Such an argument is difficult to sustain, because risky conduct is not itself a sign of nonvoluntariness, and assertions of social and cultural determinism of risky conduct are too sweeping and unsubstantiated. Nevertheless, if an individual's behavior is substantially nonvoluntary, the society may prohibit or regulate it in order to protect the individual. Beneficence supports such a policy, and neither autonomy nor justice precludes it.

Even if an individual's risk-taking is substantially voluntary, society may limit it in order to prevent the imposition of risks or costs on others, including the society. It is justifiable for the society to limit an individual's risky actions if, for example, his or her cigarette smoking or drunken driving threatens others. In many such cases, society may choose to regulate forms of conduct without prohibiting them altogether, perhaps by restricting the areas in which smoking occurs and prohibiting sales of alcohol on turnpike stops.

Another relevant nonpaternalistic consideration is protection of the financial resources of the community. Under a national health insurance scheme, we could expect increased pressure to limit individual risk-taking because citizens will argue that it is unfair to increase their premiums or taxes in order to pay for the avoidable, self-caused afflictions of others. Here again policies other than prohibition of risk-taking might be both preferable and feasible. One possible policy would be to tax risk-takers more heavily (for example, through increased taxes on alcohol and cigarettes) in order to cover their increased health costs. Such a policy may be defended on grounds of deterrence of risky conduct; but if it is defended as a way to distribute costs of health care fairly, proponents of the policy will have to show that such risky conduct really costs the society more. To be sure, concern about the rising costs of medical care has, in part, led to an emphasis on lifestyles and behavioral patterns. But some risky lifestyles and conduct may actually require less medical care. Furthermore, under a broad cost-benefit analysis (including social security and retirement programs), there may be even less reason for government intervention in some risk-taking. As Howard Leichter argues, "Over the long run, under public or private health and retirement systems, one can expect an increase rather than decrease in social expenditures as a result of avoiding health risks."[31] Thus, cost-benefit analysis may undermine such restrictive policies.

A final question is whether public policies could defensibly distinguish the risk-taker from others in the allocation and distribution of health care. Robert Veatch has argued that "it is fair . . . if persons in need of health services resulting from true, voluntary risks are treated differently from those in need of the same services for other reasons. In fact, it would be unfair if the two groups were treated equally."[32] Such an argument would count against one of the reasons frequently offered for equal access to medical care—that health needs are unpredictable, random, and undeserved. Individuals may in some cases bring their needs on themselves, and with a high degree of predictability.

Even if a limited policy of not providing medical care would be fair and just to the voluntary risk-taker, because he or she has forfeited a right to medical care for that particular need, such a policy faces insurmountable moral and practical difficulties. First, it is difficult if not impossible to pinpoint responsibility for most health needs because of the complex interactions of the "natural lottery," societal practices, and individual choices. It will rarely be possible to determine the actual role of each of these factors. For example, did a person's lung cancer result from cigarette smoking, environmental pollution, work conditions, or heredity? Second, since such a policy would require "health police" to investigate personal lifestyles and behavioral patterns, it would invite violations of moral principles and rules relating to autonomy and privacy. Third, society's sense of benevolence and compassion would probably oppose such a policy, even if it were just.

Finally, any policy focusing on individual lifestyles and behavioral patterns may be criticized on the grounds that it tends to neglect the social context of individual actions. It tends to "blame victims," rather than to "blame society." If this criticism is taken too far, it can deny all individual responsibility for risk-taking, a denial that is indefensible. Nevertheless, one central question of justice is whether to concentrate on the "natural lottery," societal practices, or individual conduct in trying to locate the *source* of health problems. Where one looks will presuppose not only a conception of health needs, but also a conception of the relation of the individual and society, and a conception of individual responsibility for conduct—all central matters of justice. For example, one would expect Marxist conceptions of justice to reject individualistic approaches to health.[33] Other theories of justice examined earlier in this chapter have similarly significant implications.

Although we have not tried in this section to identify all the important issues that emerge on the level of macroallocation, we have tried to indicate some important conflicts among various values, principles, and rules. Such conflicts pervade contemporary debates about health policy. As a result, those writers who suppose that it is possible to take an abstract theory of justice or a single principle of justice into the arena of public policy commit the same error as those who would totally exclude considerations of justice. Public policy is invariably multidimensional. Considerations of justice alone rarely determine appropriate policies of macroallocation, in part because principles of justice readily admit conflicts. Nonetheless, principles of justice are clearly relevant, and in some cases they set powerful constraints on what the government may permissibly do in health policy—just as the principle of autonomy and other moral principles act as constraints on government programs.

Microallocation

Not infrequently, health care providers, hospitals, and other institutions have to decide which persons will receive some scarce preventive or therapeutic procedure. Such microallocation decisions may have to be made after a service or good has gained acceptance through an experimental process. Insulin, penicillin, and dialysis all had such a history, and cardiac transplantation appears to be gaining acceptance. Microallocation decisions such as those involved when dialysis was scarce are particularly troubling because the disease or illness is life-threatening and the scarce resource thus offers the possibility of saving life. Here the question can escalate to, "Who shall live when not everyone can live?"[34] Unlike many contractual arrangements between patients and physicians, this question cannot be resolved by the principle of autonomy, for it is not decided *by* the patient at all. It is decided *for* the patient by others. In this section we investigate what principles of justice imply for microallocation, especially when they come into conflict with other principles and values. As we noted earlier, the anguish of "tragic choices" in microallocation may lead the society, through the government, to alter its macroallocation policies in order to increase the supply of the scarce resource, such as kidney dialysis or cardiac transplantation.

We begin with a distinction between just procedures and just outcomes. Sometimes we cannot guarantee a just outcome by any conceivable or feasible procedures, but we nevertheless remain concerned about the justice of the procedures themselves. As Rawls suggests, we may feel more secure in our judgments about just procedures than about just outcomes.[35] The common law tradition also stresses "natural justice," which tells us less about the content of a just decision than about approaches that are likely to yield just decisions. In order to obtain fair and impartial decisions, certain procedural rules are followed. For example, no party may be condemned without a hearing, the parties are entitled to know the reason for the decision, and no one may be a judge in his or her own case. Concerns about procedural due process pervade the law and are relevant to the allocation of scarce resources from both legal and moral standpoints. Indeed, both procedures and outcomes need attention: Who should make the decisions? And what should the criteria be for the selection of recipients? While distinct, these questions are, of course, interrelated. For example, if criteria of medical acceptability are used, medical experts have to play a central role in formulating and applying these criteria. A lay committee could help formulate and apply criteria of social worth, but it would have no function in a system of queuing or a lottery. (See also our discussion of decision makers in Chapter 4.)

Two sets of substantive rules and procedural rules are required. First it is necessary to formulate standards and procedures for determining the relevant pool of potential recipients, e.g., those eligible for heart transplantation. It is then necessary to develop standards and procedures for final selection, e.g., those persons actually selected to receive a heart. While these two sets of standards and procedures may overlap, it is useful to distinguish them and to consider them separately.

It is easier to secure agreement about initial inclusion and exclusion because they involve minimum standards, such as age and medical acceptability, which appear to be more objective and more easily applied than standards of final selection. Nevertheless, they sometimes incorporate arbitrary distinctions and unfounded judgments, e.g., that only people above or below a certain age can benefit from a particular treatment. The criteria of inclusion and exclusion can be arranged in three basic categories, suggested by Nicholas Rescher: the constituency factor, the progress-of-science factor, and the prospect-of-success factor.[36] The constituency factor includes clientele boundaries (e.g., veterans are served by veterans' hospitals), geographic boundaries (e.g., citizens of a state are served by a state-run hospital), and the ability to pay. It is appropriate to raise questions about all of these— especially the last—from the standpoint of justice: Which factors constitute *relevant* similarities for purposes of determining the pool from which final selection can be made?

The prospect-of-science factor may be relevant during the experimental phase of the development of a treatment, such as cardiac transplantation, because it may be important to exclude patients who have other complicating diseases in order to determine whether the experimental treatment is effective and how it can be improved. Judgments about the selection process may be influenced by judgments about the value of the experimental treatment itself. At medical centers performing cardiac transplantation, Lois Christopherson has noted,

staff members who saw the procedure as valuable and effective were more likely to believe that recipients were selected from well-educated and financially comfortable groups. Those who were particularly aware of the procedure's limitations and uncertainties were more likely to suspect that transplantation was performed disproportionately on the poor and unsophisticated.[37]

Questions about justice can be raised about selecting persons to participate in clinical research, as well as in nontherapeutic research. Neither the benefits nor the burdens of research should be unjustly distributed in society. But even the medical criteria that are relevant to and acceptable for participation in clinical research may need to be reassessed and modified when the treatment becomes more routine.

Whether the treatment is experimental or routine, the prospect-of-success factor is relevant, because a scarce medical resource should only be distributed to patients who have a reasonable chance of benefiting from it. To distribute otherwise would be an unjust use of resources. This prospect of success is usually analyzed in terms of "medical acceptability." While medical acceptability can only be formulated by medical experts, the public has a strong interest in making sure that the formulation does not incorporate covert and undefended social standards. For example, in Case #33, the Department of Health and Human Services withheld funding from heart transplants in part because the screening criteria at some institutions appeared to be "social" as well as "medical." Stanford's criteria excluded patients with "a history of alcoholism, job instability, antisocial behavior, or psychiatric illness," while requiring "a stable, rewarding family and/or vocational environment to return to posttransplant."

One useful procedural suggestion is to formulate and to apply standards of medical acceptability as though the resource were unlimited. If physicians and other health care professionals were to view scarcity as irrelevant to their determination of the initial pool, they would exclude only those candidates who could not possibly benefit from the treatment.[38] Nevertheless, the question of the relative prospect of benefit for different patients is exceedingly important, especially for such treatments as kidney or cardiac transplantation where the match between the organ and the recipient is so important.

The second stage of selection, which involves standards and procedures of final selection from the preliminary pool, has proven even more controversial. Three major approaches are in contention: (1) utilitarian principles of justice, (2) some more or less objective standards, and (3) some form of chance or queuing that expresses equality of opportunity. All of these approaches have been used for some therapies at some institutions. In the days of scarce dialysis equipment, some centers used social-worth criteria (sometimes in general terms, but sometimes in specific terms such as value to one's family), some used queuing (a first-come, first-served system), and at least one used a lottery (a randomizing system). In effect, however, all centers used one form of queuing or the first-come, first-treated rule; they did not drop patients from dialysis or refuse a second or third transplant when someone of "superior social worth" subsequently appeared. Criteria such as age were also used, especially in establishing the pool for final selection during the early years. To take other examples, in North Africa during World War II the scarce resource of penicillin was distributed to U.S. soldiers suffering from venereal disease rather than to those suffering from battle wounds (on grounds of military need); and in England polio vaccine was distributed to children by a lottery when it was scarce.

One argument in favor of the first approach—utilitarian selection—is that medical institutions and personnel are "trustees" of society. Nicholas Rescher defends utilitarian criteria (though his system is not entirely utilitarian):

In "choosing to save" one life rather than another, "the society," through the mediation of the particular medical institution in question—which should certainly look upon itself as a trustee for the social interest—is clearly warranted in considering the likely pattern of future *services to be rendered* by the patient (adequate recovery assumed), considering his age, talent, training, and past record of performance. In its allocation . . . society "invests" a scarce resource in one person as against another and is thus entitled to look to the probable prospective "return" on its investment.[39]

It is unclear, however, that society's stake in medicine necessitates viewing selection as a means to broader social goals. Indeed, society may have a stake in protecting both the patient-physician relationship and the delivery of medical care from economic considerations of investment and return. It may value the relationship of "personal care," even when it is not socially productive beyond the care provided to individuals. Were the physician to look through the patient to the society and attempt to realize society's larger goals, the relationship of personal care and trust would be radically altered.

There are many levels of responsibility in society, and not everyone should act in terms of the same standards at every level. The physician is not a policymaker. His or her primary responsibility is to the patient, and society has good reasons for insisting on the primacy of this responsibility of personal care. Physicians are to do all they can for their patients without counting society's resources and without taking into account the kinds of factors—such as statistical lives and the cost of medical research—that policymakers rightly should consider. As Howard Hiatt contends, it is

not fair to ask the physician or other medical-care provider to set them [i.e., national priorities] in the context of his or her own medical practice. A physician or other provider must do all that is permitted on behalf of his patient. In that sense, the physician is or should be responsible, with his patient and the patient's family, for setting priorities for that patient's management, within the limits available. The patient and the physician want no less, and society should settle for no less.[40]

The second approach uses "objective" criteria, such as age, life expectancy, and number of dependents. This approach would escape some of the difficulties of application that plague act-utilitarian calculations, and it would avoid the comparative evaluations of persons that many critics of utilitarian selection find disagreeable. While these more objective criteria could be fairly applied, it is not clear that they could be adequately justified. Which of the following objective criteria, for example, could be justified: age, number of dependents, or sex? Such criteria often seem arbitrarily selected, and thus appear more subjectively grounded than objectively justified. If they are not merely arbitrary, they can be reduced to either medical criteria or utilitarian criteria. We have already indicated some of the possibilities and limitations of both sorts of criteria.

Neither the first nor the second approach incorporates justice in the form of equality, fair opportunity, and equal access as well as does the third approach, which uses chance or queuing. In a situation of scarcity, especially where selection may determine life or death, equality may require queuing, lottery, or randomization—whichever procedure is the most appropriate and feasible in the circumstances.[41] ("Equality" should be here construed as "equality of opportunity," because not everyone can be treated identically.) This conclusion was also reached by the Artificial Heart Assessment Panel of the National Heart and Lung Institute:

In the event artificial heart resources are in scarce supply, decisions as to the selection of candidates for implantation of the artificial heart should be made by the physicians and medical institutions on the basis of medical criteria. If the pool of patients with equal medical needs exceeds supply, procedures should be devised for some form of random selection. Social worth criteria should not be used, and every effort should be exerted to minimize the possibility that social worth may implicitly be taken into account.[42]

In the most thorough ethical analysis of microallocation decisions in health care, Gerald Winslow "filters" various principles through Rawls's theory of justice, asking which principles rational contractors would adopt behind the "veil of ignorance."[43] He contends that they would reject or subordinate utilitarian principles to egalitarian principles and that those egalitarian principles would require queuing or random selection. In the two major cases he discusses, Winslow argues that the contractors would accept queuing in disaster medicine—probably also in the intensive care unit—and random selection for the totally implantable artificial heart after medical acceptability has been determined. Practical considerations may give priority to one mechanism over another. Nevertheless, some people may not be able to enter the queue or the lottery because of such factors as slowness in seeking help, inadequate or incompetent medical attention, delay in referral, and overt discrimination. Thus, it is necessary to determine whether the candidates for a scarce resource really had fair opportunity to enter the queue or the lottery. For example, a person's limited funds may have prevented him or her from seeking medical care until it was too late to benefit from particular therapy.

Does our argument in support of the use of chance or queuing in microallocation—after judgments of medical acceptability have been made—necessarily exclude all utilitarian calculation? Because rule-utilitarian reasoning can (but need not) support a system of chance or queuing, this question concerns whether act-utilitarian reasoning has a place within the system of microallocation. While direct act-utilitarian calculations are rarely justified in microallocation (in contrast to macroallocation where effectiveness and efficiency are central), they should be employed under some circumstances. Some defenders of utilitarian selection, or of exceptions to other systems of selection, invoke the model of *triage*, which has become common in medicine and health care. The French term "triage" means "sorting," "picking," or "choosing," and it has been applied to sorting such items as wool and coffee beans according to their quality. In the delivery of health care, triage has been practiced in war, in community disasters, and in emergency rooms where injured persons have been sorted for medical attention according to their needs and prospects. Decisions to admit and to discharge patients from Intensive Care Units often involve triage. The traditional and contemporary rationale for triage in all of these settings is "Do the greatest good for the greatest number."[44]

Yet triage decisions may take several different approaches in determining the greatest good for the greatest number. In one type of situation, victims may be sorted out according to their medical needs: those who will die without immediate help, those whose treatment may be delayed without immediate danger, those with minor injuries, and those for whom no treatment will be efficacious. Such a classification in terms of urgency of medical need and prospect of successful treatment establishes priorities of treatment that do not involve judgments about social worth.

In another type of situation we can suppose that some of the injured persons are medical personnel whose injuries are minor. These persons may, and perhaps should, be given priority of treatment so that they can be restored to help others. Similarly, in an outbreak of a disease, it seems justifiable to inoculate physicians first so that they can care for others. Such emergencies involve what Paul Ramsey calls a focused community with the clear and immediate need of either survival or maximal protection under disaster. In such focused communities, some persons may be given priority over others because they can contribute substantially to the community, just as sailors on an overloaded craft in a storm may be given priority so that they can help save the others. In a focused community, judgments about social worth are limited to the specific qualities and skills that are essential to the community's survival or protection. Although these judgments are comparative and evaluative, they do not attempt to assess the full worth of persons.[45]

The paradigm of triage suggests a way to legitimate certain presumably utilitarian exceptions within a larger system of chance or queuing. Advocates of departures from this system should appear before a lay review board and should meet the following schematic burden of proof: A patient would be given priority only if his or her contribution is indispensable to attaining a socially significant state of affairs, and only if society so values (or fears) that state of affairs that it would, for example, deny someone else a second transplant or would remove another person from the ICU (intensive care unit) in order to save this patient.[46] Perhaps the president of a country in wartime would be given priority, but in few cases would particular patients be truly indispensable to society. In genuine emergencies we are morally permitted, and perhaps even required, to depart from a system of chance or queuing, even if reluctantly. The principles of justice set a presumption in favor of a system of chance or queuing, and departures from the system must meet a heavy burden of proof. The contrast with Rescher's system is significant: His system uses utilitarian criteria until there are no major disparities in social worth among the candidates for a scarce resource; our system uses egalitarian criteria until there are major disparities in potential recipients' responsibilities and probable contributions in a social emergency. Such emergencies will probably be rare, but when they do appear, "tragic choices" may have to be made.

Conclusion

In this chapter we have examined several alternative approaches to moral problems about justice. It is not entirely clear that we must accept a single theory of justice in order to reflect constructively on these problems, for it is possible to conceive each general theory of justice as developed from a different conception of the moral life, a conception that only partially captures the diversity of that life. This may be one reason why egalitarian theories, libertarian theories, and utilitarian theories have all been skillfully defended in recent philosophy.

One widely accepted view is that these theories are irreconcilably opposed, springing as they do from rival starting points, and eventuating only in intractable and interminable disagreements. Another view is that we may be able to take the best of each theory, dispensing only with its unpalatable parts. For example, early in this chapter we noticed certain differences between egalitarian social ideals and libertarian economic ideals. Perhaps within a single political society, an economic system could be fashioned as libertarian and a social system as egalitarian, with public policies often governed by utilitarian cost-benefit considerations. But such a neat division may be politically and socially naive and unrealistic; in any event, we have no available theory at the present time to bring such diverse accounts into unity.

This crisis in moral and social thinking about justice may well stem from the very nature of such theorizing. General theories of justice attempt to introduce principles intended to order our diverse judgments about right and wrong as consistently and harmoniously as possible. The theorist starts with the broadest possible set of our considered moral judgments about justice, and then erects a theory that reflects those judgments. Because such reflections and supporting examples leave considerable latitude for choice of initial judgments, we should not be surprised if competing theories emerge. Indeed, it may not be too strong to say that at the present time there are several plausible, and perhaps equally viable, theories of justice. We shall therefore have to continue to reflect with increasing subtlety if we are to reduce the gaps between our most general theories of justice and to apply them to public policies governing the distribution of health care. In view of these competing principles of justice, it is not surprising that public policies swing back and forth, now emphasizing one, then emphasizing another.

Notes

1. *Labyrinths* (New York: New Directions, 1962), pp. 30–35.
2. See Martin Golding's "Justice and Rights: A Study in Relationship," in *Justice and Health Care*, ed. Earl E. Shelp (Boston: D. Reidel Publishing Co., 1981). The connections to certain ancient theories, including Ulpian's famous 3rd century definition, are treated in this essay. See pp. 23–35.
3. David Hume, *A Treatise of Human Nature*, ed. L. A. Selby-Bigge (Oxford: Oxford University Press, 1888), pp. 490–500.
4. *The Totally Implantable Artificial Heart: A Report of the Artificial Heart Assessment Panel of the National Heart and Lung Institute* (June 1973). DHEW Publication No. (NIH) 74-191.
5. Cf., e.g., Nicholas Rescher, *Distributive Justice* (Indianapolis, Ind.: Bobbs-Merrill, 1966), Chap. 4.
6. This case was reported by Robert E. Stevenson in the *Hastings Center Report* 10 (December 1980): 25.
7. See Norman Daniels, "Health Care Needs and Distributive Justice," *Philosophy and Public Affairs* 10 (1981): 146–79.
8. See Ronald M. Green, "Health Care and Justice in Contract Perspective," in *Ethics and Health Policy*, eds. Robert M. Veatch and Roy Branson (Cambridge, Mass.: Ballinger, 1976), pp. 111–26.
9. Cf. Charles Fried, "Equality and Rights in Medical Care," *Hastings Center Report* 6 (February 1976): 29–34.
10. Audience Survey: Symposium on Death and Dying, Southeastern Dialysis and Transplantation Association Meetings. Miami, Florida. August, 1977 (unpublished).
11. President's Commission for the Study of Ethical Problems in Medicine and Biomedical and Behavioral Research, *Compensating for Research Injuries* (Wash-

ington: Government Printing Office, 1982), Vol. I, pp. 54, 63. The Commission was ultimately more persuaded by the fairness arguments, but not *so* persuaded that they made compensation a "basic right." See p. 63.

12. W. K. Frankena, "Some Beliefs about Justice," *The Lindley Lecture*, University of Kansas (March 2, 1966), p. 10 (italics added).

13. *A Theory of Justice* (Cambridge, Mass.: Harvard University Press, 1971), p. 74.

14. Both Thomas Nagel and Robert Nozick have provided theoretical reasons to show that, as Nagel puts it, ". . . yet one probably does deserve the punishments or rewards that flow from these undeserved qualities." From "Equal Treatment and Compensatory Discrimination," *Philosophy and Public Affairs* 2 (1973), note 5. Nozick's far more radical challenge questions much of what we have argued above, but neither Nagel nor Nozick destroys the validity of the point we are making in this section. Cf. Nozick's *Anarchy, State, and Utopia* (New York: Basic Books, 1974), Chapter 7 and the first two sections of Chapter 8.

15. Rawls, *A Theory of Justice*, pp. 73f.

16. "The Idea of Equality," as reprinted in H. Bedau, *Justice and Equality* (Englewood Cliffs, N.J.: Prentice-Hall, 1971), p. 135.

17. H. Tristram Engelhardt, Jr., "Health Care Allocations: Responses to the Unjust, the Unfortunate, and the Undesirable," in *Justice and Health Care*, ed. Shelp, pp. 126–27.

18. On policies toward end-stage renal disease, see various writings by Richard Rettig, including *Formal Analysis, Policy Formulation, and End-Stage Renal Disease* (Washington: Office of Technology Assessment, 1981).

19. For a discussion of some of the main issues in macroallocation, see James F. Childress, *Priorities in Biomedical Ethics* (Philadelphia: The Westminster Press, 1981), Chapter 4, "Allocating Health Care Resources"; Tom L. Beauchamp, "Morality and the Social Control of Biomedical Technology," in *New Knowledge in the Biomedical Sciences*, eds. W. B. Bondeson, et al. (Dordrecht, Holland: D. Reidel Publishing Co., 1982); Alan Detsky, *Economic Foundations of National Health Policy* (Cambridge, Mass.: Ballinger, 1978); Robert Veatch and Roy Branson, eds., *Ethics and Health Policy*; Jay Katz and Alexander Morgan Capron, *Catastrophic Disease: Who Decides What?* (New York: Russell Sage Foundation, 1975); and Paul Ramsey, *The Patient as Person* (New Haven: Yale University Press, 1970), Chapter 7.

20. Calabresi and Bobbitt, *Tragic Choices* (New York: W. W. Norton & Co., 1978), p. 196.

21. For equal access, see especially Gene Outka, "Social Justice and Equal Access to Health Care," *Journal of Religious Ethics* 2 (1974): 11–32. For a right to a decent minimum, see Charles Fried, "Equality and Rights in Medical Care," pp. 29–34. See also several essays devoted to "Rights to Health Care," in *Journal of Medicine and Philosophy* 4 (June 1979), and H. Tristram Engelhardt, Jr., "Health Care Allocations: Responses to the Unjust, the Unfortunate, and the Undesirable," in *Justice and Health Care*, ed. Shelp, as well as other essays in this volume.

22. See Paul Ramsey, *The Patient as Person*, Chapter 7.

23. Paul Starr, "The Politics of Therapeutic Nihilism," *Hastings Center Report* 6 (October 1976): 26–30.

24. See Howard M. Leichter, *A Comparative Approach to Policy Analysis: Health Care Policy in Four Nations* (Cambridge, England: Cambridge University Press, 1979), Chapter 6.

25. In order to simplify matters, we do not consider chronic care at this point.

26. See Thomas Schelling, "The Life You Save May Be Your Own," in *Problems in Public Expenditure Analysis*, ed. Samuel B. Chase, Jr. (Washington: The Brookings Institution, 1966), pp. 127–66.

27. Outka, "Social Justice and Equal Access to Health Care," p. 24.

28. Roger W. Evans, Christopher R. Blagg, and Fred A. Bryan, Jr., "Implications for Health Policy: A Social and Demographic Profile of Hemodialysis Patients in the United States," *Journal of the American Medical Association* 245 (February 6, 1981): 478–91.

29. Oscar Salvatierra, Jr., et al., "Analysis of Costs and Outcomes of Renal Transplantation at One Center: Its Implications," *Journal of the American Medical Association* 241 (April 6, 1979): 1469–73, and Steven D. Roberts, Douglas R. Maxwell, and Thomas L. Gross, "Cost-Effective Care of End-Stage Renal Disease," *Annals of Internal Medicine* 92 (1980): Part 1, pp. 243–48.

30. For recent discussions, see Dan E. Beauchamp, "Public Health and Individual Liberty," *Annual Review of Public Health* 1 (1980): 121–36; Daniel Wikler, "Persuasion and Coercion for Health: Ethical Issues in Government Efforts to Change Lifestyles," *Milbank Memorial Fund Quarterly/Health and Society* 56 (Summer 1978): 303–17; and Robert M. Veatch, "Voluntary Risks to Health: The Ethical Issues," *Journal of the American Medical Association* 243 (January 4, 1980): 50–55; all reprinted in Tom L. Beauchamp and LeRoy Walters, eds., *Contemporary Issues in Bioethics*, 2nd ed. (Belmont, Calif.: Wadsworth Publishing Co., 1982). See also James F. Childress, *Who Should Decide? Paternalism in Health Care* (New York: Oxford University Press, 1982), Chapter 8.

31. Howard Leichter, "Public Policy and the British Experience," *Hastings Center Report* 11 (October 1981): 38.

32. Robert Veatch, "Voluntary Risks to Health: The Ethical Issues," in *Contemporary Issues in Bioethics*, 2nd ed., eds. Beauchamp and Walters, p. 462. Veatch does not apply this argument to withholding medical care but to separate funding and to prohibition.

33. See Robert Crawford, "You are Dangerous to Your Health: The Ideology and Politics of Victim Blaming," *International Journal of Health Services* 7 (1977): 663–80.

34. Much of the literature on microallocation decisions was stimulated by selection problems in kidney dialysis. See James F. Childress, "Who Shall Live When Not All Can Live?" *Soundings* 53 (1970): 339–55; Ramsey, *The Patient as Person*, Chapter 7; Katz and Capron, *Catastrophic Diseases: Who Decides What?*; Nicholas Rescher, "The Allocation of Exotic Medical Lifesaving Therapy," *Ethics* 79 (1969): 173–86; Calabresi and Bobbitt, *Tragic Choices*, esp. Chapter 7; and the literature mentioned in James F. Childress, "Rationing of Medical Treatment," in *The Encyclopedia of Bioethics*, ed. Warren T. Reich (New York: Free Press, 1978). For other issues, see also George J. Annas, "Allocation of Artificial Hearts in the Year 2002: 'Minevera v. National Health Agency'," *American Journal of Law and Medicine* 3 (Spring 1977): 59–76;

Marc D. Basson, "Choosing Among Candidates for Scarce Medical Resources," *Journal of Medicine and Philosophy* 4 (September 1979); and the thorough study by Gerald R. Winslow, *Triage and Justice: The Ethics of Rationing Life-Saving Medical Resources* (Berkeley, Calif.: University of California Press, 1982).

35. Rawls, *A Theory of Justice*.
36. Rescher, "The Allocation of Exotic Medical Lifesaving Therapy," pp. 176–77.
37. Lois K. Christopherson, "Heart Transplants," *Hastings Center Report* 12 (February 1982): 19.
38. See "Scarce Medical Resources," *Columbia Law Review* 69 (1969): 654, 656.
39. Rescher, "The Allocation of Exotic Medical Lifesaving Therapy," p. 178.
40. Howard Hiatt, "Protecting the Medical Commons: Who is Responsible?" *New England Journal of Medicine* (July 31, 1975): 235–41. See also Charles Fried, "Rights and Health Care—Beyond Equity and Efficiency," *New England Journal of Medicine* (July 31, 1975): 241–45.
41. Other reasons for using some form of chance are presented in Childress, "Who Shall Live When Not All Can Live?" and "Rationing Medical Treatment," *The Encyclopedia of Bioethics*. See also Ramsey, *The Patient as Person*, Chapter 7.
42. *The Totally Implantable Artificial Heart: A Report of the Artificial Heart Assessment Panel of the National Heart and Lung Institute*, p. 198.
43. Winslow, *Triage and Justice*.
44. *Ibid.*, Chapter 1.
45. Ramsey, *The Patient as Person*, pp. 257–58.
46. "Scarce Medical Resources," *Columbia Law Review*, p. 664.

7

Professional/Patient Relationships

So far we have developed four moral principles applicable to science, medicine, and health care. In this chapter we apply those four principles and several derivative moral rules—particularly rules of fidelity, veracity, confidentiality, and privacy—to various relationships between physicians, health care professionals, and researchers, on the one hand, and their patients or subjects, on the other. These moral rules derive from the four principles and are especially pertinent to problems that arise in professional settings. Some of these rules may be grounded in only one principle, while others may be grounded in several principles.[1]

Rules of veracity

It is commonly agreed that we have a duty of veracity, i.e., a duty to tell the truth and not to lie to or deceive others. But, as Henry Sidgwick observed many years ago, "It does not seem clearly agreed whether Veracity is an absolute and independent duty, or a special application of some higher principle."[2] Sidgwick's observation still holds. One contemporary philosopher, G. J. Warnock, includes veracity as an independent principle ranking with beneficence, nonmaleficence, and justice.[3] Others have held that rules of veracity are derived from other principles, such as respect for persons, fidelity, or utility. Whether rules of veracity are independent or derived, they express several values that merit separate treatment.

Three arguments for the duty of veracity are particularly applicable to relationships between health care professionals and patients. The first argument holds that the duty of veracity is part of the respect we owe to persons. As Alan Donagan writes:

Relations between human beings are largely carried on by means of language; and much of what is communicated in language consists of expressions of opinion about what is the case. Unless it is required by a specific moral precept, nobody has a right to know another's opinion. The respect owed to other human beings includes respect for their liberty to withhold their thoughts when it is not their duty to divulge them; but, if anybody chooses to divulge his thoughts, the respect he owes to his audience requires that the thoughts he communicates must really be his. . . .[4]

As we saw in Chapter 3, respect for persons is commonly expressed in biomedical ethics through the principle of autonomy. Not to solicit *consent* for treatment from patients or for participation in research from subjects is to violate their autonomy and to fail to respect them as persons. But consent cannot express autonomy unless it is informed, and it therefore depends on communication and ultimately on truthtelling. Thus, a duty of veracity can be derived from a principle of respect for persons or autonomy.

Second, some philosophers, including W. D. Ross, argue that the duty of veracity is an expression of the duty of fidelity or promise-keeping.[5] When we use language to communicate with others, we implicitly promise that we will speak truthfully, that we will not lie by misrepresenting our opinions, and that we will not deceive our listeners. Our participation in society and our use of shared language engender a duty of veracity because of an implicit contract. This contract generates the expectation that we will speak truthfully. Within biomedical contexts, it is sometimes possible also to point to a more specific, though still implicit, contract or promise. By entering into a relationship in the context of therapy or research, the patient or subject gains a special right to the truth regarding diagnosis, prognosis, procedures, and the like. (We examine rules of fidelity later in this chapter.)

Third, relationships of trust between human beings are necessary for fruitful interaction and cooperation. At the core of such relationships is confidence in and reliance upon others to respect rules of veracity. This argument, commonly used by rule utilitarians, holds that lying can undermine relationships of trust and produce undesirable consequences. For example, relationships between health care professionals and their patients and between researchers and their subjects ultimately depend on trust; adherence to rules of veracity is essential to maintain this trust.

Lying thus fails to show respect for persons and their autonomy, violates implicit contracts, and also threatens relationships based on trust.[6] We believe that this line of argument also flows naturally from our first six chapters. Despite this argument, the various codes of medical ethics tend to omit such rules of veracity. (See Appendix II.) The Hippocratic Oath does not impose such duties, nor does the Declaration of Geneva by the World Medical Association in 1948. The Principles of Medical Ethics of the AMA in effect from 1957 to 1980 made no mention of a duty of veracity; the physician had discretion about what to divulge to his or her patients. But in its 1980 revision of the Principles of Medical Ethics, the AMA held that the physician should "deal honestly with patients and colleagues." Nevertheless, the physician still appears to have great discretion about what to disclose, at least where consent to diagnostic or therapeutic procedures or to participation in research is not required. The AMA Judicial Council specifies disclosure requirements in obtaining informed consent, but not in other areas.[7] However, some recent studies indicate that most physicians say that they routinely disclose information about diagnosis and prognosis to terminally ill cancer patients—the most widely debated case of disclosure where consent to further procedures may not be involved.[8]

While codes of ethics in nursing also fail to specify a duty of veracity, codes and regulations of research emphasize a duty of disclosure in the research setting, where there might be a conflict between the interests of patients and the interests of society. In the context of therapy, one recent Patient's Bill of Rights (compare the American Hospital Association statement in Appendix II) holds that a patient has a right "to informed participation in all decisions involving his health care program," a right "to know what research and experimental protocols are being used" in the facility and what alternatives are available in the community, a right "to a clear, concise explanation of all proposed procedures in layman's terms, including the possibilities of any risk of mortality or serious side effects, problems related to recuperation, and probability of success," and a right "to know the identity and professional status of all those providing service."[9]

What do rules of veracity entail, and how much weight do they have? Like other duties in this volume, veracity is prima facie, not absolute. Nondisclosure, deception, and even lying can sometimes be justified when veracity conflicts with other duties. In many areas, but especially in disputes about veracity, moral debates involve the definition or description of the act as well as its justification. Consider further the meaning of "lying." We define "lying" as telling another person what one believes to be false in order to deceive the person. So defined, "lying" would only be prima facie wrong, and thus could be justified in some circumstances. If, however, "lying" is defined as intentionally withholding the truth from a person who has a right to it, then "lying" could be construed as absolutely wrong (if the right is held to be absolute rather than prima facie). The latter definition incorporates moral elements, because it holds that the truth categorically must be told to some persons. It "resolves" moral dilemmas by redefining them, for some statements that would be described as lies according to our definition would not be lies according to this definition. In Chapter 2, we discussed Case #2 in terms of both definitions of lying.

Although lying has attracted more attention and discussion than other ways of departing from rules of veracity, it is only one species of deception. Deception encompasses many acts other than lying. For example, if a physician gives a patient a placebo, he or she may or may not lie to the patient. In Case #4, the therapists intentionally deceived the patient for his benefit, but they did not lie to him. The duty of veracity requires nondeception, as well as truthtelling.

The actual number and weight of duties of veracity are still largely unresolved. However, some generalizations may be tendered. Deception that does not involve lying seems less difficult to justify than lying, because it does not as deeply threaten the relationship of trust between deceiver and deceived as does lying. Underdisclosure and nondisclosure seem still less difficult to justify in many contexts. Thus, there is a rough ordering to these distinguishable duties. By contrast to the duty not to lie and the duty not to deceive, which are broadly applicable, the duty to disclose (as examined in Chapter 3) usually depends on special relationships between the parties involved. In a clinical relationship, for example, the patient entrusts care to the clinician and generally has a right to information that the clinician would not be obligated to provide to total strangers. It is thus advisable not to conflate duties of not lying, nondeception, and disclosure, even though much of the literature views them as a single duty.

Both lies, as we have defined them, and other forms of deception are prima facie wrong and stand in need of justification; but they can sometimes be justified. We are all familiar with cases outside of medicine where nondisclosure, deception, and even lying can be justified, for veracity can easily conflict with other moral objectives or principles. In Chapter 3, we considered some of the conditions that are necessary to justify deception and incomplete disclosure in research. Those conditions were so narrowly drawn that most biomedical and social science research involving intentional deception would be unjustified. Nevertheless, we held that some important low-risk research involving minor deception could be justified if the undisclosed information would have invalidated the research had it been disclosed. (See pp. 80–83.) We shall now consider three arguments for limited disclosure and deception in *therapeutic* settings.[10]

1. The first argument for nondisclosure of some diagnoses and prognoses in the therapeutic setting represents what Henry Sidgwick called "benevolent deception." It holds that disclosure of a diagnosis of cancer, for example, would violate the duties of beneficence and nonmaleficence by causing the patient anxiety ("What you don't know can't hurt you"), by causing the patient to commit suicide, and the like. This general line of argument is found in our discussion of paternalism in Chapter 5.

One objection to this argument is based on the uncertainty of predicting consequences. As Samuel Johnson put it:

I deny the lawfulness of telling a lie to a sick man for fear of alarming him. You have no business with consequences; you are to tell the truth. Besides, you are not sure what effects your telling him that he is in danger may have. It may bring his distemper to a crisis, and that may cure him. Of all lying, I have the greatest abhorrence of this, because I believe it has been frequently practised on myself.[11]

Such an objection is especially applicable to act-utilitarian approaches to veracity. The more compelling objections to "benevolent deception" stress violations of the principles of respect for persons and fidelity, as well as the long-term threat to the relationship of trust between physicians and patients.

In Case #7, a radiologist did not warn his patients of the possibility of a fatal reaction to urography on the grounds that it would not benefit them to know and might be dangerous. He contended that if he had told the woman who died of the possible fatal reaction, she would have become upset. He would then have convinced her that the probability of benefit outweighed the slight chance of a fatal reaction. Thus, he argued, telling her would only have upset her and would not have changed the outcome. Even if such cases do not seriously threaten the relationship of trust, they involve violations of the principles of fidelity and autonomy. In particular, the radiologist denied the patient information necessary for informed consent and violated her right to make her own assessment of the risks and benefits. (Of course, not all possible information is necessary, as we argued in our discussion of informed consent and the reasonable person standard in Chapter 3.)

Case #4 represents another instance of "benevolent deception." A retired army officer was having chronic pain after several abdominal operations. He had lost weight and was depressed, unkempt, and socially withdrawn. He voluntarily entered a psychiatric ward where there was a clear expectation of reducing his reliance on Talwin to relieve his pain by substituting other forms of pain control. Nevertheless, the patient insisted that he needed his medication to control his pain. After group consultation, the therapists decided to withdraw the Talwin by gradually substituting saline, but without informing the patient. The substitution was effective, and although the patient was angry when told three weeks later, he was able to control his pain without medication and to resume relatively normal functions. The therapists justified this deceptive use of a placebo because of its "high probability of success." While it is tempting to justify the means by the ends, especially when the ends have previously been successfully realized, alternative nondeceptive means might also have worked. The prima facie duty of veracity dictates a search for available alternatives even if they sometimes require more time, energy, and money. Furthermore, on utilitarian grounds this deceptive use of a placebo may have long-term negative effects on the patient's self-image and may impair his trust in health care professionals.

2. A second argument for nondisclosure and deception is that health care professionals cannot even know, let alone communicate, the "whole truth," and if they could, many patients and subjects would not be able to comprehend and understand the "whole truth." Such an argument, however, does not undermine the duty of veracity, understood as the duty to be truthful in such cases as #7 and #8.[12] As discussed in Chapter 3, this duty requires that health care professionals disclose as fully and as completely as possible what a reasonable patient would want to know and what particular patients want to know.

3. A third argument for nondisclosure and deception is that some patients, particularly the very sick and the dying, do not really want to know the truth about their condition, despite what opinion surveys seem to reveal. According to this line of argument, neither the duty of fidelity nor the duty of respect for persons requires truthtelling, because patients indicate by various signals—if not by actual words—that they do not want to hear the truth. To the rejoinder that many, and perhaps most, patients appear to want disclosure of relevant information, proponents of this third argument for nondisclosure hold that the patients they have in mind *really* do not want to know even when they say they do. For example, such claims might be made about Cases #4–8. But claims about what patients *really* want are suspect, and there is no *moral* alternative in such cases to respecting the autonomy of competent patients by acting on their expressed wishes and wants. Also, this third argument sets dangerous precedents for paternalistic actions, even if it is a correct view of patient wishes and wants in some cases.

In some instances, of course, patients genuinely do not want to know. For example, some patients with a high risk of developing Huntington's chorea, an incurable genetic disease, indicate that they would not be interested in a simple, safe, and accurate predictive test if one were developed. In one sample, 23% of the high-risk respondents indicated that they might not take such a test.[13] In other cases, patients who suspect that they might have cancer explicitly ask not to be informed of the diagnosis and prognosis. What should health care professionals do when patients ask not to be given certain information? Some writers go so far as to suggest that a patient has a *duty* to seek and appropriate the truth—not merely a *right* to the truth.[14] But to force unwanted information on a patient is generally to act paternalistically and to violate that patient's autonomy. To force a person to confront the truth seems to be an act of disrespect, though it might on occasion be justified—e.g., in cases of weak paternalism where a person acts from false beliefs. However, respect entails allowing persons to exercise the right not to know whenever they are adequately informed and are acting autonomously.

If the disclosure of information depends in part on a duty of fidelity, what responsibility does a health care professional have when a test undertaken for a specific purpose reveals information not specifically requested by the testee, who might, however, be interested in the information? In a case discussed by Robert Veatch,[15] a forty-one-year-old woman had unexpectedly become pregnant and was referred by her physician to the Human Genetics Unit in order to determine whether her fetus might have Down's syndrome. Because of her age she was considered to be at higher risk of having a child with Down's syndrome. The woman underwent amniocentesis, in which a sample of amniotic fluid surrounding the fetus is withdrawn by a needle for purposes of a biochemical or chromosomal analysis. The test showed that the fetus did not have Down's syndrome; there was no *extra* 21st chromosome. But the sex chromosomes were abnormal: They were XYY, rather than the normal patterns of XX for female or XY for male. There is considerable debate about the significance of the extra Y chromosome. Although some studies show that XYY males tend to commit more violent crimes, other studies reject those findings. What should the genetic counselor do? Would the counselor fulfill the duties of fidelity and disclosure if he or she reported only that the fetus did not suffer from Down's syndrome? Or is the counselor also morally required to report the other findings? Does the woman have a right to this information even though she did not specifically request it? Does the fact that the correlation between the XYY chromosomes and antisocial behavior is not established make this disclosure even more risky, since it (a) could lead to an abortion or (b) could be a self-fulfilling prophecy if the woman did not abort? Should the patient have the right to make her own decision about the significance of this information? If the duty of veracity is based on respect for persons and their autonomy, a strong case can be made for disclosure, even though the woman did not specifically request this information. Attitudes toward abortion will doubtless affect the counselor's response. But if a woman has a legal right to have an abortion within the first two trimesters whatever her reasons, it seems unfair to deprive her of information that she might consider relevant. The counselor should indicate the uncertainty about the significance of the extra Y chromosome. The information should be related carefully and sensitively.

In one type of situation, the AMA Principles of Medical Ethics (see Appendix II) require disclosure of information in order to preserve trust between the public and the medical profession:

A physician shall deal honestly with patients and colleagues, and strive to expose those physicians deficient in character or competence, or who engage in fraud or deception.

Exposés by fellow physicians are, however, uncommon. On the basis of studies of professional ethics and competence, it is difficult to believe that all or most cases of deficiency in moral character or professional incompetence are disclosed to the proper bodies or to the public. The bond of loyalty to the profession, so accented in the tradition of medical ethics, makes such disclosures unlikely.

In addition to loyalty to colleagues, which may conflict with the duty to disclose information, the physician may also experience a conflict between the duty of confidentiality and the duty of veracity. Such a conflict is evident in Case #2. After tests have shown that he is histocompatible, a father decides that he does not want to donate a kidney to his five-year-old daughter who needs a transplant. Because he fears that the truth might shatter his family, he asks the physician to tell the members of his family that he is not histocompatible. The physician then tells the family that "for medical reasons," the father should not donate a kidney. Although it is possible to analyze this case in utilitarian terms—maximizing good and minimizing harm—it is possible to argue that the father's relationship with the physician was confidential and that the duty to respect confidentiality outweighed the duty of veracity in this situation. Some would argue that the duty of confidentiality justifies nondisclosure (in this case) but does not justify a lie if the wife should press the physician for an explanation of "medical reasons." This problem requires examination of the rules of confidentiality.

Rules of confidentiality and privacy

Consider the following case: The parents of a child suffering from a genetic disease insist that the physician not reveal this information to others in the family who may be at risk of having children with the same disease. Suppose, for example, that the child has Lesch-Nyhan syndrome, a disease involving uncontrollable self-mutilation. Because this disease is X-linked, the mother's sisters would be at risk. But the mother, let us suppose, dislikes her sisters, who live far away and never communicate. Furthermore, she feels the stigma of being a carrier of the disease and so wishes to conceal the information. In this case, her physician faces a conflict between a duty to respect the confidences of patients and his or her broader social responsibility. There is no way to avoid this conflict if attempts to obtain the mother's permission to disclose the information should fail. Whether this physician has a right and perhaps even a duty to disclose the information in question will depend on the basis, limits, and stringency of the rules of confidentiality.

There is widespread agreement, expressed in various ethical codes, that rules of confidentiality and privacy should prevail in relationships with patients and research subjects. The ANA code of ethics requires nurses to safeguard "the client's right to privacy by judiciously protecting information of a confidential nature," and federal regulations of research involving human subjects require protection of confidentiality and privacy. The Hippocratic Oath urges secrecy regarding what "ought not to be spoken abroad," but does not limit secrecy to what is seen or heard in professional practice. According to the current Principles of Medical Ethics (1980) of the AMA, a physician "shall safeguard patient confidences within the constraints of law." The World Medical Association International Code of Medical Ethics expressly holds even that the physician owes the patient "*absolute secrecy* on all [information] which has been confided to him or which he knows because of the confidence entrusted to him" (emphasis added). (See Appendix II.) However, most codes and general theories hold that rules of confidentiality are not absolute. In fact, it may be possible to specify several conditions under which confidentiality should not be maintained. Before we turn to the conditions for justified breaches of confidentiality, we need to inquire into the grounds of rules of confidentiality and closely related rules of privacy.

Although we may find a person who betrays secrets despicable, it is not clear that such a person violates a general moral principle or rule against telling secrets. In most instances, he or she betrays other people who entered into certain relationships counting on respect for the confidentiality of information. Under circumstances of trust, there must be confidence in and reliance upon others to respect certain principles and rules in their interactions. While some principles and rules set by professional codes are more matters of custom than morality, the patient may rightly believe that an implicit contract—to be discussed under rules of fidelity—has been broken if the professional fails to live up to these customary standards.

Rules of confidentiality can be given explicitly moral warrants, some utilitarian and others deontological. Both the majority opinion and the dissenting opinion in the Tarasoff case (see Case #1) offer a utilitarian grounding for the rule of confidentiality—as discussed in Chapter 2. Their main disagreement concerns the question of exceptions to the rule or conditions for overriding it in the psychotherapeutic relationship. According to Justice Clark's dissent, the psychiatrist does not have a duty to warn a potential victim about possible harm from a patient. Assurance of confidentiality is of paramount importance because it enables people to seek help without the stigma that would result from public knowledge: It encourages full disclosure essential for effective treatment, and it is necessary for the maintenance of trust, "the very means by which treatment is effected." Justice Clark argues that psychiatry has an important social function in the reduction of violence and that it cannot fulfill that function without the rule of confidentiality in virtually absolute form. For the state to impose a duty to warn is to undermine the rule of confidentiality and thereby to diminish psychiatry's valuable social function.

An argument that builds the right to confidentiality on the right of autonomy is often linked to deontology rather than utilitarianism. One aspect of respecting autonomy, it may be argued, is respect for a person's *privacy*. The principle of autonomy confers a right to self-determination, which, as we saw in Chapter 3, may be protected by informed consent requirements, and the right to privacy and confidentiality might be derived from this more general right to self-determination. That is, rights to privacy and confidentiality express the right to self-determination in contexts involving personal information, giving moral authority to the individual's interest in determining what will be known about him or her. If these rights were thus viewed as derivative from the principle of autonomy, controversies about privacy and confidentiality could borrow from the framework developed earlier in our discussion of autonomy and informed consent.

While this straightforward approach initially appears promising, some philosophers doubt that it provides an adequate account of privacy and confidentiality. One objection has been presented by Arthur L. Caplan, who argues that to see privacy as derived from any more basic or comprehensive moral principle is to mistake its own *fundamental* nature and importance. Caplan contends that privacy is a universal human need. All cultures allow their members at least some spheres in which the privacy of their activity is protected, and in Caplan's opinion this practice suggests that privacy is essential to the human sense of identity and well-being. Because privacy itself is a basic human need, the moral right to privacy is superior to other rights grounded in less basic ethical claims.[16]

This argument expresses an important caution, and we surely must agree that rights to privacy and confidentiality may be too diverse to be subsumed under a single moral principle. That the right to privacy is a catch-all right, encompassing many rights, is confirmed in contemporary literature on the subject. Some writers have viewed the right to privacy as primarily the right to control information about ourselves, especially insofar as that control allows us to maintain degrees of intimacy.[17] This conception of the right to privacy links it tightly to the right to confidentiality of information. Others have viewed the right to privacy as closely related to the expression of certain kinds of interests, such as security,[18] and still others have seen it as closely connected, at least by analogy, to rights of property.[19]

We take the view, however, that rights of privacy and confidentiality are most perspicuously viewed as derived from the principle of autonomy, or as some prefer to say, the principle of respect for persons. This point of view has been carefully stated by Stanley Benn: "To respect someone as a person is to concede that one ought to take account of the way in which his enterprise might be affected by one's own decisions." It follows directly from this account of respect that all persons have a right to privacy that protects unauthorized observation of and reports about their persons. Benn argues further that rules of confidentiality derive from rules protective of privacy, and that both serve as grounds for limiting the access others have to private information about individual persons.[20] While there is room for disagreement as to which rules are basic and which are derived, Benn's account seems to us to capture the central features of the relationships among these principles, rules, and rights. We thus see all our discussions in this section as intimately linked to the discussions of autonomy and informed consent in Chapter 3.

According to a landmark law review article in 1890 on the right of privacy, the individual has the right "of determining, ordinarily, to what extent his thoughts, sentiments, and emotions shall be communicated to others."[21] Whatever else privacy includes, it involves personal control over information about oneself and over access to that information. Without such personal control, important human relationships such as love, friendship, and trust would be diminished. Here the image of concentric circles is a useful illustrative device.[22] The core self with its secrets is at the center, and it chooses to grant others access to that information in accord with the relationships it desires to establish. The outer circles represent less intense and less personal relationships that require less personal information. At stake is both the *amount* and the *kind* of information. As Charles Fried suggests, while we might not mind if a person knows a general fact about us, we might believe that our privacy has been invaded if the person knows the details.[23] Similarly, we might not object if a good friend knows the nature of our illness, but we might protest that the friend has invaded our privacy if he or she observes us actually suffering from that illness.

We grant others access to information about ourselves because of such relationships as love, friendship, and trust. We may also have specific reasons for granting information to some persons. When we wish to be treated by a physician, a psychiatrist, or other health care professionals, for example, we may have to share personal information. Less may be required for the physician than for the psychiatrist or psychologist. For successful treatment by the latter, we must expose our innermost thoughts, feelings, emotions, dreams, and fantasies. We grant these health care professionals access to information about ourselves for our diagnostic and therapeutic benefit, but we generally retain control over access to that information and authorize access only when appropriate. For example, we might authorize a physician to grant an insurance company or a prospective employer access to the information. Again we see the close links between autonomy, privacy, and confidentiality.

It is not necessary, however, to choose between utilitarian and deontological defenses of rules of confidentiality. Both utility and autonomy provide a warrant for these rules and define their content under particular historical circumstances. As Richard Wasserstrom notes, it is not clear that any information as such is intrinsically private; definitions of what is private are socially contingent.[24] Thus, the line between private and public may well depend on a mix of the moral principles that we have emphasized in particular historical circumstances. Much also depends on the expectations that operate in a society at any one time.

In addition to requiring some rules of confidentiality and shaping their content, both utilitarian and deontological considerations determine the stringency or the weight of these rules. This is where the hardest questions arise. Should rules of confidentiality be viewed merely as rules of thumb? Are they absolute rules, as in the requirement of "absolute secrecy" in the International Code of Medical Ethics? Or should they be regarded as asserting prima facie duties? Parts of the majority decision in the Tarasoff case (Case #1) can be read as holding that confidentiality is only a rule of thumb. The decision as a whole, however, indicates that maintaining confidentiality is a prima facie duty, the view we defend. Even the minority dissent does not claim that confidentiality is absolute. Disagreement occurs over the range of legitimate exceptions. In both opinions, an act is prima facie wrong insofar as it violates confidentiality, but the conditions under which it is actually wrong vary in the two opinions.

Our view follows from our discussion of rules in Chapter 2: The rules of confidentiality, which could be formulated as imposing duties on health care professionals or as creating rights for patients, states a prima facie duty. Anyone who thinks that a disclosure of confidential information is morally justified or even mandatory in some circumstances bears a burden of proof. While this approach requires balancing various duties, it also establishes a structure of moral reasoning and justification. It is not enough to determine which act will respect the most duties or maximize the good, for the strong presumption against revealing confidences establishes the direction and burden of deliberation and justification.

Sometimes the health care professional has been viewed as having a "right" to violate confidences in some circumstances, but not as having a "duty" to do so. He or she is permitted, but not obligated, according to this view. Nevertheless, there are clear legal duties to divulge confidential information when necessary to report contagious diseases, gunshot wounds, child abuse, and the like. The Court held in the Tarasoff case that psychiatrists have a "duty" to warn their patient's intended victims of the patient's intention to harm or kill them. An earlier AMA code, in effect until 1980, held that the physician should not infringe the rule of confidentiality "unless he is required to do so by law or unless it becomes necessary in order to protect the welfare of the individual or of the society." Although some people have interpreted this statement as permitting but not requiring the physician to break confidences, we interpret it differently: One may not break a confidence except to fulfill another and more stringent duty—either a duty to obey the law, or a duty to protect the welfare of the patient or the community. There is no *right* to infringe confidences in such cases unless there is also a *duty* to do so. The health care professional's breach of confidentiality thus cannot be justified unless it is necessary to meet a strong conflicting duty, such as an epidemiologist's duty to protect the public's health. This conclusion does not entail that there are moral rules actually requiring one to break confidences. Rather, it means that rules protecting confidences must sometimes give way to rules protecting other interests.

Before discussing duties that may justify infringing rules of confidentiality, we should note that some breaches of confidentiality do not violate duties to the patient. For example, the company physician who informs the employers that an employee in a responsible position suffers from alcoholism may not actually violate a rule of confidentiality, for he or she may not be bound by this rule in the same way a private physician would be bound. The physician could, for example, be under contract with both the company and an employee's union to perform certain services, including the reporting of work-related information about patients. Nevertheless, both the company and the physician in such circumstances have the moral responsibility to insure that employee-patients actually understand at the outset that the traditional rule of confidentiality does not apply.

A distinction should be drawn between releasing information at the patient's *behest* and releasing it on the patient's *behalf without his or her consent.* Although the health care professional should generally release confidential information about a particular patient when the patient requests its release, he or she may encounter circumstances in which the patient refuses to authorize disclosures that would be in his or her best interests. If the patient authorizes disclosure of information—e.g., to a lawyer, court, insurance company, or family member—the health care professional does not violate the rule of confidentiality, which is designed to protect the patient's control over access to personal information. Indeed, it would be morally permissible to obtain a general waiver of confidentiality or to provide a general list of exceptions to rules of confidentiality before the patient enters the relationship. Hereafter we shall be exclusively concerned with disclosures of confidential information *without* the patient's informed authorization.

We can now broach the question, "Which duties legitimately override rules of confidentiality?" While the earlier AMA code mentioned both legal duties and actions necessary to protect patients or society, these two sets of conditions are not mutually exclusive. The law may either lay down certain conditions for the protection of the individual and society or simply allow general moral convictions to prevail. In either case, the law may not hold the health care professional accountable for a breach of confidentiality. Most instances of disclosing confidential information to protect *the patient* (rather than others) are not legally required. Some legal duties, such as the requirement to report epileptic seizures to the division of motor vehicles, may be paternalistic in some cases, but utilitarian in others. Even the legal requirement to report child abuse is not paternalistic. The health care professional has a legal duty to report child abuse in order to protect the child; duties of confidentiality apply only to the child, not to the parents, even if they are also the physician's patients. Any applicable fiduciary relationship is with the child, whose interests are primary in this context.

Legal duties to break confidentiality in order to protect *others* pose a conflict of obligations for the health care professional. On the one hand, he or she is obligated to protect a patient; on the other hand, he or she is legally obligated to act to protect the society, even if the law is unwise or unjust. There is also a *moral* obligation to obey the law, at least in a relatively just system,[25] but it again is only prima facie binding. Sometimes it may be necessary for the health care professional to infringe the duty to obey the law in order to fulfill a responsibility to his or her patient. Sometimes he or she may justifiably reason that obedience to law will result in inadequate treatment for a patient—e.g., in complicated circumstances where there is a legal duty to report venereal disease.

Infringing rules of confidentiality where there is no *legal* duty to disclose information raises additional issues. First, it is easier to justify infringements of confidentiality on grounds of the prevention of harm to others than on grounds of paternalism, especially for competent adults. The duty to report child abuse would be strong even in the absence of a statute because of the child's dependence and vulnerability. However, where competent adults are involved, breaches of confidentiality in order to protect the patient from his or her actions usually violate autonomy, and therefore increase the burden of justification. Suppose that a physician has to decide whether to disclose to a thirty-year-old woman's parents that their daughter's troubled marriage has caused her "nervous condition," which has resulted in her hospitalization. The daughter has asked the physician not to say anything to her parents, but he is convinced that her parents, also his patients, could and would help her recover. In these circumstances the alleged benefit to the patient is not of sufficient magnitude or probability to warrant overriding autonomy and rules of confidentiality. If the physician's efforts to convince the woman to tell her parents were to fail, he should maintain confidentiality even if he believes it is not in the patient's best interests.

Second, if the duty to prevent harms is more stringent than the duty to provide benefits—as it often is—then it will generally be easier to justify infringements of confidentiality in order to prevent harms to patients or others than to justify infringements in order to benefit patients. But a clear distinction cannot always be drawn between producing benefits and preventing harms; and the duty to prevent a trivial harm may not be stronger than the duty to produce a major benefit. The type of harms and benefits may also make a relevant difference. If psychiatrists have a duty to warn intended victims of violence, is the line to be drawn at threats to physical existence and integrity, such as murder and rape? Or should we extend it to include threats to property?

Third, how *probable* must the benefit or harm be before a breach of confidentiality is justified? Is a remote chance of substantial harm to many people sufficient? In the Tarasoff case the Court focused on society's interdependence: "In this risk-infested society we can hardly tolerate the further exposure to danger that would result from a concealed knowledge of the therapist that his patient was lethal."

Fourth, given normal presumptions against violating rules of confidentiality and the significance of those rules, the health care professional should seek alternative and more acceptable ways of realizing a benefit or preventing a harm, short of disclosing confidential information or infringing other important moral principles and rules. Rarely is the breach of confidentiality justified if morally and legally acceptable alternatives exist. In one case, a physician had to determine whether to disclose a patient's homosexuality to his prospective wife, who was also the physician's patient. Athough the physician chose to respect the rule of confidentiality, should he have tried to persuade the young man to tell his prospective wife? Or should he have discussed marriage and sexuality with the young woman so that she might have pressed her prospective husband for more information? Since she was his patient, the physician had a stronger obligation to disclose information to her than he would have had if she had been a stranger, and this obligation perhaps makes his complete inaction less acceptable.[26]

Finally, most interesting cases of confidentiality involve uncertainty at the time the decision must be made. Uncertainty may occur on several different levels, such as basic information, diagnosis, prognosis, and likelihood of an untoward event. For example, in one case a physician had to decide whether to inform the division of motor vehicles that his epileptic patient still suffered seizures, when this unconfirmed information came from a neighbor of the patient. In another case, a psychiatrist used hypnotic techniques to help a pilot recall suppressed information about his responsibility for the crash of a commercial plane. The information indicated that the pilot should not fly, at least temporarily. When the therapist was unable to convince the pilot that he should not fly until his problems were solved, what should the therapist have done? How much certainty did the therapist need for more vigorous action? Six months after returning to work, the pilot made an error of judgment that resulted in the crash of a transatlantic flight and the loss of many lives.[27] Suppose that a pilot of a commercial jet informs his physician that his forty-five-year-old mother was diagnosed as having Huntington's chorea. The physician has to determine whether to disclose to the airline this pilot's fifty percent risk of having the disease in the event the pilot fails to reveal it.[28] These cases involve difficult matters of judgment in determining the probability and magnitude of a harm (or a benefit) that will justify the breach of confidentiality. There can be no simple formula for deciding such cases that escapes the necessity for the risk-benefit assessments discussed in Chapter 5.

There is an important distinction between the probable effects of a disease, such as venereal disease, and the probable actions of an agent, such as a patient's threat to harm someone else. It may be easier to justify breaches of confidentiality to prevent a disease's negative effects than to prevent an agent's negative acts. Cases of doubt about whether an agent will do what he threatens to do may be harder to resolve than cases of doubt about the effects of a disease. The former cases, most of which emerge in psychiatric or psychotherapeutic relations, require more room for patient autonomy, but they do not indicate that a patient should never be committed for suicidal or homicidal tendencies. The Assembly of District Branches and the Board of Trustees of the American Psychiatric Association annotated the principles of medical ethics for psychiatry in 1973. They held (with special reference to court-ordered disclosures of confidences): "When the psychiatrist is in doubt, the right of the patient to confidentiality and, by extension, to unimpaired treatment, should be given priority."[29]

In conclusion, rules of confidentiality and privacy, based on both utilitarian and deontological considerations, establish presumptions against breaches of confidentiality and privacy. But, as we have seen, these presumptions can be rebutted if stronger duties are present. Professionals should also take care to prevent these rules from being violated through negligence—for example, through careless attention to procedures regarding computerized data or through the careless use of cases in teaching.

Rules of fidelity

According to Paul Ramsey, the fundamental ethical question in research, medicine, and health care is: "What is the meaning of the faithfulness of one human being to another?"[30] While Ramsey interprets faithfulness along such theological lines as covenant-fidelity, it is commonly expressed in philosophy in terms of fidelity or promise-keeping and in law in terms of contracts, trust, or fiduciary relations. Ramsey appears to view faithfulness, or covenant-fidelity, as the fundamental ethical principle from which all others can be derived. However, under his interpretation the principle becomes so broad as to be almost vacuous. It becomes a summary term for morality, parallel to older uses of "righteousness." Although few theologians and philosophers would concur with Ramsey in making faithfulness or fidelity the fundamental moral principle, some would accept it as one among several moral principles. An example is W. D. Ross, who viewed fidelity as one of the prima facie principles that should govern human conduct; as we saw earlier, he even derived the duty of veracity from this principle.[31]

From our standpoint, the duty of fidelity or promise-keeping is better understood in terms of rules derived from several other independent and basic moral principles. It is certainly possible to mount a rule-utilitarian argument for conventions and rules of promising and promise-keeping: Such conventions and rules promote the greatest good for the greatest number over time by facilitating human interaction and trust. But the utilitarian argument for an individual's obligation to keep promises (rather than for the institution of promise-making and promise-keeping) is strengthened when it incorporates principles such as autonomy and justice. Thus, whether one defends our basic principles because of their inherent rightness or because of their utility, some of these principles provide strong warrants for an individual's obligation to keep promises as well as for an institution of promising. For example, John Rawls contends that "the principle of fidelity is but a special case of the principle of fairness applied to the social practice of promising."[32] An appeal to respect for autonomy beyond fairness or justice appears in Charles Fried's analysis:

> The obligation to keep a promise is grounded not in arguments of utility but in respect for *individual autonomy and in trust*. Autonomy and trust are grounds for the institution of promising as well, but the argument for individual obligation is not the same. Individual obligation is only a step away, but that step must be taken. An individual is morally bound to keep his promises because he has intentionally invoked a convention whose function it is to give grounds—moral grounds—for another to expect the promised performance. To renege is to abuse a confidence he was free to invite or not, and which he intentionally did invite. To abuse that confidence now is like (but only like) lying; the abuse of a shared social institution that is intended to invoke the bonds of trust. A liar and a promise-breaker each use another person. In both speech and promising there is an invitation to the other to trust, to make himself vulnerable; the liar and the promise-breaker then abuse that trust.[33]

Fried rightly argues that, while there are similarities between fidelity to promises and veracity, it is not possible to derive fidelity from veracity (itself a derived duty in our framework). The main difference between fidelity and veracity is that upon making a promise, people create expectations on the part of others who then rely on the promise.[34] In making promises, people make morally neutral acts obligatory; they impose obligations on themselves by creating expectations in others. Promising thus changes the structure of rights and obligations.

Many relationships between professionals and patients or subjects involve duties of fidelity or promise-keeping. According to the Principles of Medical Ethics of the AMA, "a physician shall, in the provision of appropriate medical care, except in emergencies, be free to choose whom to serve, with whom to associate, and the environment in which to provide medical services." (See Appendix II.) In emergencies, as we argued in Chapter 5, physicians and other professionals may have duties to prevent or remove harm, apart from their contracts or role obligations. Nevertheless, most duties of beneficence hinge on contracts and role relations. Once a physician has established a relationship with a patient, both parties acquire duties of fidelity. The physician's duties of fidelity include a duty not to neglect the patient: "Once having undertaken a case, the physician should not neglect the patient, nor withdraw from the case without giving notice to the patient, the relatives, or responsible friends sufficiently long in advance of withdrawal to permit another medical attendant to be secured."[35] Even if such duties are legally enforceable, we should not forget their moral foundations.

As our framework implies, many moral duties are independent of our voluntary agreements, commitments, or promises to perform them. Promising can account for only a portion (though a significant portion) of our duties in research, medicine, and health care. Furthermore, other moral principles and rules limit our promises; it is commonly agreed that a promise to do what is morally wrong is not binding. Within these limits duties of fidelity may stem from the generation of expectations through words, gestures, or silence. Promises or contracts may be explicitly, implicitly, or tacitly made. Such promises or contracts are binding for physicians, other health care professionals, and researchers, except when they are overridden by stronger duties or obligations. We shall now consider some of the conflicts among contractual and role obligations, which will clarify the meaning, the limits, and the strength of duties of fidelity, particularly when some party other than the patient makes the contract.

Conflicts among contractual and role obligations

It is by now clear that rules expressing duties of fidelity, veracity, and confidentiality can be no more free of conflicts with other principles and established role obligations than the four principles discussed in Chapters 3–6. The professional-patient relationship is inherently complex, and it cannot be treated as a simple one-to-one contractual relationship in isolation from other relationships. Physicians, nurses, and hospital administrators may all find their role obligations in sharp conflict with other obligations to patients. In this final section we explore such conflicts further.

In many cases, as we have seen, the health care professional has a duty of care because of an explicit or implicit contract with the patient. In other cases, the therapeutic contract may be with a party other than the patient. The contractor may not be the beneficiary. For example, if someone promises John Doe to look after his children after his death, the promisor has an obligation to John Doe even though the children are the primary beneficiaries.[36] When parents bring a child to a physician for treatment, the physician's primary responsibility is to the child, whose interests are paramount. Courts have rightly refused to allow Jehovah's Witnesses to reject medically necessary blood transfusions for their children, even though the courts have often allowed adult Jehovah's Witnesses to reject blood transfusions for themselves (as in Case #13; but contrast Case #14).

In some cases, parents may be charged with child neglect when they fail to seek or permit highly desirable medical treatment, even if it falls short of being necessary to save the child's life. Angela Holder summarizes one such case: "A teenage boy suffered from a massive deformity of the face and neck. He was so grotesque he was excused from school attendance and was therefore illiterate. Surgery could correct the condition but could not be performed without blood transfusions. The mother objected on religious grounds to administration of blood and therefore would not consent to surgery. The court held that he was a 'neglected child' and ordered the surgery performed."[37]

In recent years there has been considerable moral debate about decisions regarding defective newborns who need surgery to sustain their lives. (See Cases #21 and 22.) In one recent case (#22), an infant with Down's syndrome needed surgery to correct a tracheoesophageal fistula—an opening between the breathing and swallowing tubes that prevents food from reaching the stomach. Surgery offered a fifty percent chance of survival. The parents refused to grant permission for the surgery, the Indiana Supreme Court declined to override their refusal, and the infant died of starvation after six days. In other cases, physicians or hospitals have gained permission from the courts to provide the medical treatment refused by the parents. Such interventions are probably more common in cases of refusal of treatment on *religious* grounds, partly because the health care professionals rarely share those beliefs. In cases where parents appeal to the best interests of the child and to familial interests, such as the prevention of disruption and strain on financial resources, physicians appear to be more willing to support the familial decision to refuse treatment. Of course, there may be major disagreements about what would be in the child's interest, or in the family's interest, but the point is that many physicians appear to be more comfortable with such judgments about interests than with refusals on religious grounds.[38] Our view is that (prima facie) physicians have a primary responsibility to the patient, even if a third party establishes the initial contract. The physician ought to act in the patient's best interests, even if it is necessary to seek a court order to authorize surgery, a blood transfusion, or the like. Other familial interests, such as avoiding the depletion of financial resources, should not be considered until a certain threshold is reached, viz., when significant patient interests would not be served by continued treatment or by a particular treatment.[39]

The above examples focus on the conflict between the interests of the patient, who is the beneficiary, and the interests of the contractor with the health care professional. In another major type of conflict it may be less clear exactly what the health care professional owes the "patient." Examples include a physician's contract to examine applicants for positions in a company or to determine whether applicants for insurance policies are good risks. In such cases, the health care professional may rightly not think of the person examined as his or her patient. The professional has certain responsibilities of due care, but they may not be as comprehensive or as stringent as the responsibilities that apply in the physician-patient relationship. They would include care in examinations so as not to injure the individual—e.g., by exposure to excessive X rays. In some jurisdictions the health care professional may not even have a legal duty to disclose the discovery of a disease to the examinee. For example, in one preemployment physical examination, X rays indicated that the woman who subsequently was hired had tuberculosis, but the physician and the employer did not disclose these findings to her. After three years, the employee became ill with tuberculosis and was hospitalized for a prolonged period. In this case, the court held that the woman's only recourse was workmen's compensation. The court disallowed her suit against her employer and the physician who examined her, on grounds that there was no established patient-physician relationship, and hence no legal duty to disclose the information to her.[40] From a moral standpoint, however, both the employer and the physician had a duty to disclose the information. This duty of disclosure stems, in part, from the broad principle of beneficence, which requires that harm be prevented.

What does the moral duty of disclosure require in conflict situations where institutional interests might be at stake? Suppose a company requires regular physical examinations of all employees by a physician. The physician's contract requires disclosure to the company about employees' health conditions that might affect their work. If the company uses materials, such as kepone or benzene, that might be hazardous to its employees, and the physician discovers symptoms of a disease that might be directly related to working conditions, what obligation does the physician have to report these findings to the employees as well as to the company? Does he or she have the same obligation if the employer expressly forbids such disclosures to employees? Health care professionals have a moral responsibility to oppose, avoid, and withdraw from contracts that would force them to withhold information of significant benefit to examinees.

In another type of situation, a health care professional may be under contract to, or otherwise obligated to, an institution to provide *care* for a group of individuals. In these cases, there can be no doubt that physicians, for example, owe "due care" to individuals who are their patients, despite the third-party contract or obligation. Examples include health care professionals in industries, prisons, and the armed services. But in these settings, care of the patient may come into conflict with institutional needs. The patient's needs generally should take precedence, but not always. Difficult cases may emerge, for example, on the battlefield. Triage in the battlefield setting may be different from triage in the peacetime emergency room. On the battlefield the needs of the military may dictate that certain patients should be given priority even when medical needs establish a different priority.

In a well-known example mentioned in Chapter 6, penicillin became available for use in North Africa in World War II, and a difficult allocation decision had to be made because the supply was severely limited. Authorities decided to give the available penicillin to soldiers suffering from venereal disease rather than to those who had been wounded on the battlefields. The former, they reasoned, could be restored to fighting capacity more easily and effectively than the latter. As we have seen in our discussion of justice and microallocation, it is not possible to generalize from the battlefield to ordinary medical practice. Moreover, even on the battlefield medical needs cannot always be wholly subordinated to military needs. For example, conventions regarding the laws of war hold that a fallen enemy soldier with medical needs is to be given equal consideration along with one's comrades.

In addition to allocation decisions that are contingent upon medical and institutional needs, health care professionals in military and other institutions sometimes make judgments about "sickness" and "health" based on institutional values. In 1966 an Air Force newsletter reported that a twenty-six-year-old staff sergeant gunner who had been on active duty in Vietnam for seven months and had flown over one hundred missions developed a fear of flying because several of his acquaintances had been killed. The diagnosis was Gross Stress Reaction, "manifested by anxiety, tenseness, a fear of death expressed in the form of rationalizations, and inability to function. His problem was 'worked through' and insight . . . was gained to the extent that he was returned to full flying duty in less than six weeks."[41] This case raises numerous questions: Which medical and psychiatric labels, if any, are appropriate in a case where the refusal could be seen as rational from the patient's standpoint but not from the military's? At what point should the psychotherapist refuse to engage in military or other service on the grounds that he or she cannot combine responsibility to patients with institutional needs in that setting? Does the physician have an obligation to inquire into the justice of a particular war before engaging in it?

Although there are borderline cases, such as the one in this Air Force newsletter, in principle physicians and psychotherapists can function in the military and can render valuable service to wounded soldiers, even in an unjust war, without violating moral principles. The rationale is that health care professionals render service to the soldier as a human being rather than to the soldier as a soldier. Thus, according to the laws of war, health care professionals are not legitimate targets for direct attack because they do not directly serve the war effort. Some actions, however, may violate canons of medical ethics and thus warrant disobedience to orders: An example is an order for a physician to help torture a prisoner in order to gain information.

Role conflicts often emerge in institutions serving multiple functions, such as caring for patients, training professionals, and conducting research. The mission of a teaching hospital is not only to care for current patients, but also to benefit future patients through the education of physicians and other professionals. The use of patients for teaching purposes may not violate the prohibition against treating persons *merely* as means, because such patients may choose to become participants and even partners in the training of professionals or the generation of scientific knowledge. Such voluntary participation or partnership presupposes a general disclosure of the functions and expectations of a teaching hospital. If patients understand the divided loyalties of teaching hospitals, are not subjected to undue risks, and are protected in other ways (for example, by the rules of privacy and confidentiality), they can be partners with teachers in the training of professionals. Indeed, some studies indicate that most patients find bedside rounds (a declining practice) to be "a positive experience that should be continued."[42]

In addition to general disclosure and consent upon entry, there should be certain specific disclosures and consents. For example, the patient should be told who will be on the surgical team and who will be in charge, even if he or she is not told that Dr. Doe will do X and Dr. Roe will do Y.[43] While patients should have the right to refuse to be used for some teaching purposes, there is reason to think that few will exercise that right if they are first educated about the importance of their role in clinical teaching, particularly when they are informed about the benefits as well as the risks. The principle of justice also requires that the burdens of such participation, even if those burdens are only minor inconveniences, not be inequitably assigned to poorer and less educated patients. The same point holds for the selection of subjects for participation in research.[44]

Similarly, the two roles of research scientist and clinical practitioner may come into conflict. As an investigator, the physician acts to generate knowledge that can lead to progress in medicine that will ultimately benefit individual patients. As a clinical practitioner, he or she may have specific contracts for care and in general must act in the present patient's best interests. Both of these roles may function to "benefit the sick"; but the scientific role aims to benefit statistical lives in the future, while the clinical role seeks to benefit particular patients now. Responsibility to future generations thus may come into conflict with "due care" for particular persons who are subjects as well as patients. The Declaration of Geneva of the World Medical Association in Appendix II affirms that "the health of my patient will be my first consideration." Can this principle be affirmed under all conditions in the context of research involving patients as subjects? If not, should it be sacrificed or at least compromised in order to benefit more people in the future?

Controlled clinical trials are important and even necessary in order to confirm that an observed effect such as reduced mortality from a particular disease is the result of a particular treatment rather than some other variable such as a widespread condition in the patient population. Among the controlled trials to determine the effectiveness and safety of treatment and procedures, the randomized clinical trial (RCT) is widely used. Instead of trying to match patients for variables so that some of the matched patients can receive A and some B, the RCT randomly assigns patients to different therapies or placebos. Randomization is to keep variables other than the treatments under examination from distorting the study. RCTs are often preferred to observational or retrospective studies on grounds that their results have a higher degree of validity because randomization eliminates bias in assignment and reduces the influence of extraneous variables. Thus, RCTs appear to offer a sound inductive technique.

But many questions can be raised about RCTs: Are they as essential as their proponents say? Can they be used without compromising acknowledged responsibilities to patients?[45] The increased probability of their results is only a matter of degree, and there might be reasons for preferring a less conclusive method if it would more adequately fulfill duties to current patients. Proponents of RCTs often argue, however, that RCTs do not violate moral duties to patients because there is genuine doubt about the merits of existing, standard, or new therapies. No patient, they note, will receive a treatment *known* to be less effective or more dangerous than another available alternative. Because current patients, in effect, are not asked to make any sacrifices, who could object to the use of RCTs, especially when they promise to benefit future patients?

A vivid recent example (see Case #28) indicates some lingering difficulties in the use of RCTs. According to one report, a controlled, double-blind experiment on a new drug, adenine arabinoside (ara-A), indicated that it is an effective treatment for herpes simplex encephalitis. Of the ten people given the placebo, seven died, one suffered severe damage, and two recovered to lead reasonably normal lives. Of the eighteen who received ara-A, five died, and six had serious brain or nerve damage, while seven recovered to lead reasonably normal lives. The ten who received the placebo were given standard treatment, which mainly consists of palliative care because no treatment prior to ara-A had been found to be effective. Critics charge that it was not necessary to have a placebo group instead of historical controls. Because ara-A had already been shown to be effective and nontoxic in some localized herpes simplex hominis infections, and because no other treatment prevented mortality and serious brain and nerve damage, moral questions were raised about giving anyone the placebo. Defenders of the research respond that we did not know the mortality rate of herpes simplex encephalitis prior to the research because the disease is so difficult to diagnose apart from brain biopsies, and that we did not know whether ara-A would be toxic when administered with large amounts of fluid to such patients. The research was stopped when the above statistics emerged, but several scientists contend that it was stopped too early, before statistically significant evidence had emerged about effectiveness and toxicity. They note that because of the small groups involved, it is misleading to say that 20% of the recipients of the placebo and 38.8% of the recipients of ara-A had reasonable recovery. If the next placebo-recipient had had reasonably normal recovery, the figures would have been much closer.[46]

Even if there are neither scientific nor ethical grounds for opposing a particular randomized clinical trial of two treatments that are roughly equal in safety and efficacy, patients may have strong preferences for one treatment or the other. Suppose two surgical procedures for treating the same disease appear to have the same survival rate (say, an average of 15 years), and suppose we propose to test their effectiveness by an RCT. The patient might have a preference if treatment A has little risk of death during the operation but a high rate of death after ten years, while treatment B has a high risk of death during the operation or postoperative recovery but a low rate of death after recovery (say, for 30 years). A patient's age, family responsibilities, and other circumstances in life might lead to a preference for one over the other.[47] While a research institution could legitimately accept only patients willing to participate in certain research projects related to their diseases, patients in other settings should be able to choose between treatments whenever both treatments are available.

Because patients commonly assume that decisions about their treatments are made in their best interests, and not in the interests of a research design, the physician-researcher should disclose all significant alternatives to patient-subjects so that they can make an informed judgment about participation. One relevant item of information is the *method* used to determine who receives a particular treatment. Some contend that disclosure of the allocation system would cause distress harmful to the patient or would lead some patients to refuse to participate in the research. They also argue that disclosure of such matters is not necessary because the patient does not need to know how the allocation is made between two treatments that appear to be equally effective and equally risky. However, because the physician-researcher is a double agent, holding dual responsibilities, he or she has a fiduciary duty to inform patient-subjects of everything directly relevant to their decisions, including conditions that might involve the physician-researcher in a conflict of interest.[48] This duty of disclosure persists throughout the period of the research and requires that the patient-subject be informed about developments that might be relevant to a decision to withdraw. (See the discussion of disclosure and informed consent in Chapter 3.)

Physician-researchers may also face difficult questions about whether to stop an experiment before its completion, and even before they have sufficient data to support the preliminary conclusion. If a physician determines that a patient's condition is deteriorating and that the patient's interests dictate withdrawal from the research, the physician should be free to act on behalf of the patient, assuming, of course, that he or she does not act in opposition to the express wishes of the patient. Some research designs take advantage of emerging evidence to alter the protocol; and some play the winner by utilizing what appear to be the best therapies until they fail. But in an RCT, particularly if it is a double-blind study, it may be difficult to determine whether the experiment as a whole should be stopped merely because some physician-researchers insist that they are satisfied by the evidence. As we noted earlier, some researchers contend that the trial of ara-A was stopped too soon, that is, before the evidence became statistically convincing. Thus, they contend, there has been no definitive determination that ara-A is superior to standard, palliative care.

One proposal to handle the ethical conflict involves a differentiation of roles; it recommends an advisory committee to determine whether to continue or stop a trial. Such a committee "must consider the impact of its decision on the treatment of future patients. Although an individual physician may only be responsible for treating his current patients, the advisory committee must act as if the care of future patients rests in their hands, because their recommendations are likely to influence therapy for the many patients to follow."[49] The differentiation of roles by using an advisory committee may be procedurally sound, but it fails to resolve the ethical questions. Instead, it relocates them. Even if occupants of different roles represent different interests—e.g., the physicians represent current patients' interests, while the scientists and the advisory committee represent future patients' interests—it is still necessary to determine when it is legitimate to impose some risks on current patients in order to benefit future ones. It must be determined whether medical knowledge and scientific progress with their undisputed benefits are optional or mandatory, whether the increased probabilities of the knowledge gained by RCTs are worth the moral costs, and whether the benefits outweigh the burdens. When the physician charged with the care of particular patients is convinced that their interests are being sacrificed for the benefit of others, he or she should not surrender the right to make a judgment to the advisory committee. He or she should remain a patient advocate. In other cases, an institutional review board may determine that the research fails to offer patient-subjects adequate protection from harm; in such cases it should demand revisions in the research protocol, and possibly even refuse to allow the research.

Some hold that the researcher-physician's commitment to the welfare of his or her patients offers the best protection, even if a research project has been authorized by an institutional review board. Others, however, contend that we should differentiate roles so that physicians do not use their own patients in research. Their point is not that a person cannot be both an investigator and a clinician, but that a person should not assume both roles for the same patient-subject.[50] A similar argument supports not allowing the physician who is to transplant a kidney from A to B to determine when A is dead. Proposals for procedures will depend in part on conceptions of human nature and convictions about the importance of reducing conflicts of interest. In many cases role-differentiation may obviate some of the moral conflicts. Nevertheless, answers to procedural questions will not be satisfactory unless we also have answers to more substantive questions. At stake is not merely who can and should protect patients' interests, but how much weight should be given to the interests of current patients and how much to future patients.

Our view is that medical knowledge and scientific progress are important, but often optional goals. Generally the duty of beneficence to future generations of patients is less stringent than the duty to "benefit the sick," who already have a special relationship with health care professionals. This conclusion should not be construed to subvert research. Rather, we should promote research methods that enable us to pursue knowledge while simultaneously protecting the interests of patients.

Perhaps in no area of health care are conflicts among duties of fidelity more pervasive and morally troubling than in nursing. There is continuity between nursing ethics and other areas of biomedical ethics because the same principles and rules apply to all health care professionals. Nevertheless, nursing ethics is distinctive. Even though the same principles and rules apply to all health care professionals, what they imply for the conduct of any particular person will depend, in part, on the structure of health care, its roles, its conventions, and its practices. For example, if we hold that a patient has a right to the truth about his or her condition, we still have to ask who, among the various possible agents, has the obligation to disclose the truth. Answers to such questions hinge, in part, on the definition of moral responsibility in nursing. Roles such as nursing are important for determining moral responsibility, that is, to whom and for what one is responsible.

The most recent codes of nursing ethics define the moral responsibility of nurses in sharply different ways from earlier codes. For example, in 1950 the first code of the American Nurses Association stressed the nurse's obligation to carry out the physician's orders, but the 1976 revision (see Appendix II) stresses the nurse's obligation to the client. While the original code emphasized the obligation to protect the reputation of associates, the later code emphasizes the obligation to safeguard the client and the public from "incompetent, unethical or illegal" practices of any person. A similar dramatic shift appears in the codes of ethics of the International Council of Nursing. An earlier code stated that "the nurse is under an obligation to carry out the physician's orders intelligently and loyally and to refuse to participate in unethical procedures." While the code recognized a clear presumption in favor of obedience to the physician's orders, it also recognized the legitimacy of not participating in "unethical procedures." It did not, however, define such procedures. The revised code of 1973 (see Appendix II) marks a definite shift: Instead of viewing the nurse as responsible primarily to the physician or to the institution, it holds that "the nurse's primary responsibility is to those people who require nursing care." Many nurses even conceive their role to be that of "patient advocate." Alterations in the codes reflect important changes in the profession of nursing, but their institutional implications have not yet been clarified or implemented in many places. Thus, nurses may have to choose between discharging a responsibility to the physician and to the institution, on the one hand, and to the patient, on the other.[51]

Consider in this connection Case #17. (Compare Case #6.) Mrs. R., who is approximately forty-five years old, a divorcee, and the mother of teenage daughters who live with her, suffers from multiple sclerosis. She often comes to the emergency room of the local community hospital for treatment of acute episodes of asthma. The physician ordered "no code" (i.e., no cardiopulmonary resuscitation) in case Mrs. R. suffered a cardiac arrest. The nurses believe that the physician made the decision without discussing it with Mrs. R. or the family, and they are not sure what Mrs. R. would want because she is often depressed when she comes to the emergency room and has not expressed her wishes. What ought a nurse to do in these circumstances?[52]

First, this case does not appear to involve a moral dilemma; it may be a conflict or dispute about moral matters without being a dilemma. Because the patient's wishes should be decisive in this sort of case, it is important to ascertain whether the patient's wishes have been determined and are being respected. There may be uncertainty about a patient's wishes without creating a moral dilemma. Thus, the first step for the nurse is to find out whether Mrs. R. competently and voluntarily requested or consented to the "no code" order. If Mrs. R. and the physician are in agreement, the "no code" order should be followed. But if Mrs. R. enters the emergency room and suffers a cardiac arrest before this information can be obtained, the nurse and others may legitimately ignore the "no code" order and provide the treatment ordinarily provided in such cases. Furthermore, if the nurse determines that the physician has ordered "no code" *against* the express wishes of Mrs. R., the nurse should not follow his orders. Because this case concerns matters of general moral principle, such as respect for patient autonomy, the nurse may not and, indeed, should not be satisfied with a refusal to carry out the "no code" order. (We will return to conscientious refusals in the next chapter.) The nurse has an obligation to seek to have the physician's order countermanded in order to protect the patient's best interests and wishes. The nurse may also have a responsibility to try to get the hospital to develop clearer and more satisfactory policies regarding CPR (cardiopulmonary resuscitation). (Such policies would cover both the substantive and the procedural matters identified in Chapter 4.)

It is beyond the scope of this book to recommend procedures to prevent or to resolve interprofessional and intrainstitutional conflicts. Nevertheless, it may be useful to note that significant conflicts between health care professionals can be expected as long as there are major differences in (1) degrees of participation in decisionmaking, and in (2) degrees of closeness and distance in the delivery of care. There will probably be political if not moral problems as long as some professionals make the decisions and order their implementation by other professionals who have not participated in the decisionmaking. For example, in several cases, nurses and other providers of care have blown the whistle on parents and physicians who have decided not to treat defective newborns.

In this chapter, we have applied the four principles of autonomy, beneficence, nonmaleficence, and justice to relationships in research, medicine, and health care. While this application has sometimes been direct, we have generally concentrated on rules derived from these principles—the rules of veracity, fidelity, confidentiality, and privacy—and their conflicts. In each instance, we explored the basis, meaning, limits, and stringency of these rules in the context of professional and patient or subject relationships. These rules, like the principles from which they are derived, are only prima facie binding, and our analysis has indicated some conditions under which they can be overridden in cases of conflict.

Morality of course includes more than these principles and rules. Any adequate ethical theory must also attend to ideals, to virtues, and to the integrity of the self, which is often expressed in terms of conscience. We turn to these matters in the final chapter.

Notes

1. Some of these derivative moral rules might be better described as derivative moral principles, but for simplicity of analysis (without oversimplification) we use the term "rules." However described, we believe they are best understood as derivative from one or more of the four basic moral principles. Furthermore, we tend to refer to them as "rules" rather than as a "rule," because they generally involve several distinct and specific requirements. Rights as well as duties are justified by principles and rules.
2. Henry Sidgwick, *The Methods of Ethics,* 7th ed. (London: Macmillan, 1907), p. 315.

3. G. J. Warnock, *The Object of Morality* (London: Methuen and Co., 1971), pp. 85–86.

4. Alan Donagan, *The Theory of Morality* (Chicago: University of Chicago Press, 1977), p. 88. See also Charles Fried, *Right and Wrong* (Cambridge, Mass.: Harvard University Press, 1978), Chapter 3.

5. See W. D. Ross, *The Right and the Good* (Oxford: Clarendon Press, 1930), Chapter 2.

6. Sissela Bok stresses the harm of lies to the one lied to, to the liar, and to social trust. See *Lying: Moral Choice in Public and Private Life* (New York: Pantheon Books, 1978), pp. 188 et passim. For discussions of utilitarianism and veracity, see David Lewis, "Utilitarianism and Truthfulness," *Australasian Journal of Philosophy* 50 (May 1972): 17–19; and Peter Singer, "Is Act-Utilitarianism Self-Defeating?", *Philosophical Review* 81 (1972): 94–104. See also Arnold Isenberg, "Deontology and the Ethics of Lying," *Philosophy and Phenomenological Research* 24 (1964): 465–80, and Roderick M. Chisholm and Thomas D. Feehan, "The Intent to Deceive," *Journal of Philosophy* 74 (March 1977): 143–59.

7. See *Current Opinions of the Judicial Council of the American Medical Association* (Chicago: American Medical Association, 1981).

8. See the analysis of various studies of truthtelling by Robert M. Veatch and Ernest Tai, "Talking about Death: Patterns of Lay and Professional Change," *Annals of the American Academy of Political and Social Science* 447 (January 1980): 29–45.

9. See also George J. Annas, *The Rights of Hospital Patients: The Basic ACLU Guide to a Hospital Patient's Rights* (New York: Avon Books, 1976). For a discussion of the duty of veracity in various codes, see Sissela Bok, "Truth-telling," *The Encyclopedia of Bioethics,* ed. Warren T. Reich (New York: The Free Press, 1978), Vol. IV. One of the earliest recognitions of rights for patients is found in the 1793 National Convention of the French Revolution.

10. See Sissela Bok's discussion of similar arguments in *Lying,* Chapter 15.

11. Boswell, *Life of Johnson,* vol. 4, p. 306, as quoted in Alan Donagan, *The Theory of Morality,* p. 89.

12. See Bok, *Lying,* Chapter 1, for a discussion of the distinction between truth and truthfulness.

13. See "Huntington's Disease: Some Prefer Not to Know," *Medical World News* 15 (April 5, 1974).

14. See Veatch, *Death, Dying, and the Biological Revolution* (New Haven, Conn.: Yale University Press, 1976), Chapter 6.

15. Robert Veatch, *Case Studies in Medical Ethics* (Cambridge, Mass.: Harvard University Press, 1977), pp. 137–39.

16. Arthur Caplan, "On Privacy and Confidentiality in Social Science Research," in *Ethical Issues in Social Science Research,* eds. Tom L. Beauchamp, et al. (Baltimore: The Johns Hopkins University Press, 1982), pp. 315–25.

17. Charles Fried, "Privacy: A Rational Context," in *Today's Moral Problems,* ed. Richard Wasserstrom (New York: Macmillan, 1975), pp. 21–33.

18. Thomas Scanlon, "Thomson on Privacy," and James Rachels "Why Privacy is Important," *Philosophy and Public Affairs* 4 (Summer 1975): 315–333.

19. Judith J. Thomson, "The Right to Privacy," *Philosophy and Public Affairs* 4 (Summer 1975): 295–314.

20. Stanley I. Benn, "Privacy, Freedom and Respect for Persons," in *Today's Moral Problems,* ed. Richard Wasserstrom, pp. 1–21. Thomson (*op.cit.*) also subsumes "the right to confidentiality" under "the right to privacy," and Hyman Gross links autonomy to privacy in his "Privacy and Autonomy," *Privacy:* Nomos XIII, eds. J. Roland Pennock and John W. Chapman (New York: Lieber-Atherton, 1971). Several courts have also viewed privacy as the foundation of confidentiality. See, for example, *Horne* v. *Patton* 291 Ala. 701, 287 So. 2d 824; reprinted in Thomas A. Shannon and Jo Ann Manfra, eds., *Law and Bioethics* (Ramsey, N.J.: Paulist Press, 1982), pp. 281–92. In this case the Alabama Supreme Court also considered the grounds of implied contract and fiduciary relations, but it emphasized privacy.

21. Samuel Warren and Louis Brandeis, "The Right of Privacy," *Harvard Law Review* 4 (1890): 193.

22. See Alan Westin, *Privacy and Freedom* (New York: Atheneum, 1967).

23. See Charles Fried, *An Anatomy of Values* (Cambridge, Mass.: Harvard University Press, 1970), p. 141.

24. Richard Wasserstrom, "The Legal and Philosophical Foundations of the Right to Privacy," in *Biomedical Ethics*, eds. Thomas A. Mappes and Jane S. Zembaty (New York: McGraw-Hill, 1981), pp. 109–16.

25. See James F. Childress, *Civil Disobedience and Political Obligation* (New Haven, Conn.: Yale University Press, 1971), and John Rawls, *A Theory of Justice* (Cambridge, Mass.: Harvard University Press, 1971), Chapter 6.

26. Harvey Kuschner, Daniel Callahan, Eric J. Cassell, and Robert M. Veatch, "The Homosexual Husband and Physician Confidentiality," *Hastings Center Report* 7 (April 1977): 15–17.

27. Bernard B. Raginsky, "Hypnotic Recall of Aircrash Cause," *International Journal of Clinical and Experimental Hypnosis* 17 (1969): 1–19.

28. Aubrey Milunsky, *The Prevention of Genetic Disease and Mental Retardation* (Philadelphia: W. B. Saunders, 1975), p. 75.

29. "The Principles of Medical Ethics with Annotations Especially Applicable to Psychiatry," *American Journal of Psychiatry* 130 (September 1974): 1063.

30. Paul Ramsey, *The Patient as Person* (New Haven, Conn.: Yale University Press, 1970), p. xii. In Robert M. Veatch's contractual perspective on biomedical ethics, the principle of keeping promises or contracts applies to several different levels. See Veatch, *A Theory of Medical Ethics* (New York: Basic Books, 1981), esp. chap. 7.

31. W. D. Ross, *The Right and the Good*, p. 21.

32. John Rawls, *A Theory of Justice*, p. 344.

33. Charles Fried, *Contract as Promise: A Theory of Contractual Obligation* (Cambridge, Mass.: Harvard University Press, 1981), p. 16.

34. Henry Sidgwick correctly observed that "the essential element of the Duty of Good Faith seems to be not conformity to my own statement [i.e., veracity], but to expectations that I have intentionally raised in others." Sidgwick, *Methods of Ethics*, p. 304. Contrast G. J. Warnock, *The Object of Morality,* chap. 7.

35. See the discussion of this rule in chapter 1, especially note 4.

36. See H. L. A. Hart's discussion in "Are There Any Natural Rights?" *Philosophical Review* 64 (1955): 175–91.

37. Summary of *In re Sampson*, 317 NYS 2d (1970), by Angela Holder, *Medical Malpractice Law* (New York: John Wiley and Sons, 1975), p. 17.

38. See, for example, Anthony Shaw, "Dilemmas of 'Informed Consent' in Children," *New England Journal of Medicine* 289 (October 25, 1973): 885–94. See also Anthony Shaw, Judson C. Randolph, and Barbara Manard, "Ethical Issues in Pediatric Surgery: A National Survey of Pediatricians and Pediatric Surgeons," *Pediatrics* 60 (October 1977): 588–99.

39. Even more complicated problems may emerge in the treatment of a pregnant woman and an unborn fetus, particularly if the fetus is viewed as a patient because of technological developments including intrauterine surgery, and if the pregnant woman's interests and the fetus' interests come into conflict. See Case #24. See also Watson A. Bowes and Brad Selgestad, "Fetal versus Maternal Rights: Medical and Legal Perspectives," *Obstetrics and Gynecology* 58 (August 1981): 209–14; John C. Fletcher, "The Fetus as Patient: Ethical Issues," *Journal of the American Medical Association* 246 (August 14, 1981): 772–3; and William R. Barclay, et al., "The Ethics of In Utero Surgery," *Journal of the American Medical Association* 246 (October 2, 1981): 1550–55.

40. Holder, *Medical Malpractice Law*, p. 19. A summary of *Lotspeich* v. *Chance Vought Aircraft Corporation*, 369 SW 2d Tex (1963).

41. *PACAF Surgeon's Newsletter* 7 (December 1966): 5, reprinted in *Hastings Center Report* 6 (February 1976): 20 (with commentary); see also Veatch, *Case Studies in Medical Ethics*, pp. 245–58. For further discussion of the physician in the military, see Robert M. Goldwyn and Victor W. Sidel, "The Physician and War," *Ethical Issues in Medicine: The Role of the Physician in Today's Society*, ed. E. Fuller Torrey (Boston: Little, Brown and Co., 1968), pp. 325–46.

42. Eugene W. Linfors and Francis A. Neelson, "The Case for Bedside Rounds," *New England Journal of Medicine* 303 (November 20, 1980): 1231.

43. According to the Judicial Council of the AMA there are strong rules against substituting a surgeon without the patient's knowledge or consent: "It is the operating surgeon to whom the patient grants consent to perform the operation." Even though this surgeon may use the assistance of residents and others, it is not appropriate for the resident or another physician to become the operating surgeon without the patient's knowledge or consent. *Current Opinions of the Judicial Council of the American Medical Association*, # 8:12.

44. See Bradford H. Gray, *Human Subjects in Medical Experimentation* (New York: Wiley-Interscience, 1975).

45. A thorough and helpful study of randomized clinical trials appears in Charles Fried, *Medical Experimentation: Personal Integrity and Social Policy* (New York: American Elsevier, 1974). For other criticisms, see Milton C. Weinstein, "Allocation of Subjects in Medical Experiments," *New England Journal of Medicine* 291 (December 12, 1974): 1278–85. For defenses of RCTs, see David P. Byar, et al., "Randomized Clinical Trials: Perspectives on Some Recent Ideas," *New England Journal of Medicine* 295 (July 8, 1976): 74–80; and several writings by Thomas Chalmers, including Thomas C. Chalmers, et al., "Controlled Studies in Clinical Cancer Research," *New England Journal of Medicine* 287 (July 13, 1972): 75–78; L. W. Shaw and T. C. Chalmers, "Ethics in Cooperative Clinical Trials," *Annals of the New York Academy of Science* 169 (1970):487–95; and Chalmers, "The Clinical Trial," *Milbank Memorial Fund*

Quarterly/Health and Society 59 (Summer 1981): 324–39. See also Robert J. Levine, *Ethics and Regulation of Clinical Research* (Baltimore: Urban and Schwarzenberg, 1981).

46. For some of the controversy, see the references listed in Case #28 in Appendix I.
47. See Weinstein, "Allocation of Subjects in Medical Experiments," p. 1280.
48. See Fried, *Medical Experimentation*, p. 71. Recently in Denmark a randomized clinical trial was conducted to assess the value of intestinal bypass in the treatment of gross obesity. One hundred and thirty patients received surgery and were compared with sixty-six patients who received medical treatment. The participants did not give informed consent to participate in the research, for relevant information was withheld and deception was used. As the researchers reported, "We did not ask for informed consent for randomisation. Patients allocated to medical treatment were told that surgery had to be postponed for an undetermined period primarily because liver-biopsy findings showed fatty infiltration. . . ." See the Danish Obesity Project, "Randomised Trial of Jejunoileal Bypass Versus Medical Treatment in Morbid Obesity," *Lancet* (December 11, 1979): 1255.
49. Byar, et al., "Randomized Clinical Trails: Perspectives on Some Recent Ideas," p. 78. These authors are commenting on a proposal by Thomas C. Chalmers, et al., "Controlled Studies in Clinical Cancer Research," pp. 75–78.
50. See Fried, *Medical Experimentation*, pp. 160–61.
51. For good discussions of these conflicts, see Martin Benjamin and Joy Curtis, *Ethics in Nursing* (New York: Oxford University Press, 1981); Stuart F. Spicker and Sally Gadow, eds., *Nursing: Images and Ideals* (New York: Springer Publishing Co., 1980), especially the articles in part 2; and Barbara Tate, *The Nurse's Dilemma: Ethical Considerations in Nursing Practice* (New York: American Journal of Nursing Co., 1977).
52. See Mila Aroskar, Josephine M. Flaherty, and James M. Smith, "The Nurse and Orders Not to Resuscitate," *Hastings Center Report* 7 (August 1977): 27–28.

8

Ideals, Virtues,
and Conscientious Actions

Throughout this book we have concentrated on acts and policies in light of the various principles and rules that determine obligations and rights. In this final chapter, we examine some other aspects of morality that also shape what people, including health care professionals, ought to do and be. These other aspects are ideals, virtues, and conscience.

Ideals

In examining ideals, it is necessary to consider two aspects or levels of morality: common moral standards within reach of everyone, and uncommon moral standards within reach only of persons who exert extraordinary effort. The first level of morality is limited to moral duties, derived from the moral principles and rules explored in the first seven chapters. In contrast to this morality of *duty*, there is a morality of *aspiration* in which agents seek to realize ideals that do not bind others. These ideals transcend ordinary, universal duties without violating them.

At the end of Albert Camus' *The Plague*, Dr. Rieux decides to make a record of those who fought the pestilence; it would be a record of "what had to be done . . . despite their personal afflictions, by all who, while unable to be *saints* but refusing to bow down to pestilences, strive their utmost to be *healers*."[1] These healers were heroes, not necessarily saints. According to J. O. Urmson, saints and heroes may either (a) do their duty where most people would not, or (b) go beyond their duty where most people would not. In the

255

first category (a), saints do their duty in situations where most people fail because of inclination, desire, or self-interest, while heroes do their duty in situations where most people succumb to fear and the desire for self-preservation. Urmson thus distinguishes between saints and heroes primarily in terms of the forces they resist but others yield to: The saint resists inclination, desire, and self-interest; the hero resists fear and the drive for self-preservation.[2]

Some features that Urmson does not emphasize are also important. Saintliness requires regular fulfillment of duty over time; it demands consistency and constancy of conduct. A final judgment about a person's saintliness cannot be made until his or her record is complete. By contrast, an agent may become a hero instantly, by a single action, such as a brief acceptance of risk while doing his or her duty. This contrast between saints and heroes may be illustrated in a medical context: A physician who works long days at low pay for several years in a poverty-stricken area may be a *saint*, though we probably would not apply that honorific title unless we thought that he or she also fulfilled other duties, such as familial duties. But however a physician may act in other settings, he or she may become a *hero* by overcoming fear about death in order to serve a few days in a plague-stricken city.

In addition to "*minor* saints and heroes" (for Urmson, those who do their duty where others would not), there are *major* saints and heroes who go beyond their duties (category b). Saint Francis is an example of a major saint, while a soldier falling on a hand grenade to save his comrades is an example of a major hero. Physicians and scientists who engage in self-experimentation can also be major heroes. For example, Daniel Carrion injected in his arm blood from a patient with verruga peruana (an unusual disease marked by many vascular eruptions of the skin and mucous membranes as well as fever and severe rheumatic pains) only to discover that it had given him a fatal disease (Oroya fever). Similarly, Werner Forssman performed the first heart catheterization on himself, walking to the radiological room with the catheter sticking in his heart.[3]

These major heroes, who voluntarily assumed significant risks for moral ends, may not have considered their actions morally optional. Many heroes (and saints) would explain their conduct in the language of "ought" and even of "necessity": "I had to act in this way." Not all moral "oughts," it seems, can be reduced to universal duties or obligations. Although the physician who heroically goes beyond his duty may say that he only did what he had to do, others would not be able to reproach him if he did not act in this way. No one could maintain that this act is a universal duty; no one could blame him for a failure to perform it—if, for example, he decided to turn around after reaching the airport on his way to the plague-stricken city.

We do not expect many persons to engage in heroic or saintly actions (at least not consistently enough to merit the appellation of saint). While such actions are *optional* from the standpoint of our ordinary moral duties, they are morally *praiseworthy*. With the addition of ideals, we have at least four categories of action: (a) actions that are right and obligatory (such as truthtelling); (b) actions that are wrong and prohibited (such as murder); (c) actions that are permissible in that they are not wrong; (d) actions that are morally optional but also supererogatory, meritorious, and praiseworthy. For most of this book, we have concentrated on (a) and (b); in this section we are concerned with (d). Actions that go beyond our duties may merit praise, but failure to perform them will not deserve blame.[4]

In claiming that some heroic actions are morally praiseworthy, we do not suggest that all heroic actions are, on balance, praiseworthy. Many factors must be considered in the evaluation of a person and his or her acts. If, for example, we think that a physician went to the plague-stricken city because of a desire to gain public recognition, or to have a set of experiences that could be the basis for a book, we are not likely to praise his or her action. Motives, the reasons for doing something, affect our judgments of persons and their actions. Furthermore, people who take risks in accord with higher, but optional, ideals sometimes do not merit our moral praise, because they also neglect certain duties in the process. On balance we might criticize them for their failure to live up to their duties rather than praise them for their heroic deeds. Imagine that a physician volunteers to take the grave risk of serving in a plague-stricken city that has attracted the world's sympathy, and suppose there are no other physicians or medical services in his own small town. Should his voluntary heroic action be praised, or should it be condemned?

Similar issues emerge in medical practice and research when physicians and others, including courts and society at large, have to decide how to respond to offers of heroic actions that go beyond ordinary duties. Such issues are especially poignant when physicians must determine whether to accept a person's offer of an organ for transplantation. Although a person's pursuit of an ideal of self-giving or assumption of risks for the sake of others may be praiseworthy, his or her donation is accepted in medical practice only if informed and voluntary. Here several questions arise of the sort explored in chapter 3: Does the prospective donor really understand the risks and benefits? What sort of information, if any, is relevant to a decision if the person understands little about the risks and benefits? Are the risks unreasonable? For our purposes two distinct cases merit consideration: an offer from a family member and an offer from a stranger.

Following Urmson, we have so far excluded cases of "natural affection" that involve assumptions of risk or sacrifices for relatives or friends (e.g., a mother going back into a burning house to rescue her child), but they are important. Suppose a mother offers to donate a kidney to her child. If there is a good match and the mother has no physical or psychological conditions that would make her donation too risky, her offer will probably be accepted. When questioned, she may indicate that she did not really calculate the probable benefits and risks but decided to be a donor even before hearing medical information about risks and benefits. She may even insist that she had no other choice. This does not mean, as some claim, that she did not make an informed choice. Even when a donor decides almost immediately upon learning that a family member needs a transplant, he or she may be acting from a sense of moral obligation and thus may have all the morally relevant information.[5] We should also verify that the donor is not being unduly influenced by familial or other pressures into making a decision against his or her wishes. (See Chapter 3.)

However, we might hesitate to allow individuals to take some risks even when we are certain that their decision is informed and voluntary. Would we, for example, be willing to remove a woman's only kidney for transplantation to her son if she had given her informed and voluntary consent? Our decision might vary according to the factual circumstances—for example, whether the mother would probably die shortly because of some other illness or whether she could probably do as well on dialysis. If, however, we consider a mother's informed and voluntary decision to give her heart to her son, we would have moral grounds for refusing to accept and act on her offer. In this case, we face not the risk, but the certainty of death. The mother may believe that her action is a moral sacrifice that she ought to make for her son. We can respect her right to her views, but we should not accept her offer. In these circumstances we should not help her be faithful to her conception of what she ought to be and do, because such an action would involve killing her. (We defended a rule against killing in medicine in Chapter 4.)

Let us now consider heroic actions by strangers. As a rule, the medical profession is suspicious of the living unrelated donor, especially the person who volunteers to donate an organ to a stranger. By the late 1960s there had been only approximately 60 living unrelated donors who were not also spouses of the recipients or who had not undergone a nephrectomy for other reasons. Since that time there have been few, if any, transplants of kidneys from living unrelated donors.[6] Some studies show that people in general do not think that the gift of an organ to a stranger is unreasonable, and they call into question the medical profession's reluctance to use living unrelated donors.[7]

This issue turns in part on the nature of reasonable risk. It is not evident that the donation of a kidney to a stranger involves so much risk to the donor that questions should be raised about his or her competence. While some opponents of a policy of donation to strangers argue that volunteers are emotionally unstable, proponents of a more permissive policy argue that giving an organ enhances the donor's self-esteem and thus is not irrational from the standpoint of risk-benefit analysis. In some circumstances, e.g., where the donor has a medical condition that would make the donation very dangerous, medical practitioners could violate their duty to do no harm by removing an organ for transplantation. Furthermore, if the donor's act would increase some risks for others, we would also have grounds for refusing the gift—for example, if a widow with three small children wanted to donate her kidney to a stranger. Similar points apply to nontherapeutic research involving human subjects.

For purposes of discussion we have stressed dramatic cases of heroic action. Such cases indicate how far principles and rules extend and where ideals of excellence appear on the moral terrain. Earlier we argued that, apart from special roles, such as lifeguard, the principle of beneficence does not impose a duty to assume significant risks in order to benefit others, even in emergencies. The *ideal* of beneficence, however, includes significant risk-taking for others. It is praiseworthy, not mandatory. While this ideal of high-risk beneficence is paradigmatic, there are other less risky moral ideals, such as giving generously, acting mercifully, forgiving others, and volunteering.[8]

Thus far we have emphasized ideal actions. Several ideals, however, concern *how* we act rather than *what* we do. They direct our attention to the manner and way of performing actions, including discharging duties.[9] Consider kindness: It is possible to discharge all the duties imposed by our principles and rules without being kindly. For example, a physician may respect a patient's autonomy and may disclose all the information the patient wants in an *unkind* way. Recognition of ideal ways or modes of acting, even in discharging duties, implies, as Urmson suggests, that there are many different ways to go beyond or to exceed one's duty without being heroic, let alone saintly. For example, a physician can be kindly, understanding, or patient without being heroic or saintly. Often it is not clear just *how* we should characterize our duty, whether in medicine or elsewhere, and it is thus not always clear what would go *beyond* the minimal requirements. What is the physician's duty to his or her patients: to spend a certain amount of time and to expend a certain amount of energy on their behalf? to perform certain acts? to accomplish certain ends? If the duty is to spend a certain amount of time with the patient, the physician can go beyond that duty by increasing his or her hours of work. If it is to perform certain tasks—such as surgery— he or she can exceed it by displaying attitudes such as kindness and gentleness. By some definitions of the physician's responsibilities, such attitudes would not exceed duty but would simply enable the physician to discharge his or her duty more completely or at a higher level.

Wherever the boundaries are drawn—for example, between lower and higher acts or between acts and attitudes—not every act or attitude that is desirable or praiseworthy is part of the physician's duty to his or her patients. A *good* physician is one who has the necessary judgmental and technical skills, who discharges duties, and who also displays moral excellence by realizing some ideals of action (including *how* as well as *what*). When we consider physicians or other health care professionals to be morally good, we usually imply that they are inclined to do what is right and to realize ideals. They are not merely motivated by a sense of "ought." They have particular virtues, i.e., dispositions to act in accord with duties and ideals. We now want to analyze virtues and character in more detail.

Virtues and character

In our discussions of right and wrong, duties and obligations, as well as ideals, we have emphasized acts rather than agents. But in addition to our judgments about right and wrong acts, obligatory and permissible acts, praiseworthy and blameworthy acts, we also make judgments about *moral goodness and badness.* We make judgments of moral value about persons, traits of character, dispositions, motives, and intentions. We talk about good and bad people, about good and bad motives, and about virtues and vices. In short, we look not only at doing but also at being, not only at duties and obligations but also at virtues, not only at conduct but also at character. We consider the moral worth of agents as well as the rightness or wrongness of their acts. Without these additional themes, our view of the moral life, in medical practice and elsewhere, would be truncated.

A good example of the place of virtue and character in medicine appears in Charles L. Bosk's *Forgive and Remember: Managing Medical Failure,* a superb ethnographic study of the way two different surgical services in "Pacific Hospital" handle medical failure, especially on the part of surgical residents.[10] Bosk found that these surgical services distinguish, at least implicitly, between different sorts of error. The first is *technical;* although the professional discharges role responsibilities conscientiously, his or her skills fall short of what the task requires. Every surgeon can be expected to make this sort of mistake some time, for surgeons are involved in an imperfectly applied science. The second sort of error is *judgmental*; a conscientious professional develops and follows an incorrect strategy. Such errors can also be expected. The third sort of error is *normative*; it violates moral or professional norms, particularly by a failure to discharge obligations conscientiously. At this point a judgment about the person enters. Bosk contends that technical and judgmental errors are subordinated to normative errors because everyone can be expected to make "honest errors" or "good faith errors." A surgeon making an honest technical or judgmental error can learn from it. While attending surgeons forgive technical or judgmental errors, they remember such errors in case a *pattern* develops. Such a pattern may indicate that a person lacks the technical and judgmental skills or the moral character to be a competent surgeon—where moral character is defined in terms of *good faith* or *conscientiousness*, that is, "doing everything possible." Attending surgeons tend not to forgive moral errors that display a resident's deficient moral character. The AMA Principles of Medical Ethics also reflect this concern for character: A physician should "strive to expose those physicians deficient in character or competence. . . ."

The word "virtue," as used in this section, should not be confused with a principle or rule about what ought to be done. Rather it is a habit, disposition, or trait that a person may possess or aspire to possess. A *moral* virtue is an acquired habit or disposition to do what is morally right or praiseworthy. It is a trait of character that disposes its possessor to act in accord with moral principles, rules, or ideals. (Any adequate general conception of virtue will also recognize that there are virtues other than moral virtues, just as there are principles, rules, and ideals that are nonmoral.)

Both deontological and utilitarian theories address the question "What ought I to *do*?" While they offer different answers to this question, theirs is a family quarrel, for they share a fairly uniform conception of the moral life: People confront dilemmas and problems that they have difficulty resolving, and the task of ethics is to deal with these problems by explicating moral principles or rules and hence duties in such situations.[11] In general, deontologists and utilitarians reject the idea that virtue could be *independent or primary* in ethics. They think we could not know which character traits to encourage unless we already subscribed to some principles. They do not deny that a study of moral virtues is important; they simply do not regard virtue ethics as making a fundamental contribution to the task of normative ethical theory.

However, several contemporary philosophers and theologians have argued that we, like the classical tradition represented by Plato and Aristotle, should take as the fundamental question, "Who should I *be*?" In their view, morality does not consist in adherence to principles and rules; rather, it is the expression of a virtuous character internal to the person—a character needing no external rules to specify right conduct.[12]

This position is attractive in many respects. Persons are not judged only by how well they live up to moral rules. Our assessments of their character are determined as much by their inner attitudes and outlooks as by their adherence to principles. Consider, for example, the virtue of charity. Whereas in Kant's view all moral worth derives from a good will attempting to meet the demands of duty, we generally have less admiration for the person who acts charitably from a sense of duty than for the person who does so spontaneously from well-formed virtues without the prod of duty. As Philippa Foot puts this point, "The man who acts charitably out of a sense of duty is not to be undervalued, but it is the other who most shows virtue and therefore to the other that most moral worth is attributed." In this regard, Foot sees Aristotle's moral theory as more acceptable than a duty-based theory, and far superior in particular to Kant's account of "moral worth."[13]

Whereas ethical theories such as Kant's find some inspiration in legal analogies and perspectives, the proponents of an agent or virtue ethics sometimes use aesthetic analogies. Judgments about persons, motives, and the like, they maintain, are closer to aesthetic judgments, while judgments about acts tend to be more akin to legal judgments.[14] Jeremy Bentham criticized concentration on the virtues, in part because of their closeness to aesthetics: "There is no marshalling them; they are susceptible of no arrangement; they are a disorderly body, whose members are frequently in hostility with one another. . . . Most of them are characterized by that vagueness which is a convenient instrument for the poetical but dangerous or useless to the practical moralist."[15]

An argument in favor of giving primacy—or at the very least independence—to virtue ethics is the following: Even though we evaluate persons through our knowledge of their actions, we do not evaluate their moral worth or goodness simply by adding up all their actions. Rather, we take account of their total set of virtues—i.e., traits of character. For example, we do not merely sum up a physician's acts in determining whether he or she is a morally good physician. A person who can never be counted on to tell the truth would hardly be said to be virtuous or to have the virtue of veracity, but not everyone who tells a lie is to be considered a liar—if the term "liar" is taken as a judgment of character. While much depends on the definition of a lie, as we have seen, some lies may be justified; and we do not call a person who tells only justified lies a liar. A physician who deceives a patient by giving a placebo (see Case #4) may not be called a liar even if we are convinced that the act is wrong. If someone tells what we consider to be an unjustified lie, we may dismiss it by saying that it was "out of character." By this attribution we mean that he or she can generally be counted on to tell the truth, to exemplify the virtue of veracity, even though he or she did not tell the truth in that situation.

If we determine that telling a lie is "in character," we appropriately consider that person a liar. Our appraisal of the agent, then, depends on whether we think that the act in question displays his or her character. Even several right or wrong acts will not necessarily lead us to declare that someone has a good or a bad character. Much depends on the particular circumstances, the person's previous acts, and the like. Most of us also have a moral character that varies over time in its strength and predictability, but even when variation results (e.g., from occasional moral weakness), we tend to retain our view of a person's typical moral behavior. Moreover, a person's character may be virtuous in some respects (e.g., he or she may be conscientious and compassionate), but suffer from deficiencies in other respects (e.g., he or she may lack patience and tolerance).

Our willingness to *trust* a health care professional will depend on what we think about that person's character. To trust others is to have confidence in and to rely upon them to act in certain ways. Trust, in contrast to control, involves putting oneself in the hands of others; it therefore entails vulnerability. It is rational only if the other is viewed as trustworthy, i.e., can be counted upon not to betray trust. A person is worthy of such trust only if he or she has displayed a character that includes several virtues.

Another argument for the primacy of virtues over action-guides appears to hold that if persons, such as health care professionals or researchers, have good motives and are virtuous, their acts will be morally acceptable. For example, Leon Kass criticizes emphasis on rules and procedures by invoking the virtues of prudence and discernment: "I increasingly believe that the attempt to replace the often inarticulate yet prudent judgments of discerning physicians with explicit rules or procedures will not lead to better decisions."[16] While conceding that it is important to obtain research subjects' informed consent, Henry Beecher, who exposed some important moral problems in research involving human subjects, insists that a "more reliable safeguard is provided by the presence of an intelligent, informed, conscientious, compassionate, responsible researcher."[17] There are, however, some problems with this approach. While we do count on morally good persons to perceive and to do what is morally right, we also know from experience that persons of good moral character sometimes fail to discern what is right. Furthermore, such persons are often the first to recognize that they do not know what ought to be done. Hence, a discussion of the morality of acts remains important, indispensable, and primary in establishing what morally good people ought to do.

A different version of this argument for the primacy of virtues concentrates not on discerning what is right and wrong, but on *desiring* to do what is right and to avoid what is wrong. Gregory Pence contends that "The ultimate argument why moral issues in medical experimentation [and other areas of medicine and health care] should be discussed in the framework of virtues, is that almost any experimenter can get around any informed consent document if he really so desires." Thus, Pence proposes that society try to "create a climate in which experimenters desire not to abuse their subjects—a point harking back to our definition of the good person as one who has the right kind of desires."[18] Even though this argument indicates why we cannot ignore the virtues and should try to inculcate them, for example, in medical education, it does not establish either the independence or the primacy of a virtue ethics. If virtues are dispositions to act in certain ways, as well as to have certain feelings, and if they harness desires and inclinations to moral actions, then it is necessary to have an independent assessment of acts in light of moral principles, rules, and ideals. Thus, if virtues are dispositions to act rightly, it remains important to determine right acts.

Because it is not possible to guarantee virtuous researchers and health care professionals, it is necessary to establish some public boundaries and limits and even to admit some sanctions, such as editorial refusals to publish reports based on unethical research. Such boundaries and limits remind us of the moral minimum expected even of morally good persons, and such sanctions may prevent morally good (but imperfect) persons from succumbing to pressures to cut corners. Even though principles, rules, and sanctions are maintained, it is not necessary to operate with presumptions of distrust of researchers, physicians, and health care professionals. A presumption of trust can be combined with a recognition that trustworthy people may sometimes fail to perceive what they ought to do and may sometimes lack sufficient virtue to do it. What Robert Dahl holds about government applies also to rules and procedures in biomedical ethics: "It seems wiser to design a government on the assumption that people will not always be virtuous and at times surely will be tempted to do evil, yet where they will not lack for the incentive and the opportunities to act according to their highest potential."[19]

In short, none of the above arguments—or any others known to us—

succeed in making judgments about persons independent of judgments about acts or in making virtue primary or sufficient for the moral life. They do, however, show very clearly why character and virtues are indispensable in the moral life and cannot be ignored in ethical theory. Moreover, utilitarians and deontologists, who focus on principles, rules, and duties, need not—and, indeed, should not—overlook character and virtues. For example, a morality of duty requires some settled *dispositions* (virtues) to act in accordance with duties, and a morality of virtues will promote dispositions to *act* in certain ways. Indeed, many moral virtues correspond to principles or rules of moral duty, and, of course, many moral vices correspond to acts prohibited by moral principles and rules. At the very least, for every principle, rule, or ideal, there is a corresponding virtue, that is, a corresponding disposition to act in a certain way. (For reasons that will be developed below, it may not be possible to say that for every moral virtue, there is a corresponding moral principle, rule, or ideal.)

This correspondence can be presented in schematic form:[20]

Theories of Duty   [correspond to]   Theories of Virtue

Common Moral Action-guides	Fundamental Principles ↓ Derivative Rules	Primary Virtues ↓ Secondary Virtues
Exceptional Moral Action-guides	Ideal Actions	Ideal Virtues

In terms of our argument in the previous chapters, there are four basic moral principles and several derivative moral rules pertinent to biomedical ethics—veracity, fidelity, confidentiality, and privacy. The following chart, which is *not* intended to be complete, indicates the correspondence or correlation between these principles and rules, on the one hand, and virtues, on the other.

Fundamental Principles	Primary Virtues
Autonomy	Respect for Autonomy
Nonmaleficence	Nonmalevolence
Beneficence	Benevolence
Justice	Justice or Fairness

Derivative Rules	Secondary Virtues
Veracity	Truthfulness
Confidentiality	Confidentialness
Privacy	Respect for Privacy
Fidelity	Faithfulness

Ideal Actions	Ideal Virtues
Forgiveness	Forgiveness
Beneficence (high risk)	Benevolence (high risk)
Acting mercifully	Mercy
Giving generously	Generosity

Obviously, these lists could be expanded to include many derivative rules and ideal actions. For example, gratitude in response to generosity might be considered either a derivative rule or an ideal action, and gratefulness would be a corresponding virtue. Instead of offering a comprehensive list of the virtues, we want to show that it is possible to bring some order to the virtues, despite Bentham's complaint, and that this order derives from a morality of principles, rules, and ideals. Nevertheless, this approach may not adequately encompass all the widely-recognized virtues. It may be more instructive to think about virtues such as courage, conscientiousness, integrity, and sincerity as connected with morality as a whole, rather than as corresponding to particular action-guides. These virtues, which tend to be more general or abstract, can be called general or "second-order virtues," in contrast to the "first-order virtues" that correspond to first-order action-guides.[21]

In addition to the primary, secondary, ideal, and general moral virtues that we have emphasized, some important virtues will be correlated with professional duties and ideals. Professional codes often stress virtues in addition to duties and ideal actions. Insisting that the medical profession's "prime objective" is to render service to humanity (reward or financial gain being a "subordinate consideration"), a recent AMA code (in effect, 1957–1980) urged the physican to be "an upright man," "pure in character and . . . diligent and conscientious in caring for the sick." It also endorsed the virtues that Hippocrates commended: modesty, sobriety, patience, promptness, and piety. In contrast to its first code in 1847, the AMA over the years has de-emphasized virtues in its various codes. Indeed, the references that remained in the 1957 version were limited, perfunctory, and marginal, and the 1980 version eliminated almost all traces of a virtue ethic, except for the admonition to "expose those physicians deficient in character or competence." Albert Jonsen and André Hellegers lament this shift away from virtues, claiming that "exhortations to virtue constitute the heart of code ethics."[22] But two points should be noted: First, the codes call for right action and hence, at least by implication, for dispositions to right action.

Second, it is possible to infer some virtues from different conceptions of health care professions. For example, if medicine is conceived in paternalistic terms, the physician's virtues will be very different than if medicine is conceived in contractual terms. In the former, virtues of benevolence, care, and compassion are dominant, while in the latter, virtues of respect and fairness are prominent. In some paternalistic conceptions of the physician's role, arrogance may be preferred to humility.[23] Leon Kass contends that the physician should be neither a master nor a slave, but rather a servant of human needs (not desires); he denies that there are any "simple rules" for balancing various considerations in patient care. He turns instead to the virtues appropriate to his conception of medicine:

Certain virtues seem to be required: *moderation* in the physician's view of what he can and cannot accomplish, *gravity* before the awesome mysteries of human being, *understanding* of the human aspects of the lives, hopes, and fears of the ill, *courage* to resist unwarranted demands for pills or procedures, and *prudent judgment* to discern the warranted from the unwarranted.[24]

The adequacy of any conception of the role of physicians and associated virtues will depend in part on its consistency with the moral principles and rules that we have presented.[25]

Virtues of nurses also hinge on conceptions of the nursing profession and its role responsibilities. As we indicated in the last chapter, conceptions of nursing have changed dramatically. In the traditional model, the nurse, as a "handmaiden" of the physician, was expected to cultivate the passive virtues of obedience and submission. In contemporary models, active virtues are more prominent. For example, if the nurse's role is perceived as patient advocacy, nurses will emphasize other virtues such as respect for rights, justice, persistence, and courage.[26] Even if the same virtue—conscientiousness, say—appears in different models, its content may be different. It may require obedience to rules in the traditional model, but constant attention to patients' rights in an advocacy model. Because claims of conscientious action pervade conflicts in health care, we consider such claims in the final section of this chapter.

In conclusion, when an agent reflects on a situation, he or she may conclude that there is no obligatory act, but may still wonder what he or she ought to do. The agent may even ask: "What would a good person do?" or "What would a good health care professional do?" ("Good" in these questions refers not to technical or judgmental skills, but to moral worth.)

Consider this example (compare Case # 11): Mr. X suffers from Huntington's chorea and believes that he would be better off dead. He carefully considers suicide in light of relevant moral principles and rules, and concludes that his suicide would not violate any duties. Nevertheless, he wonders whether a good or virtuous person would commit suicide; in particular, he worries that his act might be *cowardly*. Dr. Y, who is Mr. X's physician, also considers his responsibility in terms of moral principles and rules, concluding that Mr. X has the right to commit suicide and that it would not be wrong for Mr. X to exercise that right in his circumstances. Nevertheless, Dr. Y wonders what a good or virtuous physician would do: Would trying to persuade Mr. X not to commit suicide be *meddlesome* or *kindly*?[27] Such examples indicate the limits of moral principles and rules; rights and duties do not always fully determine what we should do and how we should do it. In particular they do not determine all forms of good, ideal, and virtuous ways of life, many of which are shaped by religious commitments and communities.[28] Such ways, however, should not violate rights and duties. If Mr. X's suicide violated his duties to others, it would probably be wrong; if Dr. Y's intervention to stop Mr. X's attempted suicide violated Mr. X's rights, it too would probably be wrong. But as long as duties and rights are discharged, there is room for moral creativity, including the pursuit and expression of good, ideal, and virtuous ways of living and acting.

Conscientious actions

Conscientiousness, we have suggested, is an important general or second-order virtue. Often agents also appeal to their consciences to interpret and justify their acts in medical practice and research. In *Death of a Man*, Lael Tucker Wertenbaker describes the last months of her husband's life and writes at one point about her husband's physician: "He would have done anything for us that was not against his own deepest conscience."[29] We are all familiar with such slogans as "Let your conscience be your guide" and "Just follow your conscience." For many who use such slogans, conscience appears to be the last recourse in moral justification. In this section we ask: What is the nature of appeals to conscience? How do they function? How much weight should we give them? And how should others respond to an agent's claim of conscience?

In Case #35, George, who is unemployed, believes that he cannot accept a position because of his moral scruples about research on chemical and biological warfare. Yet he needs this position so that his wife can stop working and they can restore family stability and better meet their children's needs. Furthermore, the other candidate for the position would uncritically pursue the research if he took the position. Thus, George has a chance to help his family and perhaps to prevent a fanatic from obtaining this position. But his conscience stands in the way.

Such claims of conscience often require nonparticipation in what an agent takes to be morally wrong. For instance, according to an international code of nursing ethics (see Appendix II), "the nurse is under an obligation to carry out the physician's orders intelligently and loyally and to refuse to *participate in unethical procedures.*" Furthermore, the nurse should expose the "incompetence or unethical conduct of associates"—although "only to the proper authority." Suppose a nurse thinks that a doctor's orders to turn off a respirator for a young patient are unethical. The nurse may think that the doctor's orders are so unethical that he or she must not only refuse to implement them but must also expose them to the proper authority. Alternatively, the nurse may think that cooperation in the doctor's orders would involve complicity in a moral wrong, although he or she is not convinced that others would act wrongly in disconnecting the machine. In this second circumstance, the nurse may not feel compelled to expose the matter to others. In effect, he or she says to the physician: "I see that the arguments you give are sufficient for you to feel that you are doing the right thing by switching off the machine. I don't doubt that *you* are acting according to your conscience, but *my* conscience tells me differently."[30] Similarly, a gynecologist may be conscientiously opposed to performing an abortion procedure, although he or she does not necessarily call into question the conscientious convictions of others. He or she may not even be opposed to a liberal abortion law, but may draw the line at material cooperation in abortion procedures.

The language of conscience can take striking forms. While testifying before the House Committee on Un-American Activities, Arthur Miller refused to answer a question about writers who were suspected of being communists: "I am trying to, and I will, protect my sense of myself . . . my conscience will not permit me to use the name of another person." A physician who refuses to perform amniocentesis for a woman who wants to determine the sex of her child so that she can abort if it is a boy may say, "I couldn't live with myself if I did that." Many expressions reflect this moral perspective: "A person has to answer to himself." "I would hate myself in the morning." "I could not look myself in the mirror." Or, as several kidney donors have exclaimed, "I had to do it. I couldn't have backed out, not that I had the feeling of being trapped, because the doctors offered to get me out. I just had to do it."[31] These statements from ordinary discourse represent appeals to conscience that include the fear of loss of integrity and wholeness if the agent acts in certain ways. Earlier in this chapter we identified "integrity" as a second-order virtue in that it disposes people to act in accord with their convictions, whatever they are. "Integrity" also provides a way to explicate the notions of conscience and conscientious action. People who hold that they cannot do X or must do Y because of their consciences are claiming that to act otherwise would undermine their integrity, their wholeness, and their sense of themselves.[32]

But what precisely is this phenomenon called conscience? In general, conscience is a mode of thought about one's acts and their rightness or wrongness, goodness or badness. It is often *retrospective*. In thinking about his or her past acts, an agent's conscience may come into play. It appears primarily as a *bad conscience*, in the form of feelings of guilt, shame, and disunity when a person believes his or her acts are wrong or bad. Hannah Arendt, however, insists that "only good people are ever bothered by a bad conscience, whereas it is a very rare phenomenon among real criminals. A good conscience does not exist except as the absence of a bad one."[33] Most often the good conscience is described by nouns such as "peace," "wholeness," and "integrity," or by adjectives such as "quiet," "clear," and "easy."

When persons appeal to their consciences or describe their acts as conscientious, they make a *prospective, hypothetical claim*. They claim that if they were to commit the act in question, they would violate their consciences. This violation would result not only in such unpleasant feelings as guilt and shame but also in a loss of integrity, wholeness, and harmony in the self. They thus make a prediction about what would happen to them if they were to commit such an act, a prediction based on the imaginative projection of concrete courses of action in light of their moral standards.

Conscience is also *personal*; it is an agent's consciousness of and reflection on his or her own acts in relation to his or her own, autonomously accepted standards or action-guides. It is a first-person claim, deriving from standards that the person may or may not also apply to the conduct of others. (These standards may be universal principles and rules or personal ideals.) When Socrates affirmed that "it is better to suffer wrong than to do wrong," he meant, as Hannah Arendt puts it, that "it was better *for him*, just as it was better for him 'to be in disagreement with multitudes than, being one, to be in disagreement with [himself].'"[34] Perhaps George in the case previously discussed would have raised moral questions about anyone's participation in research on chemical and biological welfare, and perhaps a Roman Catholic gynecologist would hold that it is morally wrong for others as well as for himself to perform abortions. But it would be odd and even absurd for either of them to say, "My conscience indicates that you should not do that."

In judging others or advising them about their conduct, we may consult our consciences by imagining what we would think and feel if we were to act in a certain way. We may then say that someone else ought not to engage in that conduct, but we *cannot logically* justify this admonition by saying "We would have guilty consciences if he did that." Perhaps we would have guilty consciences if we failed to advise him or to attempt to stop him, but our reasons for *his* abstention from that conduct must involve more than an appeal to our consciences. Our reasons must invoke the moral principles and rules that are determinative for our consciences. Our integrity, however, is not violated if someone acts in ways that we find morally unacceptable. Conscience concerns a person's own actions and inactions.

An appeal to conscience usually involves an appeal to autonomously accepted moral standards—principles, rules, or ideals—but conscience cannot itself be the sole justificatory standard. Conscience is the mode of consciousness that results from reflection on and judgment about one's past, present, or future conduct in relation to those standards. Thus, appeals to conscience do not necessarily presuppose that moral rightness and wrongness are determined by the need for moral integrity or a good conscience, as though these could serve, in effect, as the source or ground of obligation. As Thomas Nagel suggests, "If by committing murder one sacrifices one's moral purity or integrity, that can only be because there is already something wrong with murder. The general reason against committing murder cannot therefore be merely that it makes one an immoral person."[35]

We can also state this point by reference to the tiers of moral justification defended in Chapters 1 and 2: Theory—Principles—Rules—Judgments. When an agent appeals to his or her conscience to explain or to justify X, he or she has already made a judgment that X is wrong. When pressed, the agent might justify that judgment in terms of rules and principles. What then is the role of conscience? How is the action conscientious? First, the action might be conscientious in that it is maximally autonomous: The agent has carefully and scrupulously thought about the judgment in light of rules and principles, has examined all the relevant data, has discussed these matters with others, and so forth. Calling the action conscientious thus might reflect the second-order virtue of conscientiousness. But—and of utmost importance for this discussion—the agent's claim of conscience may indicate the significance for him or her of the moral judgment and its supporting principles and rules. They are held as fundamental in his or her life; they designate inviolable limits and boundaries in his or her actions. If the agent were to transgress them, he or she would experience a bad conscience—the loss of integrity or wholeness.

But if conscience emerges only after and as a consequence of moral judgments, we face some puzzles: What is it to *consult* conscience and to have a *conflict* of conscience? When a person consults his conscience, he examines his moral convictions to determine what he really thinks and feels, reconsidering principles and rules and determining their weight and relevance to the situation at hand. When he consults his conscience, it will only give him one answer: Do what you believe you ought to do. The appeal to conscience is thus only one step in the re-examination of one's moral convictions and is not morally sufficient. As we put it in Chapter 1, it provides a good but perhaps not a sufficient reason.

A "conflict of conscience" appears when a person faces two conflicting moral demands, neither of which can be met without a partial rejection of the other. The person faces a conflict of conscience because he or she has a firm judgment that both courses of action are required. George's conscience may direct him both to refuse the position because it involves immoral research on chemical and biological warfare, and to accept the position because it will prevent the research from falling into the hands of zealots and will also benefit his family. Perhaps he has misconstrued his situation and the relevant moral standards, and the only way out is to reconsider them. His apparent "conflict of conscience" may be an instance of a "doubtful conscience," unsure about the relevant standards and their weight. Perhaps, however, George faces a genuine moral tragedy. To take another example, if an agent holds certain beliefs about the fetus, he or she may feel that it is wrong either to kill the fetus or to allow the mother to die when both cannot be saved.

When agents are clear on moral grounds that they ought or ought not to do something, their appeals to conscience usually reflect several features of their situation. First, they are convinced, as we have seen, that the ethical standards at stake are so important and fundamental to them that their violation would lead to a loss of integrity and wholeness. They would experience severe guilt and/or shame. Second, this appeal to conscience usually asserts a personal sanction rather than an authority. The dictate of conscience is formal: "Do what you believe to be right, and avoid what you believe to be wrong, *or else*." The "or else" is the threat of the loss of integrity, wholeness, and peace. Third, agents claim that they will not be able to forget the deed; hence, its performance will continue to disrupt the self over time. Fourth, they cannot deny that the deed is their own. They cannot shift the responsibility for the act to someone else. For example, military doctors may be unable to plead "superior orders," if they believe that they have to answer to their medical and personal consciences first. When Captain Howard B. Levy, a military physician, refused to obey his commander's order to establish and operate a program for Special Forces Aid Men in dermatology in 1966, he argued that to obey the order would implicate him in war crimes committed by Special Forces in Vietnam and would for him, as a physician, be a violation of medical ethics.[36] Such an appeal to conscience indicates that he will not only be unable to forget the deed but that he will remember it as his own deed; he will view himself as responsible for his unjustified action. Of course, a person who makes such claims may be a victim of self-deception, or he or she might be able to forget the act, or to shift the responsibility to someone else, or even come to consider the act justified. Nevertheless, at this time conscience will not allow him or her to act.

Those who proclaim "Let your conscience be your guide" do not usually hold that conscience is an *infallible* guide. They recognize the possibility of an "erroneous conscience." Traditionally, theologians have held that it is blameworthy to act against conscience, even when conscience is mistaken. As Alan Donagan summarizes the tradition,

Christian moral theologians were not content with allowing the inculpability of impermissible actions done at the behest of conscience; they also ruled that an action done against conscience is always culpable. A man is not merely held inculpable if he does something impermissible in accordance with his conscience, he is held culpable if he does not. The reason is simple. In acting against conscience, a violation of the moral law must be intended; and such intentions are always culpable, even though, because of the agent's erroneous conscience, nothing materially wrong is done.[37]

The point is simple but important: People should do everything possible to make sure that their consciences are properly informed by relevant moral principles and rules, but finally they have to act autonomously, in accord with their consciences; to act otherwise would be to *intend to do what is believed to be morally wrong.* That intention is morally blameworthy, even if no moral wrong is done because the person happens to be mistaken about what moral principles and rules require in the circumstances.

However, it does not follow that we should simply acquiesce to the demands of conscience, our own or others', whatever their content. Conscience is not self-certifying. It may be seriously mistaken, and claims of conscience may simply be rationalizations for immoral acts. As we have argued, the second-order virtue of conscientiousness should lead us to test conscience's leadings in light of moral standards, the facts of the situation, and the judgments of others. Even so, it may be exceedingly difficult, if not impossible, for us to determine whether conscience or some other factor is dominant in motivation.[38]

In situations of conflict, agents have to determine not only how they will act in light of their consciences, but also how they will respond to the claims of conscience made by others, including their colleagues, subordinates, and patients. In general, the guidelines for response derive from our discussion of autonomy in chapter 3, because the right of self-determination rather clearly entails the right of conscientious action. The rules for justified interferences with claims of autonomy are also applicable to claims of conscience. Thus, it is possible to justify overriding a person's claim of conscientious action when his or her actions impose serious risks on others or treat others unjustly, but not when he or she is competent and no one else is harmed. For example, a person may be inoculated against his or her moral convictions in order to protect the public health.

An agent's conscience may create opposition to what others take to be *positive* or *negative duties*. For example, an agent's conscience may lead to repudiation of what others take to be the positive or affirmative duties of serving in the military, of accepting a lifesaving blood transfusion, and of being inoculated. It may also lead to a violation of what others take to be negative duties, such as refraining from certain actions, e.g., providing an FDA-banned drug to patients. Individuals and the society bear a heavy burden of proof in arguing that coercion of conscience is necessary to protect others or to preserve fairness. In some cases, the society may be able to protect an individual's conscience by pursuing its goals in other ways. In some cases, it can require other forms of service by the objector, such as the objector to military service. Occasionally, it may be able to protect the individual's conscience by performing the act in question. For example, some Jehovah's Witnesses take the view that the prohibition against taking blood forbids them from consenting to blood transfusions but does not forbid court-ordered transfusions, which would not be their responsibility.

In one case (#14), Judge J. Skelly Wright granted the Georgetown University Hospital the right to give blood transfusions to a woman without her or her husband's consent. The transfusions were necessary because she had lost two thirds of her body's blood supply from a ruptured ulcer. Judge Wright determined that neither the woman nor her husband wanted her death but that they could not consent to the blood transfusions. By granting a court order, he thought he could protect their consciences and also save her life.[39] However, this removal of responsibility by medical practitioners and the state will not work for all conscientious refusers of blood transfusions or other medical treatments. Many consciences impose strict liability. For example, some Jehovah's Witnesses hold that blood transfusions contaminate the recipients even if the responsibility belongs to the medical practitioners and the state. Although we agree with the court decision in Case #13—to allow a woman to refuse a blood transfusion while ordering it for an infant— we still have to ask what responsibility the hospital and the state have toward the child, who now may be considered an abomination by his or her family.

In medicine and health care, conflicts of conscience—within persons and between persons—sometimes emerge because people believe that role obligations or orders in a hierarchical structure are unethical. Such conflicts are especially acute when A orders B to perform an action that B believes to be wrong, as in the case of the nurse who believed it was wrong to turn off the respirator in the situation described above. It is easy to see how conflicts emerge when those who perform acts for others begin to assume moral responsibility for what they are doing. Nursing is a prime example, but not the only one.

John Lachs has used the term "mediation" to refer to "the performance of an action by some agent on behalf of another."[40] Action is mediated when B does something for A. Obviously mediation is universal and makes civilization possible, for example, through the division of labor. But mediation, Lachs insists, also has some possible negative effects: (1) manipulation of people—treatment of them merely as means to desirable ends; (2) passivity in roles—what we earlier called the passive virtues; and (3) "psychic distance"—those who perform the act experience its circumstances and its consequences, whereas those on whose behalf or at whose behest the act is performed may be insulated from it.

When a person in a role relationship believes that an act he or she is expected to perform is morally wrong, the person may claim that he or she cannot in conscience perform it. As we have noted, the person may not judge others by his or her standards. By saying "Not through me,"[41] the person may refuse to perform the act, and even withdraw from the institution. In one case, a gynecologist refused to perform a sterilization procedure. The young woman who had requested it did not like available contraceptives and did not want children. The gynecologist did not, however, try to prevent the woman from getting someone else to perform the operation.

This form of conscientious refusal or withdrawal may not be sufficient if the agent believes that others are violating fundamental and universal duties, such as nonmaleficence and justice. For instance, nurses and others might have believed that such duties were violated in Case #6—a physician refused to inform a patient that she had cancer—and Case #17—an order not to resuscitate had been written apparently without the patient's knowledge and consent. In such cases, agents may believe that it is necessary to try to ensure or prevent certain actions. After unsuccessful appeals to appropriate officials in the hierarchy, he or she may decide that it is necessary to "blow the whistle" in order to direct public attention to the actions in question. Examples include nurses, social workers, and others blowing the whistle to secure treatment for defective newborns whose physicians and families have ordered no treatment.[42]

When we encounter serious moral disagreements, or conflicts of consciences, we often fall back on procedures, e.g., in hospitals, and on second-order virtues such as conscientiousness. As John Rawls notes, "In times of social doubt and loss of faith in long established values, there is a tendency to fall back on the virtues of integrity: truthfulness and sincerity, lucidity, and commitment, or, as some say, authenticity."[43] Mutual trust within situations of serious moral conflict—for example, when a nurse feels that a physician is acting unethically—may depend on the willingness of all parties to preserve the second-order virtues and to abide by procedures. Sometimes, of course, the conflicts may be too serious or too profound to permit mutual trust. Agents may then have to take more drastic steps, while remembering that conscientiousness implies a willingness to consider and reconsider one's position.

In this chapter, we have expanded the depiction of biomedical ethics as presented in the duties and rights created by four basic moral principles and derivative moral rules. This fuller picture includes ideals that transcend duties and rights, virtues that enable agents to perceive the implications of principles and rules as well as ideals, and virtues that dispose agents to act in accord with principles, rules, and ideals. Finally, we examined conscientious actions, particularly the logic of claims of conscience. Here and throughout this book we have tried to provide a moral point of view on the activities of researchers, physicians, and other health care professionals who make important moral decisions day after day. However, ethical theory alone does not create morality. It can only cast light on morality by analyzing and appraising moral justifications. Ethics requires thought, while morality must be lived.

Notes

1. Albert Camus, *The Plague*, trans. from the French by Stuart Gilbert (New York: Random House, Vintage Books, 1972), p. 287. (Italics added.)
2. J. O. Urmson, "Saints and Heroes," *Essays in Moral Philosophy*, ed. A. I. Melden (Seattle: University of Washington Press, 1958), pp. 198–216. Other valuable

analyses of these and related issues include Joel Feinberg, "Supererogation and Rules," *Ethics* 71 (1961): 276–88, and Roderick M. Chisholm, "Supererogation and Offense: A Conceptual Scheme for Ethics," *Ratio* 5 (1963): 1–14. It should be noted that the words "saint," "saintly," "hero," and "heroic" are not always evaluative words. They are also evaluative words in contexts other than a moral one; e.g., religious, military, or athletic.

3. Jay Katz, ed., *Experimentation with Human Beings* (New York: Russell Sage Foundation, 1972), pp. 136–40.

4. See also the discussion of shame and guilt in John Rawls, *A Theory of Justice* (Cambridge: Harvard University Press, 1971), p. 484; David A. J. Richards, *A Theory of Reasons for Action* (Oxford: Clarendon Press, 1971); and Herbert Morris, ed., *Shame and Guilt* (Belmont, Calif.: Wadsworth Press, 1971).

5. See Carl H. Fellner and John R. Marshall, "Kidney Donors—The Myth of Informed Consent," *American Journal of Psychiatry* 126 (March 1970): 1245–51. On p. 1250, they write: "all relevant data are immediately available to him [i.e., the renal donor]." See also, Robert M. Eisendrath, et al., "Psychologic Considerations in the Selection of Kidney Transplant Donors," *Surgery, Gynecology and Obstetrics* 129 (August 1969): 243–48.

6. Carl H. Fellner, "Organ Donation: For Whose Sake?" *Annals of Internal Medicine* 79 (October 1973): 590.

7. See Carl H. Fellner and Shalom H. Schwartz, "Altruism in Disrepute," *New England Journal of Medicine* 284 (March 18, 1971): 582–85.

8. See Millard Schumaker, *Supererogation: An Analysis and a Bibliography* (Edmonton, Alberta: St. Stephen's College, 1977), esp. pp. 20–29. For other discussions of ideals, see R. M. Hare, *Freedom and Reason* (Oxford: Clarendon Press, 1963), chap. 8; P. F. Strawson, "Social Morality and Individual Ideal," in *Christian Ethics and Contemporary Philosophy*, ed. Ian T. Ramsey (New York: Macmillan, 1966), pp. 280–98; and A. S. Cua, *Dimensions of Moral Creativity: Paradigms, Principles, and Ideals* (University Park, Pa.: The Pennsylvania State University Press, 1978). A common objection to utilitarian theory is that it would eliminate the distinction between the obligatory and the supererogatory, because if an action in accord with ideals produces more good than any other action, then it is obligatory, not merely praiseworthy. This objection certainly holds for act utilitarianism, but the rule utilitarian can avoid it. See Tom L. Beauchamp, "Suicide," in *Matters of Life and Death*, ed. T. Regan (New York: Random House, 1980), esp. pp. 92–96; and R. M. Hare, *Moral Thinking: Its Levels, Method and Point* (Oxford: Clarendon Press, 1981), pp. 198–205.

9. See Peter A. French, *The Scope of Morality* (Minneapolis: University of Minnesota Press, 1979), esp. chap. 7.

10. Charles L. Bosk, *Forgive and Remember: Managing Medical Failure* (Chicago: University of Chicago Press, 1979). Bosk also recognizes a fourth type of error: "quasi-normative errors are eccentric and attending-specific. Each attending has certain protocols that he and he alone follows. A subordinate who does not follow these rules mocks his superordinate's authority" (p. 61).

11. Of course, ethics on this conception may also indicate that agents fail to experience some moral dilemmas because they overlook some important moral principles, rules, and ideals.

12. For an influential defense of the Aristotelian perspective, see Alasdair MacIntyre, *After Virtue* (Notre Dame: University of Notre Dame Press, 1981). For a strong statement of the primacy of character in Christian ethics, see Stanley Hauerwas' various writings, including *A Community of Character: Toward a Constructive Christian Social Ethic* (Notre Dame: University of Notre Dame Press, 1981). Gregory E. Pence has recently attempted to analyze character traits and virtues such as courage, compassion, and honesty as "an alternative framework in medical ethics—an alternative to traditional discussions of theories, conflicts, or rights." See his *Ethical Options in Medicine* (Oradell, N.J.: Medical Economics Company, Book Division, 1980).

13. Philippa Foot, *Virtues and Vices* (Oxford: Basil Blackwell, 1978), pp. 12–14.

14. See Edmund Pincoffs, "Quandary Ethics," *Mind* 80 (1971): 552–71; Lawrence C. Becker, "The Neglect of Virtue," *Ethics* 85 (January 1975): 110–22; Iris Murdoch, *The Sovereignty of Good* (New York: Schocken Books, 1971); and Stanley Hauerwas, *Vision and Virtue: Essays in Christian Ethical Reflection* (Notre Dame, Ind.: University of Notre Dame Press, 1977).

15. Jeremy Bentham, *Deontology: The Science of Morality* (London: Longman, Rees, Orme, Browne, Green & Longman, 1834), 1: 196, quoted in Arthur Flemming, "Reviewing the Virtues," *Ethics* 90 (July 1980): 587.

16. Leon R. Kass, "Ethical Dilemmas in the Care of the Ill," *Journal of the American Medical Association* 244 (October 17, 1980): 1811.

17. H. K. Beecher, "Ethics and Clinical Research," *New England Journal of Medicine* 274 (1966): 1354–60.

18. Pence, *Ethical Options in Medicine*, p. 177.

19. Robert A. Dahl, *After the Revolution? Authority in a Good Society* (New Haven: Yale University Press, 1970), p. 137. For an analysis of presumptions of trust and distrust in clinical research, see Robert J. Levine, *Ethics and Regulation of Clinical Research* (Baltimore: Urban and Schwarzenberg, 1981), esp. Chap. 13.

20. This schema has been adopted with modifications from Tom L. Beauchamp, *Philosophical Ethics* (New York: McGraw-Hill, 1982), chap. 5.

21. See William Frankena, *Ethics*, 2nd ed. (Englewood Cliffs, N.J.: Prentice-Hall, 1973), p. 64.

22. Albert R. Jonsen and André E. Hellegers, "Conceptual Foundations for an Ethics of Medical Care," in *Ethics of Health Care: Papers of the Conference on Health Care and Changing Values*, ed. Laurence R. Tancredi (Washington, D.C.: National Academy of Sciences, 1974), pp. 3–20; for a critique, see Paul Ramsey, "Commentary," in the same volume, pp. 21–29.

23. See Franz J. Ingelfinger, "Arrogance," *New England Journal of Medicine* 303 (December 25, 1980): 1507–11.

24. Leon R. Kass, "Ethical Dilemmas in the Care of the Ill," p. 1816. (Italics added.) For a longer list of virtues for physicians, see Gregory E. Pence, *Ethical Options in Medicine*, esp. pp. 202–20.

25. For an assessment of various models, see Tom L. Beauchamp and Laurence McCullough, *Medical Ethics* (Englewood Cliffs, N.J.: Prentice-Hall, 1984), especially chapter 2, and James F. Childress, *Who Should Decide? Paternalism in Health Care* (New York: Oxford University Press, 1982). Obviously, these models

of professional roles and virtues also imply patient roles and virtues. We do not here present a discussion of the "good patient."

26. For an analysis of models of nursing, see Dan W. Brock, "The Nurse-Patient Relation: Some Rights and Duties," in *Nursing: Images and Ideals*, eds. Stuart F. Spicker and Sally Gadow (New York: Springer Publishing Co., 1980), pp. 102–24.

27. These examples are influenced by James Bogen, "Suicide and Virtue," in *Suicide: The Philosophical Issues*, eds. M. Pabst Battin and David Mayo (New York: St. Martin's Press, 1980), pp. 286–92.

28. Although we have not discussed the "theological virtues," such as faith, hope, and love, religious communities frequently require their adherents to follow what the broader society might consider as ideals. In addition, such communities frequently claim additional resources, such as grace, to enable individuals to live up to those requirements. Nevertheless, some of these communities also recognize different levels of moral activity; an example is the Roman Catholic distinction between the precepts of natural law that bind all people and the counsels of perfection for those who aspire to excellence.

29. Lael Tucker Wertenbaker, *Death of a Man* (Boston: Beacon Press, 1974).

30. Alastair V.Campbell, *Moral Dilemmas in Medicine*, 2nd ed. (Edinburgh: Churchill Livingstone, 1975), p. 25. Italics added.

31. Carl H. Fellner, "Organ Donation: For Whose Sake?" *Annals of Internal Medicine* 79 (October 1973): 591.

32. For a discussion of integrity, see Peter Winch, *Moral Integrity* (Oxford: Basil Blackwell, 1968); Bernard Williams, "A Critique of Utilitarianism," in J. J. C. Smart and Bernard Williams, *Utilitarianism: For and Against* (Cambridge: Cambridge University Press, 1973), esp. pp. 108–118; and Williams, *Moral Luck: Philosophical Papers 1973–1980* (Cambridge: Cambridge University Press, 1981), esp. pp. 40–53, "Utilitarianism and Moral Self-indulgence." Because he is concerned to defend integrity against charges of moral self-indulgence, Williams insists that integrity is not a virtue, i.e., not a disposition that yields motivations, or even an executive virtue. "It is rather that one who displays integrity acts from those dispositions and motives which are most deeply his. . . ." Nevertheless, it makes sense to refer to claims of conscience as motive-statements that invoke integrity, and it is possible to do so without falling into objectionable moral self-indulgence. See James F. Childress, "Appeals to Conscience," *Ethics* 89 (July 1979): 315–35, from which many of the following points are drawn.

33. Hannah Arendt, "Thinking and Moral Considerations: A Lecture," *Social Research* 38 (Autumn 1971): 418.

34. Hannah Arendt, *Crises of the Republic* (New York: Harcourt, Brace, Jovanovich, 1972), p. 62. See Plato, *Gorgias*, 482 and 489.

35. Thomas Nagel, "War and Massacre," *Philosophy and Public Affairs* 1 (Winter 1972): 132.

36. See Robert M. Veatch's discussion of this case, *Case Studies in Medical Ethics* (Cambridge, Mass.: Harvard University Press, 1977), pp. 61–64.

37. Alan Donagan, *The Theory of Morality* (Chicago: University of Chicago Press, 1977), pp. 131–38.

38. C. D. Broad identifies some of the difficulties in assessing conscientious objec-

tion: It is difficult if not impossible to determine whether conscience as a motive in relation to other motives, such as fear, is necessary and sufficient, necessary but not sufficient, sufficient but not necessary, or neither necessary nor sufficient, to lead to the action. Determining the role of conscience in a person's action requires considering what the person would have done without conscience as a motive. See Broad, "Conscience and Conscientious Action," in *Moral Concepts*, ed. Joel Feinberg (Oxford: Oxford University Press, 1969), pp. 74–79.

39. *Application of President and Directors of Georgetown College,* 331F. 2d 1000 (D. C. Cir.), certiorari denied, 377 U. S. 978 (1964). See excerpts in Samuel Gorovitz, et al., eds., *Moral Problems in Medicine* (Englewood Cliffs, N.J.: Prentice-Hall, 1976), pp. 230–32. See also James F. Childress, "Moral Responsibility and Blood Transfusions: Ethical Issues in the Treatment of Jehovah's Witnesses," *Journal of Religion*, forthcoming.

40. John Lachs, "'I Only Work Here': Mediation and Irresponsibility," in *Ethics, Free Enterprise, and Public Policy*, eds. Richard T. DeGeorge and Joseph A. Pichler (New York: Oxford University Press, 1978), pp. 201–13.

41. See Williams, *Moral Luck*, esp. p. 50.

42. For a good analysis of professional noncompliance, especially in nursing, in terms of John Rawls's interpretation of civil disobedience, see Natalie Abrams, "Moral Responsibility in Nursing," in *Nursing: Images and Ideals*, eds. Stuart F. Spicker and Sally Gadow, pp. 148–59.

43. John Rawls, *A Theory of Justice*, p. 519.

Appendix I
Cases

Case #1

Facts in the case

On October 27, 1969, Prosenjit Poddar killed Tatiana Tarasoff. Plaintiffs, Tatiana's parents, allege that two months earlier Poddar confided his intention to kill Tatiana to Dr. Lawrence Moore, a psychologist employed by the Cowell Memorial Hospital at the University of California at Berkeley. They allege that on Moore's request, the campus police briefly detained Poddar, but released him when he appeared rational. They further claim that Dr. Harvey Powelson, Moore's superior, then directed that no further action be taken to detain Poddar. No one warned plainiffs of Tatiana's peril.

Plaintiffs, Tatiana's mother and father, . . . [allege] that on August 20, 1969, Poddar was a voluntary outpatient receiving therapy at Cowell Memorial Hospital. Poddar informed Moore, his therapist, that he was going to kill an unnamed girl, readily identifiable as Tatiana, when she returned home from spending the summer in Brazil. Moore, with the concurrence of Dr. Gold, who had initially examined Poddar, and Dr. Yandell, assistant to the director of the department of psychiatry, decided that Poddar should be committed for observation in a mental hospital. Moore orally notified Officers Atkinson and Teel of the campus police that he would request commitment. He then sent a letter to Police Chief William Beall requesting the assistance of the police department in securing Poddar's confinement.

281

Officers Atkinson, Brownrigg, and Halleran took Poddar into custody, but, satisfied that Poddar was rational, released him on his promise to stay away from Tatiana. Powelson, director of the department of psychiatry at Cowell Memorial Hospital, then asked the police to return Moore's letter, directed that all copies of the letter and notes that Moore had taken as therapist be destroyed, and "ordered no action to place Prosenjit Poddar in a 72-hour treatment and evaluation facility."

Plaintiff's second cause of action, entitled "Failure to Warn of a Dangerous Patient," . . . adds the assertion that defendants negligently permitted Poddar to be released from police custody without "notifying the parents of Tatiana Tarasoff that their daughter was in grave danger from Prosenjit Poddar." Poddar persuaded Tatiana's brother to share an apartment with him near Tatiana's residence; shortly after her return from Brazil, Poddar went to her residence and killed her.

Majority opinion in the case   TOBRINER, Justice.

We shall explain that defendant therapists cannot escape liability merely because Tatiana herself was not their patient. When a therapist determines, or pursuant to the standards of his profession should determine, that his patient presents a serious danger of violence to another, he incurs an obligation to use reasonable care to protect the intended victim against such danger. The discharge of this duty may require the therapist to take one or more of various steps, depending upon the nature of the case. Thus it may call for him to warn the intended victim or others likely to apprise the victim of the danger, to notify the police, or to take whatever other steps are reasonably necessary under the circumstances. . . .

In each instance the adequacy of the therapist's conduct must be measured against the traditional negligence standard of the rendition of reasonable care under the circumstances. . . . In sum, the therapist owes a legal duty not only to his patient, but also to his patient's would-be victim and is subject in both respects to scrutiny by judge and jury. . . . Some of the alternatives open to the therapist, such as warning the victim, will not result in the drastic consequences of depriving the patient of his liberty. Weighing the uncertain and conjectural character of the alleged damage done the patient by such a warning against the peril to the victim's life, we conclude that professional inaccuracy in predicting violence cannot negate the therapist's duty to protect the threatened victim. . . .

We recognize the public interest in supporting effective treatment of mental illness and in protecting the rights of patients to privacy . . . , and the consequent public importance of safeguarding the confidential character of psychotherapeutic communication. Against this interest, however, we must weigh the public interest in safety from violent assault.

The revelation of a communication under the above circumstances is not a breach of trust or a violation of professional ethics; as stated in the Principles of Medical Ethics of the American Medical Association (1957), section 9: "A physician may not reveal the confidence entrusted to him in the course of medical *attendance . . . unless he is required to do so by law or unless it becomes necessary in order to protect the welfare of the individual or of the community.*" (Emphasis added.) We conclude that the public policy favoring protection of the confidential character of patient-psychotherapist communications must yield to the extent to which disclosure is essential to avert danger to others. The protective privilege ends where the public peril begins. . . .

Minority opinion in the case   CLARK, Justice (dissenting).

Until today's majority opinion, both legal and medical authorities have agreed that confidentiality is essential to effectively treat the mentally ill, and that imposing a duty on doctors to disclose patient threats to potential victims would greatly impair treatment. . . .

Policy generally determines duty. Principal policy considerations include foreseeability of harm, certainty of the plaintiff's injury, proximity of the defendant's conduct to the plaintiff's injury, moral blame attributable to defendant's conduct, prevention of future harm, burden on the defendant, and consequences to the community.

Overwhelming policy considerations weigh against imposing a duty on psychotherapists to warn a potential victim against harm. While offering virtually no benefit to society, such a duty will frustrate psychiatric treatment, invade fundamental patient rights and increase violence.

The importance of psychiatric treatment and its need for confidentiality have been recognized by this court. "It is clearly recognized that the very practice of psychiatry vitally depends upon the reputation in the community that the psychiatrist will not tell. . . ."

Assurance of confidentiality is important for three reasons.

Deterrence from treatment

First, without substantial assurance of confidentiality, those requiring treatment will be deterred from seeking assistance. It remains an unfortunate fact in our society that people seeking psychiatric guidance tend to become stigmatized. Apprehension of such stigma—apparently increased by the propensity of people considering treatment to see themselves in the worst possible light—creates a well-recognized reluctance to seek aid. This reluctance is alleviated by the psychiatrist's assurance of confidentiality.

Full disclosure

Second, the guarantee of confidentiality is essential in eliciting the full disclosure necessary for effective treatment. The psychiatric patient approaches treatment with conscious and unconscious inhibitions against revealing his innermost thoughts. . . .

Successful treatment

Third, even if the patient fully discloses his thoughts, assurance that the confidential relationship will not be breached is necessary to maintain his trust in his psychiatrist—the very means by which treatment is effected. . . .

Given the importance of confidentiality to the practice of psychiatry, it becomes clear the duty to warn imposed by the majority will cripple the use and effectiveness of psychiatry. Many people, potentially violent—yet susceptible to treatment—will be deterred from seeking it; those seeking it will be inhibited from making revelations necessary to effective treatment; and, forcing the psychiatrist to violate the patient's trust will destroy the interpersonal relationship by which treatment is effected.

Violence and civil commitment

By imposing a duty to warn, the majority contributes to the danger to society of violence by the mentally ill and greatly increases the risk of civil commitment—the total deprivation of liberty—of those who should not be confined. The impairment of treatment and risk of improper commitment resulting from the new duty to warn will not be limited to a few patients but will extend to a large number of the mentally ill. Although under existing psychiatric procedures only a relatively few receiving treatment will ever present a risk of violence, the number making threats is huge, and it is the latter group—not just the former—whose treatment will be impaired and whose risk of commitment will be increased.

[This case is adapted from *Tarasoff* v. *Regents of the University of California*, California Supreme Court (17 California Reports, 3rd Series, 425. Decided July 1, 1976.) The language is that of the court. The "facts" and "majority opinion" are written by Justice Tobriner. The "dissenting opinion" is written by Justice Clark. The comments are brief excerpts from each opinion.]

Case #2

A five-year-old girl had been a patient in a medical center for three years because of progressive renal failure secondary to glomerulonephritis. She had been on chronic renal dialysis, and the possibility of a renal transplantation was considered. The effectiveness of this procedure in her case was questionable. On the other hand, it was the feeling of the professional staff that there was a clear possibility that a transplanted kidney would not undergo the same disease process. After discussion with the parents, it was decided to proceed with plans for transplantation. Tissue typing was performed on the patient; it was noted that she would be difficult to match. Two siblings, age two and four, were thought to be too young to serve as donors. The girl's mother turned out not to be histocompatible. The father, however, was found to be quite compatible with his daughter. He underwent an arteriogram, and it was discovered that he had anatomically favorable circulation for transplantation. The nephrologist met alone with the father, and gave him these results. He informed the father that the prognosis for his daughter was quite uncertain. After some thought, the girl's father decided that he did not wish to donate a kidney to his daughter. He admitted that he did not have the courage, and that, particularly in view of the uncertain prognosis, the very slight possibility of a cadaver kidney, and the degree of suffering his daughter had already sustained, he would prefer not to donate. The father asked the physician to tell everyone else in the family that he was not histocompatible. He was afraid that if they knew the truth, they would accuse him of allowing his daughter to die. He felt that this would "wreck the family." The physician felt very uncomfortable about this request. However, he agreed to tell the man's wife that "for medical reasons" the father should not donate a kidney.

[This case is reprinted by permission from Melvin D. Levine, Lee Scott, and William J. Curran, "Ethics Rounds in a Children's Medical Center: Evaluation of a Hospital-Based Program for Continuing Education in Medical Ethics," *Pediatrics* 60 (August 1977): 205.]

Case #3

Laud Humphreys, a sociologist, recognized that the public and law-enforcement authorities hold highly simplistic stereotyped beliefs about men who commit impersonal sexual acts with one another in public restrooms. "Tearoom sex," as fellatio in public restrooms is called, accounts for the majority of homosexual arrests in the United States. Humphreys decided that it would be of considerable social importance for society to gain more objective understanding of who these men are and what motivates them to seek quick, impersonal sexual gratification.

For his Ph.D. dissertation at Washington University, Humphreys set out to answer this question by means of participant observation and structured interview: He stationed himself in "tearooms" and offered to serve as "watchqueen"—the individual who keeps watch and coughs when a police car stops nearby or a stranger approaches. He played that role faithfully while observing hundreds of acts of fellatio. He was able to gain the confidence of some of the men he observed, to disclose his role as scientist, and to persuade them to tell him about the rest of their lives and about their motives. Those who were willing to talk openly with him tended to be among the better-educated members of the "tearoom trade." To avoid bias, Humphreys secretly followed some of the other men he observed and recorded the license numbers of their cars. A year later and carefully disguised, Humphreys appeared at their homes claiming to be a health-service interviewer and interviewed them about their marital status, race, job, and so on.

Humphrey's findings destroy many stereotypes. Fifty-four percent of his subjects were married and living with their wives, and superficial analysis would suggest that they were exemplary citizens who had exemplary marriages. Thirty-eight percent of Humphreys' subjects clearly were neither bisexual nor homosexual. They were men whose marriages were marked with tension; most of the 38 percent were Catholic or their wives were, and since the birth of their last child conjugal relations had been rare. Their alternative source of sex had to be quick, inexpensive, and impersonal. It could not entail any kind of involvement that would threaten their already shaky marriage and jeopardize their most important asset—their standing as father of their children. They wanted only some form of orgasm-producing action that was less lonely than masturbation and less involving than a love relationship. Of the other 62 percent of Humphreys' subjects, 24 percent were clearly bisexual, happily married, well educated, economically quite successful, and exemplary members of their community. Another 24 percent were single and were covert homosexuals. Only 14 percent of Humphreys' subjects corresponded to society's stereotype of homosexuality. That is, only 14 percent were members of the gay community and were interested primarily in personal homosexual relationships (Humphreys, 1970).

Informal inquiry (Knerr, 1977) indicated that Humphrey's research has helped persuade police departments to stop using their resources on arrest for this victimless crime. Many would count this as a social benefit.

There were also social costs. The research occurred in the middle 1960s before institutional review boards were in existence. The dissertation proposal was reviewed only by Humphreys' Ph.D. committee. Only after the research had been completed did the other members of the Sociology Department learn of it. A furor arose when some of those other members of the department objected that Humphreys' research had unethically invaded the privacy and threatened the social standing of the subjects, and they petitioned the president of Washington University to rescind Humphreys' Ph.D. degree. The turmoil resulted in numerous other unfortunate events, including a fist fight among faculty members and the exodus of about half of the department members to positions at other universities.

There was considerable public outrage as well. Journalist Nicholas von Hoffman, who was given some details of the case by one of the angered members of the Sociology Department, wrote an article about Humphreys' research and offered the following condemnation of social scientists: "We're so preoccupied with defending our privacy against insurance investigators, dope sleuths, counterespionage men, divorce detectives and credit checkers, that we overlook the social scientists behind the hunting blinds who're also peeping into what we thought were our most private and secret lives. But they are there, studying us, taking notes, getting to know us, as indifferent as everybody else to the feeling that to be a complete human involves having an aspect of ourselves that's unknown" (von Hoffman, 1970).

[This case was prepared by Dr. Joan Sieber, Visiting Research Scholar, The Kennedy Institute, 1977–78, and Professor of Psychology, California State University, Hayward. The relevant materials include:
Humphreys, L., *Tearoom Trade: Impersonal Sex in Public Places* (Chicago: Aldine Publishing Co., 1970).
Knerr, C., "What To Do Before and After the Subpoena Arrives," in Joan Sieber, ed., *Ethical Decision Making in Social Science Research* (in preparation).
von Hoffman, Nicholas, "Sociological Snoopers," *The Washington Post* B1, Col. 1 and B9, Col. 5 (January 30, 1970).]

Case #4

A 65-year-old retired army officer had several abdominal operations for gallstones, postoperative adhesions, and bowel obstructions. Because of chronic abdominal pain, loss of weight, and social withdrawal, he voluntarily entered a psychiatric ward. Although he had had a very productive military, teaching, and research career, he was now somewhat depressed and unkempt and had poor hygiene. Furthermore, he and his wife had curtailed their social activities because he could not control his pain without assuming awkward and embarrassing postures. He relied on six self-administered injections each day of Talwin (Pentazocine), which he believed to be essential to control his pain. He quoted the early literature to support his claim that Talwin is non-addictive; later studies, however, indicated that it is addictive. Having used this medication for more than two years, he had so much tissue and muscle damage that he had difficulty finding injection sites. His goal for therapy was to "get more out of life in spite of my pain."

This psychiatric ward included individual behavior therapy programs, daily group therapy, ward government, and social activities, and the staff ignored pain behaviors in order to avoid reinforcing them. Their positive procedures included relaxation techniques, covert imagery, and cognitive relabeling. Although the patient has voluntarily admitted himself to this ward where adjustment in medication was a clear expectation, he refused to allow direct modification of his Talwin dosage levels on the grounds that his experience showed that the level of medication was indispensable to control his pain. After considerable discussion with colleagues, the therapists decided to withdraw the Talwin over time without the patient's knowledge by diluting it with increasing proportions of normal saline. Although the patient experienced nausea, diarrhea, and cramps, he thought that these withdrawal symptoms were actually the result of Elavil (Amitriptyline), which the therapists had introduced to relieve the withdrawal symptoms. While the therapists did not use Elavil to deceive the patient, it served that purpose for he blamed it for his discomfort. The staff had informed the patient that his medication regime would be modified, but had not given him the details.

After three weeks of saline injections, the therapists explained what had been done. At first the patient was incredulous and angry, but he asked that the saline be discontinued and the self-control techniques continued. When he was discharged three weeks later, he reported that he experienced some abdominal pain but that he could control it more effectively with the self-control techniques than previously with the Talwin. A follow-up six months later showed that he was still using the relaxation techniques and had resumed social activities and part-time teaching.

The therapists justified this deceptive use of a placebo on grounds of its effectiveness: "We felt ethically obliged to use a treatment that had a high probability of success. To withhold the procedure may have protected some standard of openness but may not have been in his [the patient's] best interests. We saw no option without ethical problems. Although it is precarious to justify the means by the end, we felt most obliged to use a procedure designed to help the patient achieve a personally and medically desirable goal."

[Based on the description of an actual case provided by Philip Levendusky and Loren Pankratz, "Self-Control Techniques as an Alternative to Pain Medication," *Journal of Abnormal Psychology*, Vol. 84, No. 2 (1975): 165–68. In addition, several articles comment on this case report.]

Case #5

A sixty-nine-year-old male, estranged from his children and with no other living relatives, underwent a routine physical examination in preparation for a brief and much anticipated trip to Australia. The physician suspected a serious problem and ordered more extensive testing, including further blood analysis (detailing an acid phosphatase), a bone scan, and a prostate biopsy. The results were quite conclusive: The man had an inoperable, incurable carcinoma—a small prostate nodule commonly referred to as "cancer of the prostate." The carcinoma was not yet advanced, and was relatively slow growing. Later, after the disease had progressed, it would be possible to provide good palliative treatment. Blood tests and X rays showed the patient's renal function to be normal. (The physician consulted with the urologist who had performed the prostate biopsy in order to confirm the diagnosis.)

The physician had treated this patient for many years and knew that he was fragile in several respects. The man was quite neurotic and had an established history of psychiatric disease—although he functioned well in society and was clearly capable of rational thought and decisionmaking. He had recently suffered a severe depressive reaction, during which he had behaved irrationally and attempted suicide. This episode immediately followed the death of his wife, who had died after a difficult and protracted battle with cancer. It was clear that he had not been equipped to deal with his wife's death, and he had been hospitalized for a short period before the suicide attempt. Just as he was getting back on his feet, the opportunity to go to Australia materialized, and it was the first excitement he had experienced in several years.

This patient also had a history of suffering prolonged and serious depression whenever informed of serious health problems. He worried excessively and often could not exercise rational control over his deliberations and decisions. His physician therefore thought that disclosure of the carcinoma under his present fragile state would almost certainly cause further irrational behavior, and render the patient incapable of thinking clearly about his medical situation.

When the testing had been completed and the results were known, the patient returned to his physician. He asked nervously, "Am I O.K.?" Without waiting for a response, he asked, "I don't have cancer, do I?" Believing his patient would not suffer from or even be aware of his problem while in Australia, the physician answered, "You're as good as you were ten years ago." He was worried about telling such a bald lie, but firmly believed that it was justified.

[This case was prepared especially for this volume. David Bloom, M.D., was a contributing consultant.]

Case #6

Mrs. X., forty-five years of age, was diagnosed as having cancer of the colon with metastases to the lymph nodes. Miss N., a young but experienced nurse in the oncology unit, developed good rapport with Mrs. X. during the three days before the scheduled operation. Miss N. was off duty the day after surgery. When she returned, she could not locate the physician to ascertain what he had told the patient about her condition, and the associate nurse indicated that the patient had not requested or received any information from her. In talking to Mrs. X., Miss N. discovered that she did not know that the tumor was cancerous, that it had metastasized, or that her condition was serious. Mrs. X., however, was concerned about the sharp pain in her abdomen, and specifically inquired about the results of the tests. She also wondered when she might be able to return to work. The nurse avoided direct answers to these questions, and Mrs. X.'s two daughters tried to divert the conversation. When Mrs. X. asked, "Is everything all right?", no one answered.

Later Mrs. X.'s daughters, who knew the truth, asked the nurse to reassure Mrs. X. about her condition. They were worried about the possible impact of the truth, especially since Mrs. X. had recently undergone very difficult divorce proceedings. They thought that she would not be able to bear this additional burden. Although the nurse made no promises, she did try to keep the conversation with Mrs. X. as light as possible until she could talk to the attending physician—a procedure recommended by the head nurse. When the attending physician arrived in the patient's room, Mrs. X. indicated that she felt "pretty good," but asked no questions. He left after a brief examination.

Later when the nurse was finally able to talk to the physician, he indicated that no one had told Mrs. X. about her cancer because such information would only cause her unnecessary anxiety and suffering. Furthermore, he ordered Miss N. not to disclose this information, warning her that he would consider such an act a violation of the patient's best interests and a breach of professional responsibility.

After talking again to the head nurse, who recognized the dilemma but advised her to follow the doctor's orders, she decided not to disclose the information to the patient, despite her uneasy conscience.

[This case has been adapted from Rod R. Yarling, "Ethical Analysis of a Nursing Problem: The Scope of Nursing Practice in Disclosing the Truth to Terminal Patients," Parts I and II, *Supervisor Nurse* (May, 1978 and June 1978).]

Case #7

A woman had a fatal reaction during urography. The radiologist indicated that he did not warn this patient (or any other patients) of a possible fatal reaction to urography because it would not do any good. "I could have told her," he said, "that there was a chance she might have a reaction and even die. After calming her down I would then have told her that she had seen two urologists in the past week and both of them had told her she needed urography. I have done 6,000 to 8,000 urograms in the past 13 years and no one has ever had a fatal reaction. We have been doing urograms at this hospital for at least 25 years and no one has ever had a fatal reaction. Because the indications for urography were great and the chances for a reaction were remote I am sure I would have convinced Mrs. E. . . . to have the procedures. She would have then had the reaction and died and the fact that I warned her would have done Mrs. E. . . . absolutely no good." The radiologist contended that the American College of Radiology should adopt the following policy: "Our responsibility is to our patients and to do what is best for our patients medically. Informing patients of risks and possible death from urography may not be in the best interest of the patient and . . . it may be dangerous."

[Based on Robert W. Allen, "Informed Consent: A Medical Decision," *Radiology* 119 (April 1976): 233–24.]

Case #8

Ralph Cobbs was admitted to a hospital for treatment of a duodenal ulcer. He was given a series of tests and administered medication to ease his discomfort. He still, however, continued to complain of lower abdominal pain and nausea. His family physician, Dr. Jerome Sands, concluded that surgery was indicated. He discussed prospective surgery with Mr. Cobbs and advised him in general terms of the risks of undergoing a general anesthetic.

Dr. Sands then called in Dr. F. P. Grant, a surgeon, who examined Mr. Cobbs and agreed that he had an intractable duodenal ulcer and that surgery was indicated. Dr. Grant explained the nature of the operation to Mr. Cobbs, but did not discuss any of its inherent risks. Mr. Cobbs consented to the operation, which seemed successful. However, nine days later the patient began to experience intense abdominal pain. Dr. Sands advised him to return to the hospital. Two hours after his return, Mr. Cobbs went into shock and emergency surgery was performed. Internal bleeding was discovered, the result of a severed artery at the hilium of the spleen. Because of the seriousness of the hemorrhaging, Dr. Grant decided to remove the spleen, which may be taken out of an adult without adverse effects. Injuries to the spleen necessitating a subsequent operation are a risk inherent to the original type of surgery performed on Mr. Cobbs. The probability of the patient needing further surgery was approximately 5% at the time of the original operation.

A month after his second discharge from the hospital, Mr. Cobbs again experienced sharp pains in his stomach. These were traced to a developing gastric ulcer. The development of a new ulcer is another risk inherent in surgery performed to relieve a duodenal ulcer. Within four months the patient had to be rehospitalized, and a third operation was performed: a gastrectomy removing 50% of Mr. Cobbs' stomach (to reduce its acid-producing capacity). Subsequent to his discharge this time, the patient had to be readmitted because of internal bleeding caused by the premature absorption of a suture, another inherent risk of surgery. The bleeding began to abate after a week, and Mr. Cobbs was discharged for the final time.

Mr. Cobbs then brought a malpractice suit against Dr. Grant on two grounds: (1) negligent performance of the operation; (2) failure to disclose the risks of the original surgery. The Supreme Court of California used expert testimony to determine that the operation was not performed negligently; all the subsequent problems Mr. Cobbs experienced were *inherent risks* of the surgery, not the result of negligence. The second ground, however, received extensive commentary in the court's opinion. The court reasoned that this case provides a "classic illustration" of possible negligence in disclosure. While Dr. Grant had thoroughly explained the *nature* of the procedure and had performed the operation exactly as described, he had *not* discussed the possibilities of the spleen injury, of the new ulcer and ensuing gastrectomy, or of the internal bleeding resulting from the premature absorption of a suture—all "links in a chain of low probability events inherent in the initial operation." The court reasoned that this failure to inform may have constituted a violation of the physician's duty to disclose pertinent information to patients. This violation would make the physician liable for subsequent injuries, because he withheld the facts necessary for Mr. Cobbs to consent intelligently to the proposed treatment.

Dr. Grant argued that it was uncommon medical practice to disclose hazards of such low probability and that he should be held only to the standards of disclosure operative among surgeons. The court, however, quoted a precedent case (*Canterbury* v. *Spence*), which reached a different conclusion: "To bind the disclosure obligation to medical usage is to arrogate the decision on revelation to the physician alone. Respect for the patient's right of self-determination on particular therapy demands a standard set by law for physicians rather than one which physicians may or may not impose upon themselves." The court held that in this matter physician discretion cannot be reconciled with a patient's basic right to make the ultimate informed decision about his own treatment. "A mini-course in medical science is not required," the court held, but "when a given procedure inherently involves a known risk of death or serious bodily harm, a medical doctor has a duty to disclose to his patient the potential of death or serious harm. . . . The patient's right of self-decision is the measure of the physician's duty to reveal." A physician is therefore required to disclose "all information relevant to a meaningful decisional process," with respect both to the proposed therapy and its inherent risks.

Given these problems, the Supreme Court determined that a trial court should reach a judgment in this case after further analyzing the extent of "the doctor's duty to obtain the patient's informed consent."

[This case is summarized from *Cobbs* v. *Grant*, 502 P.2d 1, decided October 27, 1972. The language closely follows that of the court, and all direct quotations are from this source. The opinion was written by Justice Mosk.]

Case #9

Mrs. Catherine Lake, who was then sixty years old, suffered from chronic brain syndrome with arteriosclerosis. As a result, she had periods of confusion and mild loss of memory, interspersed with times of mental alertness and rationality. She was hospitalized after having been found wandering on a city street; when questioned she could not give her home address. During her third hospitalization, she petitioned for release on grounds of unlawful deprivation of liberty.

A psychiatrist who testified at her hearing claimed that she was unable to remember when her sister, her son, and her husband had died. She also showed what were diagnosed as paranoid tendencies, believing that government agencies had taken her pension away from her. (Her government pension had, indeed, been cut off several years earlier.) However, the psychiatrist was concerned mainly about Mrs. Lake's wandering, which presented a risk of harm to herself. She showed no tendency to harm others, nor to harm herself intentionally. Her commitment was based solely on the need for supervision because of her confused and defenseless state.

Mrs. Lake also testified at her hearing. She appeared to be fully rational, and stated that she understood her condition and the risks involved in her living outside the hospital. But she preferred to accept these risks rather than endure continued hospitalization.

The District Court, supported by the U.S. Court of Appeals, denied her petition. The court found that Mrs. Lake's family lacked the means to provide needed supervision for her. They claimed that she was "a danger to herself in that she has a tendency to wander about the streets, and is not competent to care for herself." The legal basis for her involuntary commitment was a statute providing for hospitalization of a person who "is mentally ill, and because of that illness, is likely to injure himself or others if allowed to remain at liberty." The court declared that "injure" ought to be construed broadly enough to include Mrs. Lake's situation.

However, about six months later, the Court of Appeals agreed to consider a rehearing of the case, identifying several crucial issues: How should "likely to injure himself" be interpreted? Is one who is "likely to injure himself" also automatically incompetent to choose between risk and hospitalization? Must the court consider community resources other than commitment to a mental hospital? Is equal protection denied by commitment of a person like Mrs. Lake, who would be released if her family had the means to care for her?

The case was finally returned to the District Court for an inquiry into alternative courses of treatment. The court was asked to consider whether Mrs. Lake could be released if she agreed to carry an identification card, to accept public health nursing care, to live in a foster home, or under other similar conditions. Judge Bazelon, presiding officer of the Court of Appeals, instructed the District Court that the burden of finding alternatives ought to be on the court, not on Mrs. Lake, since she lacked access to the necessary information. Bazelon referred to the position of the Department of Health, Education, and Welfare (now HHS), which mandates provision of a wide spectrum of services so that the interests of both the mentally ill person and the public will be served. He also endorsed the view of the National Council on the Aging, which recommends that "care and services be provided so as to be most satisfying to the person concerned." In line with this view, Bazelon ordered that "every effort should be made to find a course of treatment which appellant might be willing to accept." However, the lower court, after conducting a further investigation of Mrs. Lake's case, concluded that her propensity to wander aimlessly made "constant supervision . . . not only proper but required for the safety of this patient." Mrs. Lake died four years later, still confined in a mental hospital.

[This case was prepared by Carol Tauer from materials in Jay Katz, Joseph Goldstein, and Alan M. Dershowitz, *Psychoanalysis, Psychiatry, and Law* (New York: Free Press, 1967). It was expanded by James Tubbs from materials in *Lake v. Cameron*, 267 F. Supp. 155 (D.D.C. 1967) and Robert A. Burt, *Taking Care of Strangers: The Rule of Law in Doctor-Patient Relations* (New York: Free Press, 1979), chap. 2.]

Case #10

P.Z., now twenty-seven years old, is an involuntary mental patient at Lakeland State Hospital where he was committed in June 1971, after amputating his right hand. He had been previously committed to Lakeland for eight months in 1966 (after perforating his right eardrum) and for 18 months in 1969 (after removing his right eye). In all, P.Z. has spent approximately eight years in hospitals undergoing medical treatment, e.g., treatment for meningitis following the perforation of his eardrum, and for psychiatric care of a custodial and involuntary nature.

For a variety of reasons, P.Z. now wishes to leave the hospital, but his family is strongly opposed. P.Z.'s father, a factory foreman whose job is in some jeopardy due to recession layoffs, points out that the family is already in debt more than $30,000 for the medical care necessitated by P.Z.'s penchant for self-mutilation. Neither P.Z.'s parents nor his siblings can control his self-destructive outbursts at home; indeed, they are very frightened that he will turn upon them as well. P.Z., on the other hand, maintains that he has been confined long enough, that he is not dangerous, and that, in any event, there is "no treatment for me in the hospital." He states repeatedly that "I believe in God and in brotherly love" and that "One man must sacrifice himself to God for the good of all men." He believes that "it is far better for one man to believe and accept an appropriate message from God to sacrifice an eye or a hand according to the sacred scriptures rather than for the present course of the world to cause even greater loss of human life." P.Z. believes that he is the only one whom God has selected for that sacrifice and maintains that he enucleated his right eye and amputated his right hand upon "direct orders from God," and that he and God thereby established a "covenant." P.Z. now wants release from the hospital in order to "carry God's love to His children"; he emphasizes his commitment to this work by stating: "I would cut off my right foot if God told me to."

What rights does P.Z. have to determine where and how he shall live, and what mental competence does he have to assert such rights? Alternatively, what rights may be asserted by his family, or by society, to restrain, isolate, or "contain" him? If others have the right ultimately to restrain P.Z., must they also provide him with treatment beyond mere containment? If so, is custodial treatment sufficient? May society compel P.Z. to undergo more drastic, irreversible treatments, with or without his consent?

[This case was prepared by P. Browning Hoffman, M.D. for presentation in the series of Medicine and Society Conferences at the University of Virginia School of Medicine and is used by permission. The lengthy quotation has been added by the authors.]

Case #11

John K., a thirty-two-year-old lawyer, worried for several years about developing Huntington's chorea, a neurological disorder that appears in a person's thirties or forties, bringing rapid uncontrollable twitching and contractions and progressive, irreversible dementia, and leading to death in approximately ten years. John K.'s mother died from this disease, which is autosomal dominant and afflicts fifty percent of an affected parent's off-spring. Often parents have children before they are aware that one of them has the disease. John K. and his wife have a child because of contraceptive failure and an unwillingness to have an abortion because of his wife's religious convictions.

John K. has indicated to many people that he would prefer to die rather than to live and die as his mother lived and died. He is anxious, drinks heavily, and has intermittent depression, for which he sees a psychiatrist. Nevertheless, he is a productive lawyer.

John K. first noticed facial twitching three months ago, and two neurologists independently confirmed a diagnosis of Huntington's. He explained his situation to his psychiatrist and requested help in committing suicide. When the psychiatrist refused, John reassured him that he did not plan to attempt suicide any time soon.

But when he went home, he ingested all his anti-depressant medication, after pinning a note to his shirt to explain his actions and to refuse any medical assistance that might be offered. His wife, whom he had not told about the diagnosis, found him unconscious and rushed him to the emergency room without removing the note.

[This case has been adapted from Marc Basson, ed., *Rights and Responsibilities in Modern Medicine: The Second Volume in a Series on Ethics, Humanism, and Medicine* (New York: Alan R. Liss, Inc., 1981): 183–84.]

Case #12

Two sisters, sixty-eight and seventy years of age, and their husbands were searching for a schizophrenic daughter who had disappeared after her discharge from a psychiatric hospital. While their car waited for a stoplight, a nearby construction machine hit a gasoline line. The spraying gas exploded, leveling a city block and igniting the car.

The sisters arrived in our burn center two hours later. The younger sister had 91 percent full-thickness, 92 percent total-body burn, with moderate smoke inhalation; the older had 94.5 percent full-thickness, 95.5 percent total-body burn, with severe smoke inhalation. The burn team agreed that survival was unprecedented in both cases. Both women were alert and interviewed separately.

The younger sister asked about death directly, looking intently into the physician's eyes. When he answered, she replied matter-of-factly, "Well, I never dreamed that life would end like this, but since we all have to go sometime, I'd like to go quietly and comfortably, I don't know what to do about my daughter. . . ."

After she was made comfortable, the nurse obtained a description of the missing daughter and possible whereabouts. The social worker alerted the police to look for her, and telephoned relatives, informing them of the accident as gently as could be conveyed by telephone. The husbands were located at another burn unit. An attempt was made to arrange a final spousal conversation, but both husbands were intubated.

Meanwhile, the older sister doubted whether her injuries were as serious as reported. "I feel so good, wouldn't I be hurting horribly if I were going to die?" The effect of full-thickness burns on nerve endings was explained. The physician reiterated that we wished to do what she thought was best for her. She hedged, "What did my sister say? I'll go along with her decision." Since the patient seemed unsure of her decision, she was offered full therapy in the room with her sister. She then refused the therapy adamantly, but denied that she was dying.

The sisters' beds were placed next to each other so that they could see and touch each other easily. They discussed funeral arrangements and then joked, in the next breath, about the damage done to their hair. The hospital chaplain prayed with them. By active listening, he was able to convey to the older sister that her husband was not to blame for the accident as she had thought. "It's good to go out not cursing him after all our years together," she said. The younger sister died several hours later, after her sister lapsed into a coma; the older sister died the next day. The daughter was not located.

[This case is reprinted by permission from Sharon H. Imbus, R.N., M. Sc., and Bruce E. Zawacki, M.D., "Autonomy for Burn Patients When Survival is Unprecedented," in *The New England Journal of Medicine* 297 (August 11, 1977): 390.]

Case #13

Janet P., a practicing Jehovah's Witness, had refused to sign a consent for blood infusions before the delivery of her daughter. Physicians determined that the newborn infant needed transfusions to prevent retardation and possible death. When the parents refused permission for these transfusions, a hearing was conducted at the Columbia Hospital for Women to decide whether the newborn infant should be given transfusions over the parents' objections. Superior Court Judge Tim Murphy ordered a guardian appointed to sign the necessary releases, and the baby was given the transfusions. During the hearing, Janet P. began hemorrhaging, and attending physicians said she needed an emergency hysterectomy to stem the bleeding. Her husband, also a Jehovah's Witness, approved the hysterectomy but not infusions of blood. This time Judge Murphy declined to order transfusions for the mother, basing his decision on an earlier D.C. Court of Appeals ruling. Janet P. bled to death a few hours later. Her baby survived.

[This case is based on a news report by Martha M. Hamilton in *The Washington Post*, November 14, 1974. It was prepared by James J. McCartney.]

Case #14

Mrs. Jones was brought to the hospital by her husband for emergency care, having lost two thirds of her body's blood supply from a ruptured ulcer. She had no personal physician, and relied solely on the hospital staff. She was a total hospital responsibility. It appeared that the patient, age twenty-five, mother of a seven-month-old child, and her husband were both Jehovah's Witnesses, the teachings of which sect, according to their interpretation, prohibited the injection of blood into the body. When death without blood became imminent, the hospital sought the advice of counsel, who applied to the District Court in the name of the hospital for permission to administer blood. Judge Tamm of the District Court denied the application, and counsel immediately applied to me [Judge J. Skelly Wright], as a member of the Court of Appeals, for an appropriate writ.

I called the hospital by telephone and spoke with Dr. Westura, Chief Medical Resident, who confirmed the representations made by counsel. I thereupon proceeded with counsel to the hospital, where I spoke to Mr. Jones, the husband of the patient. He advised me that, on religious grounds, he would not approve a blood transfusion for his wife. He said, however, that if the court ordered the transfusion, the responsibility was not his. I advised Mr. Jones to obtain counsel immediately. He thereupon went to the telephone and returned in ten or fifteen minutes to advise that he had taken the matter up with his church and that he had decided that he did not want counsel.

I asked permission of Mr. Jones to see his wife. This he readily granted. Prior to going into the patient's room, I again conferred with Dr. Westura and several other doctors assigned to the case. All confirmed that the patient would die without blood and that there was a better than fifty percent chance of saving her life with it. Unanimously they strongly recommended it. I then went inside the patient's room. Her appearance confirmed the urgency which had been represented to me. I tried to communicate with her, advising her again as to what the doctors had said. The only audible reply I could hear was "Against my will." It was obvious that the woman was not in a mental condition to make a decision. I was reluctant to press her because of the seriousness of her condition and because I felt that to suggest repeatedly the imminence of death without blood might place a strain on her religious convictions. I asked her whether she would oppose the blood transfusion if the court allowed it. She indicated, as best I could make out, that it would not then be her responsibility. . . .

I . . . signed the order allowing the hospital to administer such transfusions as the doctors should determine were necessary to save her life. . . .

[This case is taken from *Application of the President and Directors of Georgetown College*, 331 F.2d 1000 (D.C. Cir.), certiorari denied, 377 U.S. 978 (1964).]

Case #15

A doctor aged sixty-eight was admitted to an overseas hospital after a barium meal had shown a large carcinoma of the stomach. He had retired from practice five years earlier, after severe myocardial infarction had left his exercise tolerance considerably reduced. The early symptoms of the carcinoma were mistakenly thought to be due to myocardial ischaemia. By the time the possibility of carcinoma was first considered, the disease was already far-advanced; laparotomy showed extensive metastatic involvement of the abdominal lymph nodes and liver. Palliative gastrectomy was performed with the object of preventing perforation of the primary tumor into the peritoneal cavity, which appeared to the surgeon to be imminent. Histological examination showed the growth to be an anaplastic primary adenocarcinoma. There was clinical and radiological evidence of secondary deposits in the lower thoracic and lumbar vertebrae.

The patient was told of the findings and fully understood their import. In spite of increasingly large doses of pethidine, and of morphine at night, he suffered constantly with severe abdominal pain and pain resulting from compression of spinal nerves by tumor deposits.

On the tenth day after the gastrectomy the patient collapsed with classic manifestations of massive pulmonary embolism. Pulmonary embolectomy was successfully performed in the ward by a registrar. When the patient had recovered sufficiently he expressed his appreciation of the good intentions and skill of his young colleague. At the same time, he asked that if he had a further cardiovascular collapse no steps should be taken to prolong his life, for the pain of his cancer was now more than he would needlessly continue to endure. He himself wrote a note to this effect in his case records, and the staff of the hospital knew his feelings.

His wish notwithstanding, when the patient collapsed again, two weeks after the embolectomy—this time with acute myocardial infarction and cardiac arrest—he was revived by the hospital's emergency resuscitation team. His heart stopped on four further occasions during that night and each time was restarted artificially. The body then recovered sufficiently to linger for three more weeks, but in a decerebrate state, punctuated by episodes of projectile vomiting accompanied by generalized convulsions. Intravenous nourishment was carefully combined with blood transfusion and measures necessary to maintain electrolyte and fluid balance. In addition, antibacterial and antifungal antibiotics were given as prophylaxis against infection, particularly pneumonia complicating the tracheotomy that had been performed to ensure a clear airway. On the last day of his illness, preparations were being made for the work of the failing respiratory centre to be given over to an artificial respirator, but the heart finally stopped before this endeavor could be realized.

[This case is reprinted by permission from W. St. C. Symmers, Sr., "Not Allowed to Die," *British Medical Journal* 1 (1968): 442.]

Case #16

Mr. C. was a 51-year-old white male lawyer who had suffered from emphysema, a severe, chronic, and irreversible lung disease, for over twenty years. Throughout he saw himself engaged in a desperate and unremitting struggle; he was even known to attempt to jog with an oxygen tank strapped to his back. He had applied to Stanford University Medical Center for a still experimental, total heart-lung transplant, only to be turned down because of his age. No patients were accepted who were over 50 years old.

Eventually Mr. C.'s lungs failed him, and he was brought to Public Service University Medical Center—where he characteristically attempted to carry on his legal practice from his hospital bed. Assistants brought him materials, and he dictated briefs in bed. Despite treatment, his condition worsened rapidly and he was soon transferred to the intensive care unit (ICU) of the hospital.

Shortly after the transfer, a meeting was held between Mr. and Mrs. C., Mr. C.'s own doctor, and Dr. K., the attending physician in charge of the ICU. At that meeting the physicians explained to the C.s that Mr. C.'s condition was irreversible and terminal. Soon he would lose the ability to breathe without assistance. Mechanical assistance was available, tubes could be inserted into his lungs (intubation), and a mechanical ventilator could breathe for him. However, both physicians advised against intubation because it was a painful and costly process that would merely prolong the process of dying. Despite this advice, Mr. C. *insisted* that he be intubated, if intubation offered him any chance of surviving or prolonging life. At that point, according to Dr. K. "the three of us looked at each other, and it was very clear the message that he was giving. And the decision was made at that point that we would be very aggressive with him and that we would treat him the way that he wanted."

Dr. K. then wrote a note in Mr. C.'s chart explaining that he and Mr. C. had made an agreement that Mr. C. was to be a "Full code and should be intubated" when this treatment became necessary. ("Full code" means that the entire battery of resuscitative therapy will be employed should Mr. C. experience a cardio or pulmonary arrest. "No-code" means that no cardio-pulmonary resuscitation is to be given.) The agreement was reached on Friday. His respiratory status deteriorated markedly over the weekend, and it became obvious Monday morning that he was soon going to arrest. At this point Mrs. C. began to reconsider her views on intubation. Dr. K. described what then happened: "His wife was concerned about putting him on the ventilator. And I explained to her that we really had no choice. It wouldn't be fair to him to go back on [our agreement]—even though all the evidence suggested that it was hopeless."

Nonetheless Dr. K. put the question to the seven staff members with whom he discussed the case on rounds that morning. They took a straw vote on what to do. Four (including Dr. K.) voted to intubate Mr. C., and four voted against. Three of the no votes were made by anesthesiology fellow A., surgery resident, S., and Nurse N. When interviewed about their votes they gave the following explanations:

Dr. S.: "We really are concerned with two sets of patients here, the wife and two children, and Mr. C. We couldn't do anything more for Mr. C., but we could help the wife and children. So I voted not to intubate him."

Nurse N.: "We took a vote on morning rounds, and we were evenly divided on whether to put him on the ventilator. I voted no. It wasn't justifiable. We couldn't make him any better. . . . What were we going to accomplish by putting him on the ventilator?"

Anesthesiologist A.: "I am not in agreement with the decision to put him on the ventilator. . . . he was only on the ventilator for two days. . . . So I don't feel that anything outrageous was done. . . . It simply was not the right way. . . . It was pointed out by all the people involved . . . that this case is as clear cut as can be imagined in terms of the inability of us to contribute medically in any way to a reversal of the disease or to a meaningful prolongation of his life. . . . This is not even a gray area in this particular area. . . . You have to respect the patient's wishes—and yet—the patient's wishes, in effect, involve him getting ineffective medical therapy. And in this particular case . . . it is medical therapy that is *outrageously* expensive. He was on a Bear ventilator, and Bear ventilators are scarce. We might have needed his bed and the Bear for other patients—what would have happened if he had lingered for weeks. . . . This is a major intervention. I am not willing to do it simply to cater to the patient's wishes."

The decision to intubate held, however, and *Dr. K.* reports: "So we put him on the ventilator Monday. It was a very difficult technically complicated maneuver. . . . Once the decision was made it became a challenging technical and medical exercise . . . to do this to someone with this degree of lung disease. . . . We did. . . . We finally accomplished it—putting him on the ventilator—and it was obvious that the things we said were absolutely right—i.e., that the intubation was useless. . . . Wednesday afternoon it was obvious that we were not going anywhere, and we wrote a note." The patient was then no-coded (i.e., an order was written not to resuscitate the patient, and not to give him any new therapy).

The next day, *Dr. T.* assumed responsibility for the ICU. He understood the case as follows: "A contract was made with Mr. C. that when the time came he would be intubated, even though this was not the advice of his private physician or of the attending physician. When I came on the service he had become so severe that he could not give informed consent to anything." Dr. T. surveyed the situation and discussed it with Mr. C.'s private physician [who] agreed that . . . our therapy was causing more suffering than anything else. . . . His family wanted us to end this aggressive therapy. . . . They wanted us to remove the mechanical ventilator and cut his oxygen down to 21% and let him pass on in peace. And so what I did was . . . give him more and more morphine. . . . They were there when I disconnected the ventilator, and they stayed with him until he expired 15 minutes later." [Note: Withdrawal of therapy is a more radical procedure than no coding; morphine is a respiratory depressant; the combination of morphine and withdrawal almost certainly guaranteed a quick death, especially since Mr. C. was then put on a T-piece, which is a less effective means of respiratory support.]

[This case was recorded as part of the Moral Methodologies of Intensive Care Units project, funded by an EVIST program (NEH-NSF) directed by R. Baker. The medical unit involved was a medical-surgical intensive care unit at a large well-established private university hospital located in a major metropolitan area. The interviews with the medical staff involved were held on the two days following the death of Mr. C. All quotations are taken directly from the tape without modification.]

Case #17

Mrs. R., a forty-five-year-old housewife, has multiple sclerosis and suffers frequent asthma attacks that require treatment in the emergency room of the local community hospital. The physician has written a "no code" order for Mrs. R. This means that no efforts will be made to resuscitate her if she were to suffer a cardiac arrest during an acute asthma attack in the hospital. As far as the nurses know, the physician's decision was made without discussion with the patient or the patient's family. Mrs. R's husband, a middle-management executive in a local firm, divorced her several years earlier, and Mrs. R. has been responsible for two teen age daughters (ages 14 and 16), who live at home.

According to some of the nurses, Mrs. R's medical condition and situation at home are "intolerable." They even feel that they "certainly wouldn't want to live under those conditions." There is, however, no evidence that Mrs. R. feels this way. She usually seems depressed when she comes into the emergency room, but she has not expressed her views to the nurses. The nurses wonder what they should do if Mrs. R. suffers a cardiac arrest when they are on duty.

[This case has been adapted from Anne J. Davis and Mila A. Aroskar, *Ethical Dilemmas and Nursing Practice* (New York: Appleton-Century-Crofts, 1978), pp. 207–08.]

Case #18

By 1976, sixty-seven-year-old Joseph Saikewicz had lived in state institutions for over forty years. His I.Q. was ten, and his mental age was approximately two years and eight months. He could communicate only by gestures and grunts, and he responded only to gestures or physical contacts. He appeared to be unaware of dangers and became disoriented when removed from familiar surroundings.

His health was generally good until April, 1976, when he was diagnosed as having acute myeloblastic monocytic leukemia, which is inevitably fatal. In approximately 30 to 50 percent of cases of this type of leukemia, chemotherapy can bring about temporary remission which usually lasts between two and thirteen months. The results are poorer for patients older than sixty. In addition, chemotherapy often has serious side effects including anemia and infections.

At the petition of the Belchertown State School, where Saikewicz was located, the Probate Court appointed a guardian *ad litem* with authority to make the necessary decisions concerning the patient's care and treatment. The guardian *ad litem* noted that Saikewicz's illness was incurable, that chemotherapy had significant adverse side effects and discomfort, and that Saikewicz could not understand the treatment or the resulting pain. For all these reasons he concluded "that not treating Mr. Saikewicz would be in his best interests." The Supreme Judicial Court of Massachusetts upheld this decision on July 9, 1976 (although its opinion was not issued until November 28, 1977). Mr. Saikewicz died on September 4, 1976.

[This case is drawn from *Superintendent of Belchertown* v. *Saikewicz*, Mass. 370 N.E. 2d 417 (1977).]

Case #19

In November, 1977, 78-year-old Earle Spring suffered a mild scratch on the instep of his foot. A fiercely independent outdoorsman, he left the cut unattended until his foot finally became gangrenous. Hospitalization was followed by pneumonia and then a diagnosis of kidney failure. After undergoing three five-hour dialysis sessions a week, Spring soon improved enough to return home. Meanwhile his mental deterioration, which had been diagnosed before his injury as "chronic organic brain syndrome," became markedly pronounced.

After more than a year of treatment, the nephrologist informed Spring's son, Robert, that his father was not benefiting from dialysis. He suggested it may have been a mistake to have initiated it on a man his age, and that it might be best if the treatments were ended. The son and the wife agreed with the physician and requested that the treatments be stopped. However, because of the Massachusetts Supreme Judicial Court's 1977 *Saikewicz* ruling [Case #18 in this Appendix], decisions of such significance in that state have to be made by courts rather than by families and physicians.

On January 25, 1979, Robert Spring, who had been appointed temporary guardian, petitioned the Franklin County Probate Court for an order to terminate the hemodialysis treatments. They began a full adversary hearing in which the guardian *ad litem*, an attorney appointed by the court to represent the best interests of the patient, had the responsibility for presenting "all reasonable arguments in favor of administering treatment to prolong the life of the individual involved."

Mark I. Berson, Spring's guardian *ad litem*, insisted (contrary to *Saikewicz*) that the court could not render a "substituted judgment" (a statement of what Spring himself would have wanted) without some evidence from Spring's lucid moments on that subject. On May 15, 1979, Judge Keedy entered a judgment permitting the temporary guardian, Robert Spring, "to refrain from authorizing further life-prolonging medical treatment" for his father. Attorney Berson was not satisfied there was sufficient evidence that Spring would have wanted to terminate the treatments, and he appealed. Judge Keedy vacated his original order and on July 2 entered a new one to the effect that Spring's wife and son, together with the attending physician, were to make the decision. Again Berson appealed.

The Court of Appeals upheld the probate court's action. It rejected Berson's's position on the need for an express statement of intent to withhold treatment. In its words, "Such a contention would largely stifle the very rights of privacy and personal dignity which the *Saikewicz* case sought to secure for incompetent persons." Berson appealed.

On January 10, the Supreme Judicial Court (SJC) heard the case. It concluded that the trial judge's finding that Earle Spring "would, if competent, choose not to receive the life prolonging treatment" was correct. But unlike the trial judge and the Court of Appeals, the SJC found that the facts "bring the case within the rule of *Saikewicz*." It therefore held "it was an error to delegate the decision to the attending physician and the ward's wife and son." Once again, Spring's guardian was directed by the probate court to "refrain from authorizing any further life prolonging treatment" for his father.

Meanwhile, it was becoming clear that the staff of the Holyoke Geriatric Center were, in their own words, "appalled over the decision to stop the dialysis treatment." Two nurses on the 3 to 11 shift asked Spring if he wanted to die. Reportedly, he replied, "No." Although a psychiatrist had previously evaluated Spring as "incompetent," the nurses taking his statement as proof of Spring's desires brought their story to a local newspaper, which used it as headline news. Berson responded immediately. On the basis of an affidavit filed by a right-to-life group, he petitioned Judge Keedy to reinstate the dialysis treatments until new evidence of Spring's competence could be gathered. The right-to-life activists hired a lawyer to petition the probate court to admit them as parties to the case. In the sixth judicial determination on Spring's case, Judge Keedy denied the petition to reinstate dialysis treatment. Berson appealed once more.

This appeal was granted by the SJC, which then appointed five psychiatrists and geriatric specialists to determine Spring's mental status. During that time Spring had been admitted to the hospital suffering from an infection and pneumonia. He responded to medical treatment and returned to the nursing home on March 25, but in an extremely weakened condition. The following Sunday, the day before the competency hearing was scheduled, Earle Spring died. The next day the five court-appointed physicians filed their report: Spring "was suffering from such profound mental impairment that he had no idea where he was or what was going on. The dementia was not related to the kidney failure, was untreatable, and irreversible." Had he not died the day before, the responsibility for deciding to stop the dialysis treatments would have rested where it had fourteen months previously— with the court.

[This case was prepared by John J. Paris, S. J. It derives from his "Death, Dying, and the Courts: The Travesty and Tragedy of the Earle Spring Case," *Linacre Quarterly* 49 (February, 1982): 26–41.]

Case #20

Phillip Becker is a Down's syndrome child born with a ventricular septal defect (a hole between the two pumping chambers of the heart, which results in increased pressure in the pulmonary artery and a diminished life expectancy). Phillip has never lived with his parents and has been institutionalized since birth. He is described as "near the top level" of intelligence for a

Down's child. He has good manual and motor skills, can dress himself and write his name, is toilet trained, and takes part in school and Boy Scout activities. His school psychologist believes that Phillip could be placed in the county's sheltered workshop following his schooling.

In 1978, when Phillip was 11 years old, his parents were charged with not providing him with the "necessities of life" because they had refused permission for cardiac surgery to correct his septal defect. When the case first came to court, the Beckers argued that their primary reason for refusing consent was that they do not want Phillip to outlive them. They stated that geriatric care in this country is seriously inadequate and that Phillip's "quality of life would be poor" after their deaths. Mere life, they claimed, "is not what it's all about." Phillip's cardiologist testified that life expectancy for someone with Phillip's condition, left uncorrected, is thirty years, that perhaps one-fourth of such persons would die suddenly and that most others would slowly deteriorate, during which time they would suffer from fainting spells and cyanosis because of a lack of oxygenated blood. He also pointed out that this condition makes its victims a constant worry for caretakers. He put the risk of death from surgery itself at 3 to 5 percent (another cardiologist put the surgical risk for a Down's child at 5 to 10 percent), and noted a less than 1 percent chance that Phillip might require a cardiac pacemaker after surgery.

In his opinion on the case Judge Eugene M. Premo found the proposed surgery "elective" and not "a life-saving emergency." He decided not to order it against the parents' wishes. The case was appealed by the California Attorney General's office. The appeals court found that the surgery would be more risky than average because of Phillip's pulmonary vascular changes and because he was a Down's syndrome child. Thus, it held, the lower court's opinion was justified.

During his years of institutionalization Phillip had become the special friend of Herbert and Patsy Heath. The Heaths visited him often and took him into their home for weekends. In 1981 the Heaths sought legal guardianship of Phillip, claiming that they had become his psychological parents (he had come to know them as "Dad" and "Mom") and that it would be in Phillip's best interests to be placed in their care. They promised to reconsider the surgery decision. After hearing the guardianship case, Judge William J. Fernandez found that Phillip had never received constancy of affection, nurturing, or the opportunity to develop basic confidence and trust from his natural parents. (The Beckers claimed to have visited Phillip 5 or 6 times a year, but institutional officials said they came only twice a year.) By contrast, the Heaths had maintained a constant and growing relationship with him since he was 5 years old. While the Beckers viewed Phillip as permanently retarded and with no "hope of living in society," the Heaths perceived him as communicative, educable, and possessed of many basic skills. On this basis, Judge Fernandez concluded that "psychological parenting between the Heaths and Phillip exists" and awarded guardianship to the Heaths. His stated purpose in this decision was to provide Phillip "a chance to secure a life worth living." Judge Fernandez's ruling allowed for medical tests to determine whether heart surgery for Phillip is now desirable; some physicians had testified during the trial that he may be too old for the surgery and that its risks may now outweigh its benefits. The California Court of Appeal upheld Judge Fernandez's ruling.

[This case was prepared by James B. Tubbs from two articles by George J. Annas: "Denying the Rights of the Retarded: The Phillip Becker Case," *Hastings Center Report* 9 (December 1979): 18–20; and "'A Wonderful Case and an Irrational Tragedy': The Phillip Becker Case Continues," *Hastings Center Report* 12 (February 1982): 25–6. See also: "Parents Bar Surgery and Lose Son's Custody," *The New York Times*, August 9, 1981; "'Psychological' Parents Win," *The Washington Post*, October 22, 1981; and "A New 'Right-to-Life' Battleground Opens Over Mentally Retarded Child," *The Washington Post*.]

Case #21

Baby girl Betsy Novick had immediately apparent physical malformations when she was born. A diagnosis of Seckel or "bird-headed" dwarfism was made. She had, in addition to low birth weight and length, large eyes, a large, beaklike nose, narrow face, receding lower jaw, strabismus, and a club foot. Seckel dwarfism, an autosomal recessive genetic disease, had affected Mr. Novick's brother as well. Life expectancy is good, but a much simplified gross cerebral structure is related to mental retardation. It was apparent that institutionalization would be necessary. The Novicks were of modest means and the vivid memory of the devastating impact of Mr. Novick's brother immediately convinced him that the child could not be cared for at home.

The Novicks lived in the state that has the lowest per capita income spent on institutions for the retarded. Although court action promised some marginal improvements in the institutions, they promised to be bleak, under-staffed, custodial institutions for the foreseeable future. The fact that Betsy had rather peculiarly repulsive features led the parents to fear that she would receive particularly poor care, yet they saw no alternative.

In the next two months Betsy developed a persistent pyloric stenosis, a narrowing of the pylorus between the stomach and intestines causing projectile vomiting that did not respond to phenobarbital, atropine, or special diet. If not surgically treated, death by starvation would result. The parents, at first stunned by the additional severe medical problem, considered the alternatives. They envisioned the virtually certain, severe burden and suffering to be placed on the child in any institutions conceivably available in the next decade or two. They decided that it was a burden the child should not bear, even though in principle they knew society should be providing better support for them. They decided against the surgery. The child died after two weeks of deterioration.

[This case was prepared by Robert M. Veatch and is used by permission.]

Case #22

On May 18, 1982, the U.S. Department of Health and Human Services issued a letter to 6,800 hospitals receiving federal funding, reminding the recipients that under Section 504 of the Rehabilitation Act of 1973, "it is unlawful . . . to withhold from a handicapped infant nutritional sustenance or medical or surgical treatment required to correct a life-threatening condition if: (1) the withholding is based upon the fact that the infant is handicapped; and (2) the handicap does not render treatment or nutritional sustenance medically contraindicated." H. H. S. Secretary Richard Schweiker noted further that, "In providing this notice . . . we are reaffirming the strong commitment of the American people and their laws to the protection of human life."

The occasion for this reminder was the death, one month earlier, of a Bloomington, Indiana infant identified to the public only as "Infant Doe." Baby boy Doe was born with Down's syndrome (trisomy 21) and with a tracheoesophogeal fistula (an opening between the breathing and swallowing tubes that prevents passage of food to the stomach). The baby's parents were informed that surgery to correct his fistula would have "an even chance of success." Left untreated, the fistula would soon lead to the baby's death from starvation or pneumonia (induced by stomach secretions reaching the lungs). The parents, who also have two healthy children, chose to withhold food and treatment and "let nature take its course."

Court action to remove the infant from his parents' custody (and permit the surgery) was sought by the county prosecutor. Such action was denied by the court, and the Indiana Supreme Court declined to review the lower court's ruling. Infant Doe died, at six days of age, as Indiana authorities were seeking intervention from the U.S. Supreme Court. The parents' lawyer commented that the mother was with her child to the end—"It wasn't a case of abandonment. It was a case of love."

[This case was adapted by James Tubbs from Fred Barbash and Cristine Russell, "The Demise of 'Infant Doe': Permitted Death Gives Life to an Old Debate," *The Washington Post*, April 17, 1982, and from the *HHS News*, May 18, 1982.]

Case #23

The patient, a 40-year-old nullipara with an 18-month history of infertility, underwent genetic amniocentesis at 17 weeks' gestation for the indication of advanced maternal age. Her medical history was unremarkable except for hypothyroidism, for which she had received dessicated thyroid extract, 3 g daily, since 1960. An ultrasound scan before the procedure revealed a twin pregnancy with biparietal diameters of both fetuses compatible with 17.5 weeks' gestation, two clearly defined amniotic sacs, and one placenta on the posterior uterine wall. Amniotic fluid from each sac obtained separately for chromosomal studies revealed two male fetuses. Twin A had a normal male karyotype (46, XY), but chromosomal analysis of Twin B indicated trisomy 21 (47, XY + 21).

Presented with the diagnosis of carrying one normal and one affected fetus, the parents were confronted with the difficult task of making one of two decisions: to induce abortion and lose both fetuses, or to continue the pregnancy. The mother desperately wanted to have the normal child but could not face the burden of caring for an abnormal child for the rest of her life. Having been made aware of the case report from Sweden in which selective termination of an abnormal twin had been successfully performed even though the unaffected twin was delivered prematurely, she asked if a similar procedure could be offered to her. If it had been refused, she would have chosen to abort both fetuses. At that point, she was referred to us.

Extensive medical and legal counseling and an explanation of the many risks were provided. These risks included abortion of both fetuses, premature delivery of the surviving fetus, performing the procedure on the wrong twin since markers for sac A or B were lacking, and the development of disseminated intravascular coagulation in the mother as a result of fetal death in utero. After careful consideration, the patient decided to undertake the procedure anyway. In view of the fact that the procedure had never been performed in this country, we decided, out of an abundance of caution, to obtain confirmation from a court of law of the parents' right to consent on behalf of the normal fetus.

[This case is reprinted with permission from *New England Journal of Medicine* 304 (June 18, 1981): 1525, where it appeared in Thomas D. Kerenyi and Usha Chitkara, "Selective Birth in Twin Pregnancy with Discordancy for Down's Syndrome."]

Case #24

A 33-year-old unmarried white woman, gravida 2, para 1, was admitted to the hospital in labor at 0730. The patient had received no prenatal care, and although the expected date of confinement was uncertain she was thought to be near term. Membranes had ruptured spontaneously 2 hours before admission. Early in the pregnancy the patient had been hospitalized twice for gallbladder disease, at which time cholecystectomy and subsequent reexploration for removal of a common duct stone were performed. While the patient recovered uneventfully from both of these procedures, it was not recognized that she was pregnant. Significant past history included the delivery of twins 3 years before admission and a lifelong problem of morbid obesity (estimated weight 157.5 kg).

The patient was noted to be angry and uncooperative. Vital signs included blood pressure, 140/100 mmHg; pulse, 100 beats/min; and temperature, 36.5C. With the exception of obesity, the general physical findings were essentially normal. Estimated fetal weight was 3000 g, regular contractions were occurring every 5 to 7 minutes, and fetal heart tones were 140 beats/min. The cervix was 2 cm dilated and not well effaced, and amniotic fluid was clear, but the exact presentation and position of the fetus were difficult to ascertain because of the high and unidentifiable presenting part.

. . . Ninety minutes after admission the amniotic fluid was noted to be meconium stained. Later the fetal heart rate (FHR) tracing demonstrated late decelerations, which were confirmed by internal FHR monitoring showing a loss of baseline variability as well. Because of these findings suggesting fetal hypoxia, the high station of the fetal presenting part, and the desultory progress of labor, the patient was advised of the dangers to the infant, and delivery by cesarean section was recommended. Because of her fear of surgery, the patient refused; furthermore, she requested permission to leave the hospital against medical advice. The patient's mother and sister, with whom she lived, and the father of the baby were fully informed of the circumstances. All involved attempted to persuade the patient to accept the advice of the physicians, but to no avail. The obstetric psychiatric consultant interviewed the patient and was convinced that she was neither delusional nor mentally incompetent. The patient was capable of understanding the circumstances and making a rational decision.

At this point the hospital administration was advised of the situation, and the hospital attorney interviewed the patient. Convinced of the intransigence of the patient's position and advised by the physicans that there was evidence of persistent, even worsening, fetal distress, the legal staff requested intervention by the juvenile court. Attorneys were appointed by the court to represent the patient and the unborn infant, and a hearing was convened in the patient's room with the judge presiding. Testimony from the professional staff and from the patient, including cross-examination by the attorneys for the mother and the fetus, was heard, after which the court found that the unborn baby of the patient was a dependent and neglected child within the meaning of the Colorado Children's Code. It was then ordered that a cesarean section be performed to safeguard the life of the unborn child.

Following the court's decision, the patient, although still reluctant, became more cooperative and agreed to the induction of general anesthesia. At 1830 hours, 11 hours after admission, a 3500-g female infant was delivered by low transverse cesarean section. . . .[1]

The infant responded promptly to resuscitation, which included direct endotracheal suctioning to remove meconium. Except for transient respiratory distress, attributed to intrapartum asphyxia, the infant had an uneventful neonatal course and at 8 months of age was growing and developing normally. The patient's postoperative recovery was uncomplicated except for delayed healing of the superficial portion of the abdominal incision.

Following the delivery, the physicians, nurses, social workers, and consultants from the Department of Psychiatry met on a regular basis to discuss concerns about this patient's relationship with her newborn infant. Initially the patient demonstrated affectionate and caring behavior toward the infant. Several months later, however, the court assigned all 3 of her children to foster care when case workers found significant evidence of neglect of the infant and siblings. The court's decision to remove the children from the custody of the mother was independent of events that occurred in the second pregnancy.

[This case is reprinted by permission from Watson Bowes, Jr. and Brad Selgestad, "Fetal Versus Maternal Rights: Medical and Legal Perspectives," *Obstetrics and Gynecology* 58 (August 1981): 209–211.]

[1]Apgar scores were 2 and 8 at 1 and 5 minutes, respectively; umbilical artery blood gases (cord specimen) were pH, 7.20; PCO_2, 59 mmHg; PO_2, 4 mmHg; and base excess, —7.

Case #25

A forty-year-old widow with chronic glomerulonephritis has been on maintenance hemodialysis for ten years. Over the past two years she has been progressively deteriorating from multiple complications which have included severe renal osteodystrophy, inability to obtain adequate blood access, and malnutrition from intermittent depression. Peritoneal dialysis cannot be accomplished because of multiple abdominal surgical procedures with adhesions. Her physician has recommended transplantation because he feels she will not survive over four to six months on dialysis.

The patient has four children (ages eleven to fourteen years) and wants a transplant to allow her to live and provide for the future well-being of her children.

The patient's forty-four-year-old brother is a farmer with eight children. He refused to donate or be tissue typed. The patient has a forty-two-year-old sister who was willing to donate but was not tissue typed because she has been an insulin-requiring diabetic for ten years.

The patient also has a thirty-five-year-old mentally retarded brother who has been institutionalized since age eight. This brother is an A match with four antigens being identified. He is so severely retarded that he cannot comprehend or understand any of the risks of nephrectomy. He is able to take care of his own personal needs and ambulate with guidance. He neither recognizes his own family members nor interacts with medical staff. The patient would regularly drive 300 miles to see her brother four times per year until twelve years ago, when her own personal and family needs reduced the frequency to one to two times per year. She has not seen her brother for three years, because of her own medical illnesses. At the present time she feels she has a duty to her brother but there is no particular closeness.

Her fourteen-year-old daughter would like to donate a kidney, even though she is a 2-antigen mismatch. The daughter has demonstrated a perceptive, thorough, and reasonably unemotional grasp of her mother's situation and needs, and of the seriousness of her own potential donation. ABO blood types for the retarded brother and the daughter are compatible.

The patient's older brother and sister feel the donor should be the younger, mentally retarded brother. The diabetic sister is the legal guardian of the retarded brother. Both parents are dead. She has been on the cadaveric transplant waiting list for two years.

The following statements are reasonable projections based on known data:

	2-yr. kidney survival	2-yr. patient survival
Retarded brother to patient	70%	85%
Minor child to patient	60%	75%
Cadaveric to patient	40%	65%

[This case was written from a case history at St. Francis Hospital, Honolulu, by Dr. Arnold W. Siemsen, Institute of Renal Diseases, St. Francis Hospital.]

Case #26

In June of 1978, Robert McFall, thirty-nine years old and a Pittsburgh asbestos worker, entered Mercy Hospital with an uncontrollable nosebleed. Physicians diagnosed his condition as aplastic anemia, a rare and usually fatal disease in which the bone marrow fails to produce enough red and white blood cells and platelets. McFall's physician recommended a bone-marrow transplant on the ground that it would increase his patient's chance of surviving for one year from 25 percent to 40 to 60 percent. The search for a compatible transplant donor began with McFall's six brothers and sisters. After they were located in various parts of the country, none turned out to be compatible.

The search continued and McFall's first cousin, David Shimp, aged forty-three, agreed to undergo some preliminary tests. He was a perfect match for tissue compatibility; but then suddenly he refused to be tested for genetic compatibility. He had decided that he would not donate bone marrow to his cousin, even if he was a perfect match. Apparently, some family discussions and disagreements had influenced Shimp's decision. He told his cousin that his wife was angry because he had undergone the first tests without telling her. Shimp's mother also appeared to be bitter about a decades-old disagreement in the family, and she too asked him to stop the testing.

Friends and other of McFall's relatives believed that disagreements of the past should not affect the present, and they tried to persuade Shimp to change his mind. When McFall called his cousin and told him "You're killing me," Shimp responded that his wife had to come first. Even Shimp's four children tried to persuade him that he would be responsible for his cousin's early death, and they volunteered to be tested themselves; but Shimp would not be moved.

McFall then filed suit to compel his cousin to undergo the bone-marrow transplant. McFall's attorney argued in court that the procedure is essentially harmless to the donor and that the marrow would be replenished, just as blood is replenished after donation. He also cited English common law, dating back to the thirteenth century, which upheld society's right to force an individual "to help secure the well-being of other members of society." Shimp's attorney argued that his client's right to refuse could not be invaded, and that "no one could be forced to submit to an operation." Shimp told reporters that he refused to be a donor because he was afraid of becoming paralyzed during the procedure and feared that his marrow might fail to regenerate.

Judge John Flaherty denied McFall's request to force Shimp to undergo the transplant. The judge based his decision on United States common law precedents, which do not recognize a legal duty to take action to save another person's life. "This would defeat the sanctity of the individual," he argued. "Our society is based on the right and sanctity of the individual. It would require forcible submission to the medical procedure. Forcible extraction of bodily tissues causes revulsion to the judicial mind. The rights of the individual must be upheld, even though it appears to be a harsh decision." The judge also declared irrelevant the argument by McFall's attorney that in English law, court-ordered transplants are permitted. Although he thus held that Shimp had no legal obligation to donate his marrow, Judge Flaherty nevertheless called Shimp's refusal "morally indefensible."

After the ruling, McFall told the press, "I feel sorry for my cousin because he and I are friends and he was under a lot of pressure." Shimp made no comment, but his mother said, "He's not a coward the way they are trying to make him out to be. When you get on the table there is no guaranteeing how much bone marrow they will take. It could be my son's death sentence. The doctors don't care about the donors; they care about patients."

On August 10, 1978, Robert McFall died of a cranial hemorrhage. His last request was that his family forgive his cousin, whose actions he found understandable even if not justifiable. A hospital spokesperson said that cranial hemorrhage is a common complication for people with aplastic anemia and that it might have occurred even with the bone-marrow transplant. The day after his cousin died, Shimp said, "I could throw up right now. I feel terrible about Robert dying, but he asked me for something I couldn't give. That's all I can say now. I feel sick."

[Sources for this case include Barbara J. Culliton, "Court Upholds Refusal to Be Medical Good Samaritan," *Science* 201 (Aug. 18, 1978): 596–597; "Bone Marrow Transplant Plea Rejected," *American Medical News* 21: 31 (Aug. 11, 1978): 13;

"Anemia Victim Dies, Asks Forgiveness for Cousin," *International Herald Tribune* (Aug. 12–13, 1978); "Judge Upholds Transplant Denial," *The New York Times* (July 27, 1978), p. A10; Dennis A. Williams and Lawrence Walsh, "The Law: Bad Samaritan," *Newsweek* 92: 6 (Aug. 7, 1978): 35; Alan Meisel and Loren H. Roth, "Must a Man Be His Cousin's Keeper?" *Hastings Center Report* 8 (October 1978): 5–6. The case is *McFall* v. *Shimp*, NO. 78-17711 In Equity (C.P. Allegheny County, Penn., July 26, 1978).]

Case #27

The Willowbrook State School is an institution for mentally retarded children on Staten Island, New York. The population of Willowbrook increased from 200 in 1949 to over 6,000 in 1963. Hepatitis was first noticed among residents of Willowbrook in 1949, and in 1954 Dr. Saul Krugman and his associates, Dr. Joan Giles, Dr. Jack Hammond et al., began to study the disease there. Of the 5,200 residents at Willowbrook during one part of their study, 3,800 were severely retarded with I.Q.s of less than 20. In addition, at least 3,000 of the children were not toilet-trained. Since infectious hepatitis is transmitted via the intestinal-oral route, and since susceptible children were constantly being admitted to the institution, there was a persistent and continuing endemic situation of contagious hepatitis. In fact, virtually all susceptible children became infected within the first six to twelve months of residence at the institution. This strain of hepatitis, however, was especially mild in the three to ten age range.

In an attempt to develop an effective prophylactic agent, Krugman and his associates did a number of different studies, some of which involved artificially exposing children to the Willowbrook strain of hepatitis infection. Of the 10,000 admissions to Willowbrook since 1956, approximately 750–800 children were admitted to Krugman's special hepatitis unit. These study groups included only children whose parents gave written consent. Originally, information was conveyed to individual parents by letter or personal interview. In later studies the group technique, i.e., discussing the project in detail with a group of prospective consenting parents, was employed. Children who were wards of the state or children without parents were never included in the studies.

Studies were carried out in a special unit with optimum isolation facilities to protect the children from other infectious diseases. Even when over-crowding forced the institution to stop further admissions for awhile in 1964, room was available in this special unit for children whose parents "volun-teered" them for this project. One direct benefit of the study to the children themselves was that, in addition to being protected from other infectious diseases, they also frequently developed immunity from hepatitis itself after contraction of the mild form administered by Krugman. These studies were reviewed and sanctioned by various local, state, and federal agencies.

[This case was prepared by James J. McCartney.]

Case #28

On August 11, 1977, Whitley, et al. reported in *The New England Journal of Medicine* that a new drug, adenine arabinoside (ara-A), had been tested and found to be highly useful in the treatment and cure of biopsy-proved herpes simplex encephalitis, a disease that often leads to severe brain and nerve damage or death. Prior to ara-A, standard treatment consisted mainly of palliative care and was not considered effective. Some critics of the research insisted that it is not necessary to have a randomized clinical trial of therapy for a disease that has such high rates of mortality and severe damage and that is currently treated by ineffective therapy. In such cases, they argue, it is sufficient to use historical controls. Furthermore, they insist, in previous tests ara-A had been found to be effective in treating some herpes infections and to have no demonstrable hepatic, renal or hematologic toxicity. They claim that scientific knowledge did not require a controlled trial, which deprived some patients of a promising drug. Furthermore, they note, brain biopsy may be risky for such seriously ill patients and perhaps put the control group at greater risk than standard treatment would have.

Defenders of the research respond that prior to this research, scientists did not know the mortality and long-term morbidity rates of herpes simplex encephalitis because it is difficult to diagnose with certainty apart from a brain biopsy, and that scientists did not know whether ara-A would have serious toxic effects when administered in large doses along with large volumes of intravenous fluid to patients suffering from this disease.

The collaborative study, supported by the National Institute of Allergy and Infectious Disease, was a controlled, double-blind trial. Of the twenty-eight patients involved, ten received the placebo, i.e., standard treatment, while the others received the experimental drug.

Recipients of ara-A

Number of recipients	18
Deaths	5
Severe damage	6
Reasonably normal recovery	7

Recipients of the placebo

Number of recipients	10
Deaths	7
Severe damage	1
Reasonably normal recovery	2

The trial was stopped when these statistics emerged because of the apparently greater chance of surviving the disease with ara-A. All patients were then treated with ara-A. Several scientists, however, contend that the research was stopped too soon because the data are not statistically significant. They note that the number of recipients of both treatments is very small and that the figures about reasonably normal recovery may be misleading: 38.8% for recipients of ara-A and 20% for recipients of the placebo. If the next recipient of the placebo had recovered to a reasonably normal level, the figures would have then been much closer. As I. J. Good, a statistician, notes, "if having severe sequelae is regarded as just as bad as being dead, the ara-A treatment is barely significantly better than the placebo." Thus, some critics claim, the research did not definitely establish the superiority of ara-A in the treatment of herpes simplex encephalitis.

[This case was prepared on the basis of information in the following sources: Richard J. Whitley, et al, "Adenine Arabinoside Therapy of Biopsy-proved Herpes Simplex Encephalitis," *New England Journal of Medicine* 297 (August 11, 1977): 289–294; Correspondence, *New England Journal of Medicine* 297 (December 8, 1977): 1288–90; James J. McCartney, "Encephalitis and Ara-A: An Ethical Case Study," *Hastings Center Report* 8 (December 1978): 5–7; Correspondence, *Hastings Center Report* 9 (August 1979): 4, 44–47; and I. J. Good, "Adenine Arabinoside Therapy," *Journal of Statistical Computation and Simulation* 6 (1978): 314–15.]

Case #29

Recently the Center for Disease Control (CDC) had to decide what to do in followup of individuals who participated in a measles vaccine field trial coordinated by CDC in the early 1960s.

The study involved 5,210 schoolchildren in five different areas (Buffalo, New York: Cincinnati, Ohio; Seattle, Washington; Rochester, New York; and DeKalb County, Georgia). Approximately one-half of these received a placebo, one-quarter received three doses of killed measles virus vaccine (KMV), at monthly intervals, and one-quarter received two doses of KMV followed by a dose of live measles virus vaccine 1 month later. Approximately one-third of those in the study were immune to measles at the time of the study; the remainder were susceptible. The study indicated that protection from the three doses of KMV was temporary. At the end of the trial, those who had received placebos were offered the more effective course of KMV followed by live virus vaccine.

Several investigators have subsequently reported that individuals who received KMV (either by itself or in a series followed by live virus vaccine within 3 months of the completion of the series) could develop an unusual syndrome when subsequently exposed to wild measles virus. This syndrome has come to be called "atypical measles syndrome" (AMS), and it has been seen almost exclusively in those who received KMV. Although morbidity can be severe, often including pneumonia, only one instance has been reported of death possibly due to AMS. The condition is generally viewed as being noninfectious, with only one instance reported of possible transmission arising from a case of AMS. For several years, the Public Health Service Immunization Practices Advisory Committee (and the American Academy of Pediatrics Committee on Infectious Diseases) has recommended that those who previously received KMV be revaccinated with live measles virus vaccine. It is difficult to determine the degree of compliance with these recommendations.

No special effort has been taken to follow up participants in the CDC field trials to offer revaccination with live vaccine. The primary issue, therefore, is whether or not CDC should undertake special efforts to identify participants in the 1961–62 KMV field trials to recommend revaccination with live measles virus vaccine. If the answer to his question is yes, a secondary issue relates to the types of steps that should be undertaken.

In considering the most appropriate course of action with study participants, several other factors should be mentioned.

1. Revaccination might not prevent the occurrence of AMS.
2. There may be an increased reaction rate following administration of live measles virus vaccine to previous recipients of KMV.
3. Likelihood of exposure to natural measles in participants.
4. Difficulties in identifying and locating participants in the field trial.
5. Calculations indicate that, of the original 5,210 study participants, only 189 are still susceptible to measles, and 23 of them probably might be expected to develop AMS at some time in the future.
6. Prevention of all these anticipated cases would require identification and followup of each of the field trial participants. Based on experience with other long-term followup studies carried out by CDC, the best estimate is that no more than 20 percent could be reached through telephone calls, once records were found. With individual field followup, a higher proportion could be reached (probably over 50 percent) with an average expenditure of effort of one person-day per participant contacted. Using GS-11 or 12 Public Health Advisors, this would mean an expenditure of approximately $92.50 per participant contact, which would translate to a cost of approximately $20,000 per case of AMS prevented.

[This case was prepared from materials submitted by CDC to a panel of consultants regarding possible CDC followup of participants in the Killed Measles Vaccine Field Trial.]

Case #30

State Bill 529 calls for the establishment of community-based homes for the care and education of the mentally retarded. The bill provides one home for every fifteen persons presently institutionalized in four state institutions for the mentally retarded at a cost of $55.8 million. The estimated costs for the new care for the present population of 7,600 will be $70 million a year.

The bill was introduced by Representative John Sheehan who spoke in favor of it. He painted a dismal picture of antiquated institutions bereft of basic human necessities or amenities. Thousands of human beings, many unclothed, spend their lives huddled in dark, drab rooms, where they are supervised by an overworked staff, many of whom have no professional training. Sheehan, who has the support of the parents' organization, the State Department of Mental Health, the local ACLU, and the religious leadership, concluded his case by pleading, "Justice requires that we extend this token contribution to these citizens, burdened by physical and psychological suffering, and by the degradation of our society's past inhumanity to its fellow humans."

Representative James Hudson and Dr. Robert Simmons, while emphasizing their concern for care of the retarded, spoke in opposition to the bill. Representative Hudson, noting that he was the elected representative of all the citizens in his district, argued that he had an obligation to examine the alternative uses for the $14 million in additional funds called for by the bill. But first, he pointed out that the new total sum of $70 million equalled 1.5 percent of the state's budget, a budget raised by all its citizens, while the institutionalized population equalled only one-tenth of one percent of the state's population. The proposed increase of $14 million could buy hot lunches for all the state's school children; it could also provide job training for productive members of society. Hudson argued that the fairest thing to do would be to spread the money evenly among those who would be productive. "Our task as legislators," he concluded, "must be to serve the greatest good of the greatest number."

Dr. Simmons, as a physician, argued that the money could be used more efficiently in providing health care for three groups: normal or more nearly normal children (thousands of whom could be reached for every mentally retarded child), those potentially engaged in productive labor, and pregnant women. He showed that much mental retardation can be eliminated, through prenatal diagnosis which he estimated to cost $200 per case for Down's syndrome compared to $60,000 for each institutionalized child. Even allowing that some of the institutionalized retarded might be gainfully employed if they were in high-quality, community-based homes, the savings from spending the funds on detection rather than on more expensive forms of institutionalized care are enormous.

The legislative committee must now make its decision on the bill.

[This case, written by Robert M. Veatch, appeared as Case #529 in "Who Has First Claim on Health Care Resources?" *Hastings Center Report* (August 1975): 13 and is used by permission.]

Case #31

Thomas Merriam was Director of Budget Planning at the National Institutes of Health and chief advisor to the Assistant Secretary on the congressional message on the 1976 fiscal year NIH budget. He was under a great deal of pressure from Dr. Alan Sanders, Director of the National Institute of Arthritis, Metabolism, and Digestive Diseases, to increase the budget for research on arthritis.

Dr. Sanders argued that in 1974 3,377,000 persons in the United States suffered from arthritis severe enough that their activity was limited. There were almost 4 million hospital days attributable to arthritis and 57 million days of bed disability. There was anger in Dr. Sanders' voice during the meeting Merriam had with the Institute director. It was as if he could not get anyone to take arthritis seriously. He claimed that because there were virtually no deaths attributable to arthritis, the government policy analysts were grossly underemphasizing the disease that produced the second largest number of persons with limitation of activity in the United States. The suffering was enormous, yet the planners were using formulas that calculated number of days of life likely to be added for research dollar invested. This meant that arthritis would receive virtually no funding if Merriam and his associates relied exclusively on the formula.

Sanders claimed that the National Cancer Institute and the Heart and Lung Institute were getting more money than they could use because of the excessive emphasis on death prevention rather than suffering prevention. Sanders conceded that cancer and heart disease also produce some disability. The cancer institute was less the target of his attack since the cancer budget was not part of the NIH planning, it being separated out by the Nixon administration as part of the war on cancer. He emphasized the inequity between the heart institute and the funds for arthritis. The number of persons with limitation of activity is about the same in the two cases (3.9 million for heart disease compared with 3.4 million for arthritis). Yet the heart institute budget was $290,511,000, while the arthritis portion of Sanders' institute's budget was only $14,076,000. Expressed in days of disability, there were 93 million days for heart disease and 57 million for arthritis. How, Sanders asked, can that difference justify the much larger difference in the budgets?

Merriam was frustrated after his conversation with Sanders. He wanted an objective, statistically certain way of allocating the research funds between a condition like heart disease that produces some disability, but is the primary cause of death, and a condition like arthritis that is also a serious debilitator, but causes no death. He considered his options:

1. Use cost/benefit ratios to maximize the number of days of life added per dollar invested.
2. Use cost/benefit analysis to calculate the dollars lost to the economy from

work lost from the two conditions, and use that ratio to propose funds for the two programs.

3. Use cost/benefit analysis to calculate both costs of the diseases and costs of the potential research, and use dollars most efficiently.

4. Survey people asking them how they would like their money to be spent, and allocate the funds by calculating the average apportionment.

5. Allocate funds in proportion to the number of people suffering from the two conditions regardless of deaths, costs of treatment, costs of research, or any other variables.

6. Ask experts working on research in the two areas what the likelihood of a breakthrough might be, and use those estimates as a basis for allocating funds.

7. Turn the matter over to the politicians to decide what the priorities ought to be.

Merriam needed a principle for dealing with Dr. Sanders's complaint. What should he do?

[This case is based on actual data, but does not reflect actions or positions taken by actual employees of the National Institutes of Health during the period described in this case. It is Case 570: *Arthritis and Heart Disease: Where Should Research Funds Go?* prepared by Robert M. Veatch and is used by permission.]

Case #32

The totally implantable artificial heart is a blood pump constructed of synthetic materials, driven by a motor and a power source, all of which are totally and permanently implanted within the body in place of the natural heart. Such a device is now being developed at the National Heart and Lung Institute, and, through NIH contracts, in various research centers and corporations. The first phase of its development, the design, engineering, and testing of components, is substantially complete, and preparations are being made for extensive animal experimentation. Three alternative power systems are being contemplated: an electric motor powered by a biological fuel cell, an electric motor powered by rechargeable batteries, or a nuclear engine powered by 53 grams of Plutonium 238. The pump must be made of materials that are compatible with blood and are sufficiently durable to meet work demands. The power system must be responsive to physiological needs of the body. Candidates for this artificial heart would be persons whose own diseased heart is incapable of cardiac output sufficient to sustain life. The diseased natural heart would be totally removed and replaced by the aritifical pump, controls, and power source. It has been estimated that between 17,000 and 50,000 patients annually might benefit from such a device. The total costs for medical care, hospitalization, the device itself, and the energy source will be in the order of $15,000 to $25,000, and probably more for the nuclear-powered heart. (Later estimates are that the costs will run $50,000 to $75,000/implantation.)

Case #33

In 1967 Dr. Christian Barnard performed the first heart transplant on a human being. There subsequently have been more than two hundred cardiac transplantations in the United States, where the centers at Stanford University and at the Medical College of Virginia have been the most active and successful. Stanford carefully screens potential recipients and reports that 65% of its transplant recipients can expect to survive at least one year. The chance of surviving five years is considered better than fifty percent. One Stanford patient has survived over eleven years, and one Medical College of Virginia patient has survived over seven years. Because of these successes, proponents of cardiac transplantation argue that it should be made widely available, but others are not convinced that the problem of tissue rejection has been sufficiently solved or that the benefits of cardiac transplantation outweigh its costs.

On February 1, 1980, the twelve lay trustees of the Massachusetts General Hospital announced that they had voted not to permit heart transplants at that institution "at the present time." Their explanatory statement noted that "to turn away even one potential cardiac transplantation patient is a very trying course to follow," but that "in an age where technology so pervades the medical community, there is a clear responsibility to evaluate new procedures in terms of the greatest good for the greatest number." In June of 1980, Patricia Harris, then Secretary of the Department of Health and Human Services, withdrew an earlier tentative authorization for Medicare to cover heart transplants. She held that authorization of funds no longer can depend solely on the safety, effectiveness, and acceptance of a technology by the medical community. In addition, a technology must be evaluated in terms of its "social consequences." Cost is one factor, and the specter of another program like the one for kidney dialysis and transplantation has created bureaucratic and congressional caution. For example, heart transplants at Stanford now average over $100,000 per patient. If 2,000 transplants were performed, the cost would thus be over 200 million dollars. If 30,000 transplants were performed, the cost would be over 3 billion dollars. Estimates vary, but some reports suggest that each year in the United States there may be 30,000 to 75,000 victims of heart disease whose condition is hopeless without cardiac transplantation and who could possibly benefit from cardiac transplantation (if we assume that it would be possible to locate enough hearts for transplantation).

The Department of Health and Human Services was also concerned about Stanford's screening criteria, which include "a stable, rewarding family and/or vocational environment to return to posttransplant; a spouse, family member or companion able and willing to make the long-term commitment to provide emotional support before and after the transplant; financial resources to support travel to and from the transplant center accompanied by a family member for final evaluation." "Contraindications" for selection as a cardiac recipient at Stanford include "a history of alcoholism, job instability, antisocial behavior, or psychiatric illness." While some of these criteria may be medically relevant, others have been accused of incorporating unarticulated, undefended, and even indefensible criteria of "social worth."

As a result of the uncertainty surrounding cardiac transplantation, DHHS ordered a two-year study (with an outside cost of two-million dollars) to assess the "social consequences" before deciding whether to provide funds to pay for the operation.

[This case has been prepared from the following sources: Alexander Leaf, "The MGH Trustees Say No to Heart Transplants," *New England Journal of Medicine* 302 (May 8, 1980): 1087–88; Richard A. Knox, "Heart Transplants: To Pay or Not to Pay," *Science* 209 (August 1, 1980): 570–75; and Lois K. Christopherson, "Heart Transplants," *Hastings Center Report* 12 (February 1982): 18–21.]

Case #34

In the mid-1970s two professors at Harvard, Milton Weinstein and William B. Stason, became interested in facts and policies pertaining to high blood pressure in American society. Few people in the United States know about, or pay much attention to, the fact that they themselves may have high blood pressure. The Harvard researchers noted that 17 percent of the adult American population, or 24 million persons, have problems with high blood pressure, that even minimally adequate treatment for these persons would cost over $5 billion annually (if all were treated), that close to 50 percent of the affected population are not even aware of the fact that they have problems, and that only about one-sixth of that group are receiving proper medical treatment and control.

The investigators became concerned with determining the most cost-effective way to tackle the problem of controlling hypertension in the American population. Data from screening programs that identify people who do not know that they have high blood pressure revealed that it is not cost-efficient to try to inform persons of their problem unless they are already under a physician's care. In general, people who were informed of their condition through massive screening and education programs were not likely to report to a physician for treatment. Among those who did subsequently see a physician, adherence to the recommended therapy turned out to be extremely poor.

As they further developed their research, Weinstein and Stason discovered (somewhat surprisingly) that, rather than to launch a communitywide campaign, it is more cost-effective to treat three classes of persons in the attempt to reduce the general public health problem of high blood pressure: (1) younger men, (2) older women, and (3) those patients with very high blood pressure. When the researchers combined these findings with their previous findings that large-scale, public screening and informational programs are not medically effective (and not cost-effective), they were led to conclude: "A community with limited resources would probably do better to concentrate its efforts on improving adherence of known hypertensives, even at a sacrifice in terms of the numbers screened. This conclusion holds even if such proadherence interventions are rather expensive and only moderately effective, and even if screening is very inexpensive. . . . Finally, screening in the regular practices [of physicians] is more cost-effective than public screening."

These investigators were bothered by their own recommendation because it implicitly meant that, if acted on by public policy experts in the government, the poorest sector of the country, which is also in greatest need of medical attention, would not be provided with any benefits of high blood pressure education and management. Public screening would be sacrificed in order to do a larger good for the whole community, where only persons known to have high blood pressure who were already in contact with a physician about their problem would be recontacted and new educational attempts made. These investigators were concerned because there seemed to them to be a possible injustice in excluding the poor and minorities by a public health endeavor aimed expressly at the economically better-off sector of society. Yet their statistics were very compelling: No matter how carefully planned the efforts, nothing worked except programs directed at those already in touch with physicians. They also discovered that a certain amount of money devoted to the education of physicians was quite cost-effective. Moreover, they knew that it was most unlikely, and perhaps undeserved in light of other health needs, that there would be new allocations of public health money to control high blood pressure. Yet it would take massive new allocations even to begin to affect the poorer sections of society.

These investigators therefore recommended what they explicitly referred to as a "utilitarian" set of criteria for allocation.

[This case was prepared by consulting Milton Weinstein and William B. Stason, *Hypertension* (Cambridge: Harvard University Press, 1976) and their articles in *New England Journal of Medicine* 296 (1977): 716–21, and *Hastings Center Report* 7 (October 1977): 24–29.]

Case #35

Having recently completed his Ph.D. degree in chemistry, George has not been able to find a job. His family has suffered from his failure since they are short of money, his wife has had to take a full-time job, and the small children have been subjected to considerable strain, uncertainty, and instability. An established chemist can get George a position in a laboratory that pursues research in chemical and biological warfare. Despite his perilous financial and familial circumstances, George feels that he cannot accept this position because of his conscientious opposition to chemical and biological warfare. The older chemist notes that while he is not enthusiastic about this project, the research will continue whatever George decides. Furthermore, if George does not take the position it will be offered to another young man who would probably pursue the research with alacrity and promptitude. Indeed, the older chemist confides, his concern about this other candidate's nationalistic fervor and uncritical zeal for research in chemical and biological warfare in part led him to recommend George. George's wife is puzzled and hurt by George's reaction since she sees nothing wrong with such research. She is mainly concerned about the instability of their family and their children's problems.

[Adapted from Bernard Williams, "A Critique of Utilitarianism," in J. J. C. Smart and Bernard Williams, *Utilitarianism For and Against* (Cambridge: Cambridge University Press, 1973), pp. 97–98.]

Appendix II

Codes of Ethics

The Hippocratic Oath
World Medical Association, Declaration of Geneva
American Medical Association, Principles of Medical Ethics
International Council of Nurses, Code for Nurses
American Nurses' Association Code for Nurses
World Health Organization, Constitution
American Hospital Asociation, A Patient's Bill of Rights
The Nuremberg Code
World Medical Association, Declaration of Helsinki
Department of Health and Human Services, Basic HHS Policy
   for Protection of Human Research Subjects

The Hippocratic Oath

I swear by Apollo Physician and Asclepius and Hygieia and Panaceia and all the gods and goddesses, making them my witnesses, that I will fulfil according to my ability and judgment this oath and this covenant:

To hold him who has taught me this art as equal to my parents and to live my life in partnership with him, and if he is in need of money to give him a share of mine, and to regard his offspring as equal to my brothers in male lineage and to teach them this art—if they desire to learn it—without fee and covenant; to give a share of precepts and oral instruction and all the other learning to my sons and to the sons of him who has instructed me and to pupils who have signed the covenant and have taken an oath according to the medical law, but to no one else.

I will apply dietetic measures for the benefit of the sick according to my ability and judgment; I will keep them from harm and injustice.

I will neither give a deadly drug to anybody if asked for it, nor will I make a suggestion to this effect. Similarly I will not give to a woman an abortive remedy. In purity and holiness I will guard my life and my art.

I will not use the knife, not even on sufferers from stone, but will withdraw in favor of such men as are engaged in this work.

Whatever houses I may visit, I will come for the benefit of the sick, remaining free of all intentional injustice, of all mischief and in particular of sexual relations with both female and male persons, be they free or slaves.

What I may see or hear in the course of the treatment or even outside of the treatment in regard to the life of men, which on no account one must spread abroad, I will keep to myself holding such things shameful to be spoken about.

If I fulfil this oath and do not violate it, may it be granted to me to enjoy life and art, being honored with fame among all men for all time to come; if I transgress it and swear falsely, may the opposite of all this be my lot.

[Reprinted by permission of the publisher from Ludwig Edelstein, *Ancient Medicine*, edited by Oswei Temkin and C. Lillian Temkin (Baltimore: Johns Hopkins University Press, 1967.)]

The World Medical Association Declaration of Geneva

Physician's Oath

At the time of being admitted as a member of the medical profession:

I solemnly pledge myself to consecrate my life to the service of humanity;

I will give to my teachers the respect and gratitude which is their due;

I will practice my profession with conscience and dignity; the health of my patient will be my first consideration;

I will maintain by all the means in my power, the honor and the noble traditions of the medical profession; my colleagues will be my brothers;

I will not permit considerations of religion, nationality, race, party politics or social standing to intervene between my duty and my patient;

I will maintain the utmost respect of human life from the time of conception, even under threat, I will not use my medical knowledge contrary to the laws of humanity;

I make these promises solemnly, freely and upon my honor.

[Adopted by the General Assembly of the World Medical Association, Geneva, Switzerland, September 1948 and amended by the 22nd World Medical Assembly, Sydney, Australia, August 1968. Reprinted by permission.]

American Medical Association Principles of Medical Ethics

Preamble

The medical profession has long subscribed to a body of ethical statements developed primarily for the benefit of the patient. As a member of this profession, a physician must recognize responsibility not only to patients, but also to society, to other health professionals, and to self. The following Principles adopted by the American Medical Association are not laws, but standards of conduct which define the essentials of honorable behavior for the physician.

  I. A physician shall be dedicated to providing competent medical service with compassion and respect for human dignity.

 II. A physician shall deal honestly with patients and colleagues, and strive to expose those physicians deficient in character or competence, or who engage in fraud or deception.

III. A physician shall respect the law and also recognize a responsibility to seek changes in those requirements which are contrary to the best interests of the patient.

 IV. A physician shall respect the rights of patients, of colleagues, and of other health professionals, and shall safeguard patient confidences within the constraints of the law.

  V. A physician shall continue to study, apply and advance scientific knowledge, make relevant information available to patients, colleagues, and the public, obtain consultation, and use the talents of other health professionals when indicated.

VI. A physician shall, in the provision of appropriate patient care, except in emergencies, be free to choose whom to serve, with whom to associate, and the environment in which to provide medical services.

VII. A physician shall recognize a responsibility to participate in activities contributing to an improved community.

[Adopted by the American Medical Association in 1980 and reprinted with permission.]

International Council of Nurses
Code for Nurses: Ethical Concepts Applied to Nursing

The fundamental responsibility of the nurse is fourfold: to promote health, to prevent illness, to restore health and alleviate suffering.

The need for nursing is universal. Inherent in nursing is respect for life, dignity and rights of man. It is unrestricted by considerations of nationality, race, creed, color, age, sex, politics or social status.

Nurses render health services to the individual, the family and the community and coordinate their services with those of related groups.

Nurses and People

The nurse's primary responsibility is to those people who require nursing care.

The nurse, in providing care, promotes an environment in which the values, customs and spirtual beliefs of the individual are respected.

The nurse holds in confidence personal information and uses judgment in sharing this information.

Nurses and Practice

The nurse carries personal responsibility for nursing practice and for maintaining competence by continual learning.

The nurse maintains the highest standards of nursing care possible within the reality of a specific situation.

The nurse uses judgment in relation to indivdual competence when accepting and delegating responsibilities.

The nurse when acting in a professional capacity should at all times maintain standards of personal conduct which reflect credit upon the profession.

Nurses and Society

The nurse shares with other citizens the responsibility for initiating and supporting action to meet the health and social needs of the public.

Nurses and Co-Workers

The nurse sustains a cooperative relationship with co-workers in nursing and other fields.

The nurse takes appropriate action to safeguard the individual when his care is endangered by a co-worker or any other person.

Nurses and the Profession

The nurse plays the major role in determining and implementing desirable standards of nursing practice and nursing education.

The nurse is active in developing a core of professional knowledge.

The nurse, acting through the professional organization, participates in establishing and maintaining equitable social and economic working conditions in nursing.

[Adopted by the International Council of Nurses, May 1973 and reprinted by permission.]

American Nurses' Association Code for Nurses

Preamble

The *Code for Nurses* is based on belief about the nature of individuals, nursing, health, and society. Recipients and providers of nursing services are viewed as individuals and groups who possess basic rights and responsibilities, and whose values and circumstances command respect at all times. Nursing encompasses the promotion and restoration of health, the prevention of illness, and the alleviation of suffering. The statements of the *Code* and their interpretation provide guidance for conduct and relationships in carrying out nursing responsibilities consistent with the ethical obligations of the profession and quality in nursing care.

Code for Nurses

1. The nurse provides services with respect for human dignity and the uniqueness of the client unrestricted by considerations of social or economic status, personal attributes, or the nature of health problems.

2. The nurse safeguards the client's right to privacy by judiciously protecting information of a confidential nature.

3. The nurse acts to safeguard the client and the public when health care and safety are affected by the incompetent, unethical, or illegal practice of any person.

4. The nurse assumes responsibility and accountability for individual nursing judgments and actions.

5. The nurse maintains competence in nursing.

6. The nurse exercises informed judgment and uses individual competence and qualifications as criteria in seeking consultation, accepting responsibilities, and delegating nursing activities to others.

7. The nurse participates in activities that contribute to the ongoing development of the profession's body of knowledge.

8. The nurse participates in the profession's efforts to implement and improve standards of nursing.

9. The nurse participates in the profession's efforts to establish and maintain conditions of employment conducive to high quality nursing care.

10. The nurse participates in the profession's effort to protect the public from misinformation and misrepresentation and to maintain the integrity of nursing.

11. The nurse collaborates with members of the health professions and other

citizens in promoting community and national efforts to meet the health needs of the public.

[Adopted by the American Nurses' Association in 1976 and reprinted by permission.]

Constitution of the World Health Organization

The States Parties to this Constitution declare, in conformity with the Charter of the United Nations, that the following principles are basic to the happiness, harmonious relations and security of all peoples:

Health is a state of complete physical, mental and social well-being and not merely the absence of disease or infirmity.

The enjoyment of the highest attainable standard of health is one of the fundamental rights of every human being without distinction of race, religion, political belief, economic or social condition.

The health of all peoples is fundamental to the attainment of peace and security and is dependent upon the fullest co-operation of individuals and States.

The achievement of any State in the promotion and protection of health is of value to all.

Unequal development in different countries in the promotion of health and control of disease, especially communicable disease, is a common danger.

Healthy development of the child is of basic importance; the ability to live harmoniously in a changing total environment is essential to such development.

The extension to all peoples of the benefits of medical, psychological and related knowledge is essential to the fullest attainment of health.

Informed opinion and active co-operation on the part of the public are of the utmost importance in the improvement of the health of the people.

Governments have a responsiblity for the health of their peoples which can be fulfilled only by the provision of adequate health and social measures.

Accepting these principles, and for the purpose of co-operation among themselves and with others to promote and protect the health of all peoples,

the Contracting Parties agree to the present Constitution and hereby establish
the World Health Organization as a specialized agency within the terms of
Article 57 of the Charter of the United Nations.

[Reprinted from *World Health Organization: Basic Documents*, 26th ed. (Geneva:
World Health Organization, 1976), p. 1.]

American Hospital Association
A Patient's Bill of Rights

The American Hospital Association presents a Patient's Bill of Rights with
the expectation that observance of these rights will contribute to more
effective patient care and greater satisfaction for the patient, his physician,
and the hospital organization. Further, the Association presents these rights
in the expectation that they will be supported by the hospital on behalf of its
patients, as an integral part of the healing process. It is recognized that a
personal relationship between the physician and the patient is essential for
the provision of proper medical care. The traditional physician-patient
relationship takes on a new dimension when care is rendered within an
organizational structure. Legal precedent has established that the institution
itself also has a responsibility to the patient. It is in recognition of these
factors that these rights are affirmed.

1. The patient has the right to considerate and respectful care.

2. The patient has the right to obtain from his physician complete current
information concerning his diagnosis, treatment, and prognosis in terms
the patient can be reasonably expected to understand. When it is not
medically advisable to give such information to the patient, the information
should be made available to an appropriate person in his behalf. He has the
right to know, by name, the physician responsible for coordinating his care.

3. The patient has the right to receive from his physician information
necessary to give informed consent prior to the start of any procedure
and/or treatment. Except in emergencies, such information for informed
consent should include but not necessarily be limited to the specific procedure
and/or treatment, the medically significant risks involved, and the probable
duration of incapacitation. Where medically significant alternatives for care
or treatment exist, or when the patient requests information concerning
medical alternatives, the patient has the right to such information. The
patient also has the right to know the name of the person responsible for the
procedures and/or treatment.

4. The patient has the right to refuse treatment to the extent permitted by law and to be informed of the medical consequences of his action.

5. The patient has the right to every consideration of his privacy concerning his own medical care program. Case discussion, consultation, examination, and treatment are confidential and should be conducted discreetly. Those not directly involved in his care must have the permission of the patient to be present.

6. The patient has the right to expect that all communications and records pertaining to his care should be treated as confidential.

7. The patient has the right to expect that within its capacity a hospital must make reasonable response to the request of a patient for services. The hospital must provide evaluation, service, and/or referral as indicated by the urgency of the case. When medically permissible, the patient may be transferred to another facility only after he has received complete information and explanation concerning the needs for and alternatives for such a transfer. The institution to which the patient is to be transferred must first have accepted the patient for transfer.

8. The patient has the right to obtain information as to any relationship of his hospital to other health care and educational institutions insofar as his care is concerned. The patient has the right to obtain information as to the existence of any professional relationships among individuals, by name, who are treating him.

9. The patient has the right to be advised if the hospital proposes to engage in or perform human experimentation affecting his care or treatment. The patient has the right to refuse to participate in such research projects.

10. The patient has the right to expect reasonable continuity of care. He has the right to know in advance what appointment times and physicians are available and where. The patient has the right to expect that the hospital will provide a mechanism whereby he is informed by his physician or a delegate of the physician of the patient's continuing health care requirements following discharge.

11. The patient has the right to examine and receive an explanation of his bill regardless of source of payment.

12. The patient has the right to know what hospital rules and regulations apply to his conduct as a patient.

No catalog of rights can guarantee for the patient the kind of treatment he has a right to expect. A hospital has many functions to perform, including the prevention and treatment of disease, the education of both health professionals and patients, and the conduct of clinical research. All these activities must be conducted with an overriding concern for the patient, and, above all, the recognition of his dignity as a human being. Success in achieving this recognition assures success in the defense of the rights of the patient.

[Approved by the American Hospital Association House of Delegates, February 6, 1973, and reprinted by permission of the American Hospital Association.]

The Nuremberg Code

The great weight of the evidence before us is to the effect that certain types of medical experiments on human beings, when kept within reasonably well-defined bounds, conform to the ethics of the medical profession generally. The protagonists of the practice of human experimentation justify their views on the basis that such experiments yield results for the good of society that are unprocurable by other methods or means of study. All agree, however, that certain basic principles must be observed in order to satisfy moral, ethical and legal concepts:

1. The voluntary consent of the human subject is absolutely essential.

This means that the person involved should have legal capacity to give consent; should be so situated as to be able to exercise free power of choice, without the intervention of any element of force, fraud, deceit, duress, over-reaching, or other ulterior form of constraint or coercion; and should have sufficient knowledge and comprehension of the elements of the subject matter involved as to enable him to make an understanding and enlightened decision. This latter element requires that before the acceptance of an affirmative decision by the experimental subject there should be made known to him the nature, duration, and purpose of the experiment; the method and means by which it is to be conducted; all inconveniences and hazards reasonably to be expected; and the effects upon his health or person which may possibly come from his participation in the experiment.

The duty and responsibility for ascertaining the quality of the consent rests upon each individual who initiates, directs or engages in the experiment. It is a personal duty and responsibility which may not be delegated to another with impunity.

2. The experiment should be such as to yield fruitful results for the good of society, unprocurable by other methods or means of study, and not random and unnecessary in nature.

3. The experiment should be so designed and based on the results of animal experimentation and a knowledge of the natural history of the

disease or other problem under study that the anticipated results will justify the performance of the experiment.

4. The experiment should be so conducted as to avoid all unnecessary physical and mental suffering and injury.

5. No experiment should be conducted where there is an *a priori* reason to believe that death or disabling injury will occur; except, perhaps, in those experiments where the experimental physicians also serve as subjects.

6. The degree of risk to be taken should never exceed that determined by the humanitarian importance of the problem to be solved by the experiment.

7. Proper preparations should be made and adequate facilities provided to protect the experimental subject against even remote possibilities of injury, disability, or death.

8. The experiment should be conducted only by scientifically qualified persons. The highest degree of skill and care should be required through all stages of the experiment of those who conduct or engage in the experiment.

9. During the course of the experiment the human subject should be at liberty to bring the experiment to an end if he has reached the physical or mental state where continuation of the experiment seems to him to be impossible.

10. During the course of the experiment the scientist in charge must be prepared to terminate the experiment at any stage, if he has probable cause to believe, in the exercise of the good faith, superior skill and careful judgment required of him that a continuation of the experiment is likely to result in injury, disability, or death to the experimental subject.

[Reprinted from *Trials of War Criminals before the Nuernberg Military Tribunals under Control Council Law No. 10*, vol. 2 (Washington, D.C.: U.S. Government Printing Office, 1949), pp. 181–82.]

The World Medical Association Declaration of Helsinki

Introduction

It is the mission of the medical doctor to safeguard the health of the people. His or her knowledge and conscience are dedicated to the fulfillment of this mission.

The Declaration of Geneva of the World Medical Association binds the doctor with the words, "The health of my patient will be my first consideration," and the International Code of Medical Ethics declares that, "Any act or advice which could weaken physical or mental resistance of a human being may be used only in his interest."

The purpose of biomedical research involving human subjects must be to improve diagnostic, therapeutic and prophylactic procedures and the understanding of the aetiology and pathogenesis of disease.

In current medical practice most diagnostic, therapeutic or prophylactic procedures involve hazards. This applies *a fortiori* to biomedical research.

Medical progress is based on research which ultimately must rest in part on experimentation involving human subjects.

In the field of biomedical research a fundamental distinction must be recognized between medical research in which the aim is essentially diagnostic or therapeutic for a patient, and medical research, the essential object of which is purely scientific and without direct diagnostic or therapeutic value to the person subjected to the research.

Special caution must be exercised in the conduct of research which may affect the environment, and the welfare of animals used for research must be respected.

Because it is essential that the results of laboratory experiments be applied to human beings to further scientific knowledge and to help suffering humanity, The World Medical Association has prepared the following recommendations as a guide to every doctor in biomedical research involving human subjects. They should be kept under review in the future. It must be stressed that the standards as drafted are only a guide to physicians all over the world. Doctors are not relieved from criminal, civil and ethical responsibilities under the laws of their own countries.

I. Basic principles

1. Biomedical research involving human subjects must conform to generally accepted scientific principles and should be based on adequately performed laboratory and animal experimentation and on a thorough knowledge of the scientific literature.

2. The design and performance of each experimental procedure involving human subjects should be clearly formulated in an experimental protocol which should be transmitted to a specially appointed independent committee for consideration, comment and guidance.

3. Biomedical research involving human subjects should be conducted only by scientifically qualified persons and under the supervision of a clinically competent medical person. The responsibility for the human subject

must always rest with a medically qualified person and never rest on the subject of the research, even though the subject has given his or her consent.

4. Biomedical research involving human subjects cannot legitimately be carried out unless the importance of the objective is in proportion to the inherent risk to the subject.

5. Every biomedical research project involving human subjects should be preceded by careful assessment of predictable risks in comparison with foreseeable benefits to the subject or to others. Concern for the interests of the subject must always prevail over the interests of science and society.

6. The right of the research subject to safeguard his or her integrity must always be respected. Every precaution should be taken to respect the privacy of the subject and to minimize the impact of the study on the subject's physical and mental integrity and on the personality of the subject.

7. Doctors should abstain from engaging in research projects involving human subjects unless they are satisfied that the hazards involved are believed to be predictable. Doctors should cease any investigation if the hazards are found to outweigh the potential benefits.

8. In publication of the results of his or her research, the doctor is obliged to preserve the accuracy of the results. Reports of experimentation not in accordance with the principles laid down in this Declaration should not be accepted for publication.

9. In any research on human beings, each potential subject must be adequately informed of the aims, methods, anticipated benefits and potential hazards of the study and the discomfort it may entail. He or she should be informed that he or she is at liberty to abstain from participation in the study and that he or she is free to withdraw his or her consent to participation at any time. The doctor should then obtain the subject's freely-given informed consent, preferably in writing.

10. When obtaining informed consent for the research project the doctor should be particularly cautious if the subject is in a dependent relationship to him or her or may consent under duress. In that case the informed consent should be obtained by a doctor who is not engaged in the investigation and who is completely independent of this official relationship.

11. In case of legal incompetence, informed consent should be obtained from the legal guardian in accordance with national legislation. Where physical or mental incapacity makes it impossible to obtain informed consent, or when the subject is a minor, permission from the responsible relative replaces that of the subject in accordance with national legislation.

12. The research protocol should always contain a statement of the ethical

considerations involved and should indicate that the principles enunciated in the present Declaration are complied with.

II. Medical research combined with professional care (clinical research)

1. In the treatment of the sick person, the doctor must be free to use a new diagnostic and therapeutic measure, if in his or her judgment it offers hope of saving life, reestablishing health or alleviating suffering.

2. The potential benefits, hazards and discomfort of a new method should be weighed against the advantages of the best current diagnostic and therapeutic methods.

3. In any medical study, every patient—including those of a control group, if any—should be assured of the best proven diagnostic and therapeutic method.

4. The refusal of the patient to participate in a study must never interfere with the doctor-patient relationship.

5. If the doctor considers it essential not to obtain informed consent, the specific reasons for this proposal should be stated in the experimental protocol for transmission to the independent committee (1, 2).

6. The doctor can combine medical research with professional care, the objective being the acquisition of new medical knowledge, only to the extent that medical research is justified by its potential diagnostic or therapeutic value for the patient.

III. Non-therapeutic biomedical research involving human subjects (non-clinical biomedical research)

1. In the purely scientific application of medical research carried out on a human being, it is the duty of the doctor to remain the protector of the life and health of that person on whom biomedical research is being carried out.

2. The subjects should be volunteers—either healthy persons or patients for whom the experimental design is not related to the patient's illness.

3. The investigator or the investigating team should discontinue the research if in his/her or their judgment it may, if continued, be harmful to the individual.

4. In research on man, the interest of science and society should never take precedence over considerations related to the wellbeing of the subject.

[Adopted by the 18th World Medical Assembly, Helsinki, Finland, 1964, and as revised by the 29th World Medical Assembly, Tokyo, Japan, 1975. Reprinted by permission.]

Department of Health and Human Services Basic HHS Policy for Protection of Human Research Subjects (Excerpts)

§46.111 Criteria for IRB [Institutional Review Board] Approval of Research.

(a) In order to approve research covered by these regulations the IRB shall determine that all of the following requirements are satisfied:

(1) Risks to subjects are minimized: (i) By using procedures which are consistent with sound research design and which do not unnecessarily expose subjects to risk, and (ii) whenever appropriate, by using procedures already being performed on the subjects for diagnostic or treatment purposes.

(2) Risks to subjects are reasonable in relation to anticipated benefits, if any, to subjects, and the importance of the knowledge that may reasonably be expected to result. In evaluating risks and benefits, the IRB should consider only those risks and benefits that may result from the research (as distinguished from risks and benefits of therapies subjects would receive even if not participating in the research). The IRB should not consider possible long-range effects of applying knowledge gained in the research (for example, the possible effects of the research on public policy) as among those research risks that fall within the purview of its responsibility.

(3) Selection of subjects is equitable. In making this assessment the IRB should take into account the purposes of the research and the setting in which the research will be conducted.

(4) Informed consent will be sought from each prospective subject or the subject's legally authorized representative, in accordance with, and to the extent required by § 46.116.

(5) Informed consent will be appropriately documented, in accordance with, and to the extent required by § 46.117.

(6) Where appropriate, the research plan makes adequate provision for monitoring the data collected to insure the safety of subjects.

(7) Where appropriate, there are adequate provisions to protect the privacy of subjects and to maintain the confidentiality of data.

(b) Where some or all of the subjects are likely to be vulnerable to coercion or undue influence, such as persons with acute or severe physical or mental illness, or persons who are economically or educationally disadvantaged, appropriate additional safeguards have been included in the study to protect the rights and welfare of these subjects.

§ 46.116 General Requirements for Informed Consent.

Except as provided elsewhere in this or other subparts, no investigator may involve a human being as a subject in research covered by these regulations unless the investigator has obtained the legally effective informed consent of the subject or the subject's legally authorized representative. An investigator shall seek such consent only under circumstances that provide the prospective subject or the representative sufficient opportunity to consider whether or not to participate and that minimize the possibility of coercion or undue influence. The information that is given to the subject or the representative shall be in language understandable to the subject or the representative. No informed consent, whether oral or written, may include any exculpatory language through which the subject or the representative is made to waive or appear to waive any of the subject's legal rights, or releases or appears to release the investigator, the sponsor, the institution or its agents from liability for negligence.

(a) Basic elements of informed consent. Except as provided in paragraph (c) or (d) of this section, in seeking informed consent the following information shall be provided to each subject:

(1) A statement that the study involves research, an explanation of the purposes of the research and the expected duration of the subject's participation, a description of the procedures to be followed, and identification of any procedures which are experimental;

(2) A description of any reasonably foreseeable risks or discomforts to the subject;

(3) A description of any benefits to the subject or to others which may reasonably be expected from the research;

(4) A disclosure of appropriate alternative procedures or courses of treatment, if any, that might be advantageous to the subject;

(5) A statement describing the extent, if any, to which confidentiality of records identifying the subject will be maintained;

(6) For research involving more than minimal risk, an explanation as to whether any compensation and an explanation as to whether any medical

treatments are available if injury occurs and, if so, what they consist of, or where further information may be obtained;

(7) An explanation of whom to contact for answers to pertinent questions about the research and research subjects' rights, and whom to contact in the event of a research-related injury to the subject; and

(8) A statement that participation is voluntary, refusal to participate will involve no penalty or loss of benefits to which the subject is otherwise entitled, and the subject may discontinue participation at any time without penalty or loss of benefits to which the subject is otherwise entitled.

(b) Additional elements of informed consent. When appropriate, one or more of the following elements of information shall also be provided to each subject:

(1) A statement that the particular treatment or procedure may involve risks to the subject (or to the embryo or fetus, if the subject is or may become pregnant) which are currently unforeseeable;

(2) Anticipated circumstances under which the subject's participation may be terminated by the investigator without regard to the subject's consent;

(3) Any additional costs to the subject that may result from participation in the research;

(4) The consequences of a subject's decision to withdraw from the research and procedures for orderly termination of participation by the subject;

(5) A statement that significant new findings developed during the course of the research which may relate to the subject's willingness to continue participation will be provided to the subject; and

(6) The approximate number of subjects involved in the study.

(c) An IRB may approve a consent procedure which does not include, or which alters, some or all of the elements of informed consent set forth above, or waive the requirement to obtain informed consent provided the IRB finds and documents that:

(1) The research is to be conducted for the purpose of demonstrating or evaluating: (i) Federal, state, or local benefit or service programs which are not themselves research programs, (ii) procedures for obtaining benefits or services under these programs, or (iii) possible changes in or alternatives to these programs or procedures; and

(2) The research could not practicably be carried out without the waiver or alteration.

(d) An IRB may approve a consent procedure which does not include, or which alters, some or all of the elements of informed consent set forth above, or waive the requirements to obtain informed consent provided the IRB finds and documents that:

(1) The research involves no more than minimal risk to the subjects;

(2) The waiver or alteration will not adversely affect the rights and welfare of the subjects;

(3) The research could not practicably be carried out without the waiver or alteration; and

(4) Whenever apropriate, the subjects will be provided with additional pertinent information after participation.

(e) The informed consent requirements in these regulations are not intended to preempt any applicable federal, state, or local laws which require additional information to be disclosed in order for informed consent to be legally effective.

(f) Nothing in these regulations is intended to limit the authority of a physician to provide emergency medical care, to the extent the physician is permitted to do so under applicable federal, state, or local law.

§ *46.117 Documentation of Informed Consent.*

(a) Except as provided in paragraph (c) of this section, informed consent shall be documented by the use of a written consent form approved by the IRB and signed by the subject or the subject's legally authorized representative. A copy shall be given to the person signing the form.

(b) Except as provided in paragraph (c) of this section, the consent form may be either of the following:

(1) A written consent document that embodies the elements of informed consent required by § 46.116. This form may be read to the subject or the subject's legally authorized representative, but in any event, the investigator shall give either the subject or the representative adequate opportunity to read it before it is signed; or

(2) A "short form" written consent document stating that the elements of informed consent required by § 46.116 have been presented orally to the subject or the subject's legally authorized representative. When this method is used, there shall be a witness to the oral presentation. Also, the IRB shall approve a written summary of what is to be said to the subject or the representative. Only the short form itself is to be signed by the subject or the representative. However, the witness shall sign both the short form and a copy of the summary, and the person actually obtaining consent shall sign a copy of the summary. A copy of the summary shall be given to the subject or the representative, in addition to a copy of the "short form."

(c) An IRB may waive the requirement for the investigator to obtain a signed consent form for some or all subjects if it finds either:

(1) That the only record linking the subject and the research would be the consent document and the principal risk would be potential harm resulting from a breach of confidentiality. Each subject will be asked whether the subject wants documentation linking the subject with the research, and the subject's wishes will govern; or

(2) That the research presents no more than minimal risk of harm to subjects and involves no procedures for which written consent is normally required outside of the research context.

In cases where the documentation requirement is waived, the IRB may require the investigator to provide subjects with a written statement regarding the research.

Bibliography of Suggested Readings

Original Texts (Ethical Theory)

Beauchamp, Tom L. *Philosophical Ethics: An Introduction to Moral Philosophy.* New York: McGraw-Hill, 1982.

Benditt, Theodore M. *Rights.* Totowa, N.J.: Rowman and Littlefield, 1982.

Brandt, Richard B. *A Theory of the Good and the Right.* Oxford: Clarendon Press, 1979.

Donagan, Alan. *The Theory of Morality.* Chicago: University of Chicago Press, 1977.

Feinberg, Joel. *Social Philosophy.* Englewood Cliffs, N.J.: Prentice-Hall, 1973.

Frankena, William K. *Ethics.* 2nd Edition. Englewood Cliffs, N.J.: Prentice-Hall, 1973.

Gert, Bernard. *The Moral Rules.* New York: Harper and Row, 1970.

Hare, R. M. *Moral Thinking: Its Levels, Method and Point.* Oxford: Clarendon Press, 1981.

MacIntyre, Alasdair. *After Virtue: A Study in Moral Theory.* Notre Dame, Ind.: University of Notre Dame Press, 1981.

——. *A Short History of Ethics.* New York: Macmillan, 1966.

Mackie, J. L. *Ethics: Inventing Right and Wrong.* Harmondsworth, Eng.: Penguin Books, 1977.

Rawls, John. *A Theory of Justice.* Cambridge, Mass.: Harvard University Press, 1971.

Singer, Peter. *Practical Ethics.* Cambridge: Cambridge University Press, 1979.

Taylor, Paul. *Principles of Ethics: An Introduction.* Encino, Calif.: Dickenson Publishing Co., 1975. (Belmont, Calif.: Wadsworth Publishing Co.).

Original Texts (Biomedical Ethics)

Barber, Bernard. *Informed Consent in Medical Therapy and Research.* New Brunswick, N.J.: Rutgers University Press, 1980.

Benjamin, Martin, and Curtis, Joy. *Ethics in Nursing.* New York: Oxford University Press, 1981.

Brody, Howard. *Ethical Decisions in Medicine.* 2nd edition. Boston: Little, Brown and Company, 1981.

Burt, Robert A. *Taking Care of Strangers: The Rule of Law in Doctor-Patient Relations.* New York: The Free Press, 1979.

Campbell, Alastair V. *Moral Dilemmas in Medicine.* 2nd ed. Edinburgh: Churchill-Livingston, 1975.

Childress, James F. *Priorities in Biomedical Ethics.* Philadelphia: The Westminster Press, 1981.

Culver, Charles M., and Gert, Bernard. *Philosophy in Medicine: Conceptual and Ethical Issues in Medicine and Psychiatry.* New York: Oxford University Press, 1982.

Fletcher, Joseph. *Morals and Medicine.* Boston: Beacon Press, 1960.

Fried, Charles. *Medical Experimentation: Personal Integrity and Social Policy.* New York: American Elsevier Publishing Co., 1974.

Glover, Jonathan. *Causing Death and Saving Lives.* New York: Penguin Books, 1977.

Jonsen, Albert R., Siegler, Mark, and Winslade, William J. *Clinical Ethics: A Practical Approach to Ethical Decisions in Clinical Medicine.* New York: Macmillan Publishing Co., Inc., 1982.

Levine, Robert J. *Ethics and Regulation of Clinical Research.* Baltimore: Urban and Schwarzenberg, Inc., 1981.

McCormick, Richard A. *How Brave a New World? Dilemmas in Bioethics.* Garden City, N.Y.: Doubleday, 1981.

Pellegrino, Edmund D., and Thomasma, David C. *A Philosophical Basis of Medical Practice: Toward a Philosophy and Ethic of the Healing Professions.* New York: Oxford University Press, 1981.

Pence, Gregory E. *Ethical Options in Medicine.* Oradell, N.J.: Medical Economics Company, 1980.

Ramsey, Paul. *Ethics at the Edges of Life.* New Haven: Yale University Press, 1978.

———. *The Patient as Person.* New Haven: Yale University Press, 1970.

Veatch, Robert M. *A Theory of Medical Ethics.* New York: Basic Books, Inc., 1981.

———. *Death, Dying, and the Biological Revolution: Our Last Quest for Responsibility.* New Haven: Yale University Press, 1976.

Anthologies

Abernethy, Virginia, ed. *Frontiers in Medical Ethics: Applications in a Medical Setting.* Cambridge, Mass.: Ballinger Publishing Company, 1980.

Beauchamp, Tom L., and Walters, LeRoy, eds. *Contemporary Issues in Bioethics.* 2nd edition. Belmont, Calif.: Wadsworth Publishing Co., 1982.

Gorovitz, Samuel, et al., eds., *Moral Problems in Medicine.* 2nd edition. Englewood Cliffs, N.J.: Prentice-Hall, 1983.

Humber, James M., and Almeder, Robert F., eds. *Biomedical Ethics and the Law.* 2nd edition. New York: Plenum Press, 1976.

Hunt, Robert, and Arras, John, eds. *Ethical Issues in Modern Medicine.* Palo Alto, Calif.: Mayfield Publishing Co., 1977.

Katz, Jay, comp. *Experimentation with Human Beings: The Authority of the Investigator, Subject, Professions and State in the Human Experimentation Process.* New York: Russell Sage Foundation, 1972.

Mappes, Thomas, and Zembaty, Jane, eds. *Biomedical Ethics.* New York: McGraw-Hill, 1981.

Reiser, Stanley Joel, Dyck, Arthur J., and Curran, William J., eds. *Ethics in Medicine: Historical Perspectives and Contemporary Concerns.* Cambridge, Mass.: MIT Press, 1977.

Robison, Wade L., and Pritchard, Michael S., eds. *Medical Responsibility: Paternalism, Informed Consent, and Euthanasia.* Clifton, N.J.: The Humana Press, 1979.

Shannon, Thomas A., ed. *Bioethics: Basic Writings on the Key Ethical Questions That Surround the Major Modern Biological Possibilities and Problems.* Rev. edition. New York: Paulist Press, 1981.

Shannon, Thomas A., and Manfra, Jo Ann, eds. *Law and Bioethics: Texts with Commmentary on Major U.S. Court Decisions.* New York: Paulist Press, 1982.

Shelp, Earl E., ed. *Beneficence and Health Care* (*Philosophy and Medicine*; v. 11). Dordrecht, Holland: D. Reidel Publishing Company, 1982.

———, ed. *Justice and Health Care* (*Philosophy and Medicine*; v. 8). Dordrecht, Holland: D. Reidel Publishing Company, 1981.

Veatch, Robert, and Branson, Roy, eds. *Ethics and Health Policy.* Cambridge, Mass.: Ballinger Publishing Co., 1976.

Reference Works

Levine, Carol, and Veatch, Robert M. *Cases in Bioethics from the Hastings Center Report.* Hastings-on-Hudson, N.Y.: The Hastings Center, 1982.

Reich, Warren T., ed. *Encyclopedia of Bioethics.* New York: Macmillan and Free Press, 1978. Vols. 1–4.

Sollitto, Sharmon and Veatch, Robert M., comps. *Bibliography of Society, Ethics and the Life Sciences.* Hastings-on-Hudson, N.Y.: Institute of Society, Ethics, and the Life Sciences. Updated periodically.

Veatch, Robert M. *Case Studies in Medical Ethics.* Cambridge, Mass.: Harvard University Press, 1977.

Walters, LeRoy, ed. *Bibliography of Bioethics*, Vols. 1– . Detroit: Gale Research Co. Issued annually.

Journals

We here offer a list of only some of the more significant journals, arranged according to their various emphases.

There are a few journals that deal primarily, if not exclusively, with issues of biomedical ethics. Among these are *Ethics in Science and Medicine, The Hastings Center Report, The Journal Of Medical Ethics,* and *IRB: A Review of Human Subjects Research.* Other journals deal both with the history and philosophy of medicine and biomedical ethics. Journals such as *The Bulletin of the History of Medicine, The Journal of Medicine and Philosophy, Ethics and Values in Health Care,* and *Perspectives in Biology and Medicine* are representative.

Some journals with a more general ethical orientation frequently include articles that apply basic ethical principles to problems raised by contemporary biology and medicine. Such journals include *Ethics, The Journal of Religious Ethics,* and *Philosophy and Public Affairs.* In addition, several medical and legal journals frequently publish articles dealing with biomedical ethics. Representative are *The American Journal of Law and Medicine, The Journal of Legal Medicine, The Journal of Thanatology, The Journal of the American Medical Association, Lancet, The New England Journal of Medicine,* and *Obstetrics and Gynecology.*

Index

353